298
Current Topics in Microbiology and Immunology

Editors

R.W. Compans, Atlanta/Georgia
M.D. Cooper, Birmingham/Alabama
T. Honjo, Kyoto · H. Koprowski, Philadelphia/Pennsylvania
F. Melchers, Basel · M.B.A. Oldstone, La Jolla/California
S. Olsnes, Oslo · M. Potter, Bethesda/Maryland
P.K. Vogt, La Jolla/California · H. Wagner, Munich

E. Vivier and M. Colonna (Eds.)

Immunobiology of Natural Killer Cell Receptors

With 27 Figures and 8 Tables

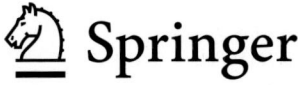

Eric Vivier, DVM, PhD.
Laboratory of NK Cells and Innate Immunity
Centre d'Immunologie de Marseille-Luminy (CIML)
CNRS-INSERM-Université de la Méditerranée
Campus de Luminy, Case 906
13288 Marseille Cedex 09
France

e-mail: vivier@ciml.univ-mrs.fr

Marco Colonna, M.D.
Department of Pathology and Immunology
Washington University School of Medicine
West Building, Rooms 4724, Box 8118
660 South Euclid Ave
St. Louis, MO 63110
USA

e-mail: mcolonna@pathology.wustl.edu

Cover illustration: Natural Killer (NK) cell activation results from a dynamic equilibrium between complementary and sometime antagonist forces, such as that initiated by activating receptors recognizing stress-induced self (e.g. NKG2D ligands) and inhibitory receptors recognizing constitutively-expressed self (e.g. MHC class I molecules).

Library of Congress Catalog Number 72-152360

ISSN 0070-217X
ISBN-10 3-540-26083-8 Springer Berlin Heidelberg New York
ISBN-13 978-3-540-26083-7 Springer Berlin Heidelberg New York

This work is subject to copyright. All rights reserved, whether the whole or part of the material is concerned, specifically the rights of translation, reprinting, reuse of illustrations, recitation, broadcasting, reproduction on microfilm or in any other way, and storage in data banks. Duplication of this publication or parts thereof is permitted only under the provisions of the German Copyright Law of September, 9, 1965, in its current version, and permission for use must always be obtained from Springer-Verlag. Violations are liable for prosecution under the German Copyright Law.

Springer is a part of Springer Science+Business Media
springeronline.com
© Springer-Verlag Berlin Heidelberg 2006
Printed in Germany

The use of general descriptive names, registered names, trademarks, etc. in this publication does not imply, even in the absence of a specific statement, that such names are exempt from the relevant protective laws and regulations and therefore free for general use.
Product liability: The publisher cannot guarantee the accuracy of any information about dosage and application contained in this book. In every individual case the user must check such information by consulting the relevant literature.

Editor: Simon Rallison, Heidelberg
Desk editor: Anne Clauss, Heidelberg
Production editor: Nadja Kroke, Leipzig
Cover design: design & production GmbH, Heidelberg
Typesetting: LE-TEX Jelonek, Schmidt & Vöckler GbR, Leipzig
Printed on acid-free paper   SPIN 11332404   27/3150/YL – 5 4 3 2 1 0

List of Contents

Strategies of Natural Killer Cell Recognition and Signaling 1
    C. A. Stewart, E. Vivier, and M. Colonna

Signal Transduction in Natural Killer Cells 23
    A. W. MacFarlane IV and K. S. Campbell

Transcriptional Regulation of NK Cell Receptors 59
    S. K. Anderson

Extending Missing-Self? Functional Interactions Between Lectin-like
Nkrp1 Receptors on NK Cells with Lectin-like Ligands 77
    B. F. M. Plougastel and W. M. Yokoyama

The CD2 Family of Natural Killer Cell Receptors 91
    M. E. McNerney and V. Kumar

Immunobiology of Human NKG2D and Its Ligands 121
    S. González, V. Groh, and T. Spies

NKG2 Receptor-Mediated Regulation of Effector CTL Functions
in the Human Tissue Microenvironment 139
    B. Jabri and B. Meresse

Dendritic Cell–NK Cell Cross-Talk: Regulation and Physiopathology 157
    L. Zitvogel, M. Terme, C. Borg, and G. Trinchieri

NK Cell Activating Receptors and Tumor Recognition in Humans 175
    C. Bottino, L. Moretta, and A. Moretta

NK Cell Recognition of Mouse Cytomegalovirus-Infected Cells 183
    S. M. Vidal and L. L. Lanier

NK Cell Receptors Involved in the Response to Human
Cytomegalovirus Infection 207
    M. Gumá, A. Angulo, and M. López-Botet

The Impact of Variation at the *KIR* Gene Cluster on Human Disease 225
  M. Carrington and M. P. Martin

NK Cells in Autoimmune Disease 259
  S. Johansson, H. Hall, L. Berg, and P. Höglund

Subject Index 279

List of Contributors

(Addresses stated at the beginning of respective chapters)

Anderson, S. K.   59
Angulo, A.   207

Berg, L.   259
Borg, C.   157
Bottino, C.   175

Campbell, K. S.   23
Carrington, M.   225
Colonna, M.   1

González, S.   121
Groh, V.   121
Gumá, M.   207

Höglund, P.   259
Hall, H.   259

Jabri, B.   139
Johansson, S.   259

Kumar, V.   91

Lanier, L. L.   183
López-Botet, M.   207

MacFarlane IV, A. W.   23
Martin, M. P.   225
McNerney, M. E.   91
Meresse, B.   139
Moretta, A.   175
Moretta, L.   175

Plougastel, B. F. M.   77

Spies, T.   121
Stewart, C. A.   1

Terme, M.   157
Trinchieri, G.   157

Vidal, S. M.   183
Vivier, E.   1

Yokoyama, W. M.   77

Zitvogel, L.   157

Strategies of Natural Killer Cell Recognition and Signaling

C. A. Stewart[1] (✉) · E. Vivier[1] · M. Colonna[2]

[1] Lab of NK Cells and Innate Immunity, Centre d'Immunologie de Marseille-Luminy, INSERM-CNRS-Univ. Méditerranée, Campus de Luminy, 13288 Marseille cedex 09, France
stewart@ciml.univ-mrs.fr

[2] Department of Pathology and Immunology, Washington University School of Medicine, St. Louis, MO 63110, USA

1	Introduction	2
2	Themes of NK Cell Recognition	2
3	Inhibitory Recognition and Signaling	3
3.1	Inhibitory Receptors for MHC Class I	3
3.2	Inhibitory Receptors for Non-MHC Ligands	6
4	Activating Recognition and Signaling	6
4.1	Some ITAM-Based Receptors	6
4.2	NKG2D	7
4.3	Activating Homologs of Inhibitory MHC Class I Receptors	7
5	The NK Cell Activation Cascade: From Surface Triggers to Effector Function	8
6	Complexities in NK Cell Activation	10
6.1	Consequences of ITIM Phosphorylation	10
6.2	2B4 Inhibition and Activation	10
6.3	Roles of Adhesion	11
6.4	Cytotoxicity and Cytokine Responses	12
7	A Challenge for the Future: Understanding the Integration of Signals by NK Cells	13
	References	14

Abstract The participation of natural killer (NK) cells in multiple aspects of innate and adaptive immune responses is supported by the wide array of stimulatory and inhibitory receptors they bear. Here we review the receptor-ligand interactions and subsequent signaling events that culminate in NK effector responses. Whereas some receptor-ligand interactions result in activation of both NK cytotoxicity and cytokine production, others have more subtle effects, selectively activating only one pathway or having distinct context-dependent effects. Recent approaches offer ways to unravel how the integration of complex signaling networks directs the NK response.

1
Introduction

Natural killer (NK) cells are large granular lymphocytes of the innate immune system. They are widespread throughout the body, being present in both lymphoid organs and nonlymphoid peripheral tissues (Cooper et al. 2004; Ferlazzo and Munz 2004). NK cells are involved in direct innate immune reactions against viruses, bacteria, parasites, and other triggers of pathology, such as malignant transformation, all of which cause stress in affected cells (Moretta et al. 2002; Raulet 2004). Importantly, NK cells also link the innate and adaptive immune responses, contributing to the initiation of adaptive immune responses (see chapter by Zitvogel et al., this volume) (Martin-Fontecha et al. 2004) and executing adaptive responses with the CD16 FcγRIIIA immunoglobulin Fc receptor. Such responses are mediated through two major effector functions, the direct cytolysis of target cells and the production of cytokines and chemokines. We focus here on the nature of recognition events by NK cells and address how these events are integrated to trigger these distinct and graded effector functions.

2
Themes of NK Cell Recognition

The dissection of NK cell innate recognition strategies was initiated by the discovery that NK cell cytotoxicity inversely correlates with the level of major histocompatibility complex (MHC) class I expression on target cells (Karre et al. 1986). The missing self hypothesis elegantly provided an explanation for this phenomenon and led to the discovery of multiple inhibitory receptors that block activating signals by recruitment of protein tyrosine phosphatases to their intracytoplasmic immunoreceptor tyrosine-based inhibition motifs (ITIMs) (Long 1999; Vivier and Daëron 1997). Opposing this inhibitory signaling, innate stimulatory recognition by NK cells can be classified in three general modes: recognition of constitutively expressed self molecules, recognition of motifs upregulated by stressed cells, and direct recognition of infectious pathogen components (Raulet 2004; Vivier and Malissen 2005). Together, the numerous receptors carrying out these functions allow NK cells to discriminate between target and non-target cells (Fig. 1) (Cerwenka and Lanier 2001; Vilches and Parham 2002; Vivier and Biron 2002; Yokoyama 1998). Only a minority of these receptors, such as the natural cytotoxicity receptors (NCR), are truly NK cell specific, with many being found on other hematopoietic cells. The question of how all the signals are integrated from multiple, redundant and opposing, simultaneously engaged pathways to culminate in graded NK cell responses, that is, cytotoxicity and/or cytokine production, serves to illustrate the complex and dynamically balanced nature of cell activation (Lanier 2003; Vivier et al. 2004).

3
Inhibitory Recognition and Signaling

3.1
Inhibitory Receptors for MHC Class I

Multiple families of receptors in mouse and human recognize MHC class I products and transmit inhibitory signals when engaged. CD94/NKG2 receptors are heterodimers of C-type lectin type II transmembrane proteins that recognize the nonclassical MHC class I molecules HLA-E (human leukocyte antigen-E, in human) and Qa-1^b (in mouse) (Borrego et al. 1998; Braud et al. 1998; Lee et al. 1998; Vance et al. 1998). Of the NKG2 family members that associate with CD94 (including NKG2A, C, and E), NKG2A contains ITIMs in its cytoplasmic domain conferring inhibitory function. Recognition of HLA-E or Qa-1^b by CD94/NKG2 requires the presence of peptides in the peptide binding grooves of these class I molecules. Many of these peptides are derived from the leader sequences of classical MHC class I molecules (Braud et al. 1997; Kraft et al. 2000), thus making CD94/NKG2A a sensor of active MHC class I biosynthesis and presentation. CD94/NKG2 is unique in both its high evolutionary conservation and its means of recognizing classical MHC class I as a "proxy" sensor.

Members of other NK cell MHC class I receptor families directly bind to classical MHC class I molecules. In the mouse and rat, NK cell recognition of subsets of MHC class I allotypes is mediated by members of the Ly49 family of C-type lectin type II transmembrane proteins. In contrast, human NK cells use immunoglobulin domain-containing type I transmembrane proteins for the same function. The immunoglobulin-like transcript 2 (ILT2, or LIR1) receptor recognizes a broad range of both classical and nonclassical MHC class I molecules (Chapman et al. 1999; Colonna et al. 1997), whereas members

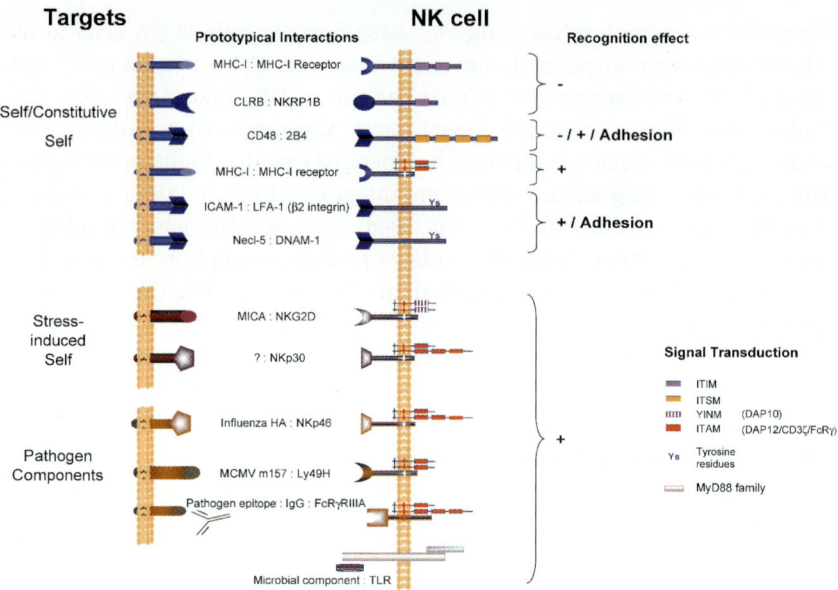

Fig. 1 Themes in NK cell recognition and signaling. NK receptors can be classified according to their recognition of ligands expressed by self cells, stressed cells, or pathogens. Prototypical receptor-ligand interactions that are described in the text are shown. Additional ligands are known for a number of the receptors shown. Effects of these interactions are detailed as inhibitory (−), activating (+), or involved in adhesion. The motifs used by membrane receptors or associated signaling adaptor molecules are shown for each receptor. These serve to illustrate the association of many NK activating receptors with specialized signaling transmembrane adaptor proteins that contain ITAMs (immunoreceptor tyrosine-based activation motifs) or YINM motifs in their cytoplasmic tails. These adaptors form homodimers or heterodimers through disulfide bonding and associate with membrane receptors using charged amino acids in the transmembrane domain (*stars*; *white* indicates positive charge, *red* indicates negative charge). Other motifs including ITIM (immunoreceptor tyrosine-based inhibitory motif) and ITSM (immunoreceptor tyrosine-based switch motif) are found within the cytoplasmic domains of NK receptors. The FcγRIIIA (CD16) receptor could be classified as recognizing constitutive self, stressed self, or pathogen-expressed moieties depending on a particular IgG antibody. As IgG antibodies recognizing constitutive self molecules are frequently avoided through processes of immune tolerance, FcγRIIIA is classified here as recognizing pathogen components. The figure includes both human and murine molecules that are not always found in the other species. Other important abbreviations: *MHC*-I, major histocompatibility complex class I molecule; *MICA*, MHC class I chain-related protein A; *Influenza HA*: influenza virus hemagglutinin; *MCMV*, murine cytomegalovirus; *TLR*, Toll-like receptor. Direct interaction and inhibitory modulation of NKp30 by pp65 of human cytomegalovirus has been described (Arnon et al. 2005). Therefore, NKp30 may also be defined as recognizing pathogen components

of the killer immunoglobulin-like receptor (KIR) family are much more specific. Primate KIR show MHC class I allotype specificity and appear to be functional homologs of rodent Ly49 despite their diverse evolutionary origin. Hitherto-studied mammalian species segregate into those with an expansion of *KIR* genes or *Ly49* genes (Parham 2005). An interesting feature of both KIR and Ly49 recognition of MHC class I is sensitivity to peptides bound in the MHC class I groove. Many KIR and some Ly49 receptors are sensitive to peptide changes (Franksson et al. 1999; Hanke et al. 1999; Hansasuta et al. 2004; Peruzzi et al. 1996; Rajagopalan and Long 1997; Zappacosta et al. 1997), but this sensitivity is far less pronounced and specific than that underpinning T cell antigen recognition. The different roles of peptide are also reflected in the binding kinetics of NK and T cell MHC class I receptors. Although both types of receptor have similar affinities, KIRs have fast on and off rates with favorable binding entropy whereas T cell receptors (TCR) have slower kinetics (Maenaka et al. 1999; Vales-Gomez et al. 1998). The slow on rate of the TCR is relatively peptide independent and may reflect an energetically unfavorable transition state in which peptide-independent TCR-MHC contacts are made. Peptide has a large influence on the off rate, however, reflecting its importance in complex stability and role in T cell signaling (Wu et al. 2002).

NK recognition of individual allotypes of MHC class I could play an important role in innate immunity against viruses or tumorigenic processes that result in the loss of expression of specific MHC class I allotypes (Garcia-Lora et al. 2003). In addition, the polymorphic nature of both NK receptors and their MHC ligands suggests that a population effect may be at work, with NK receptors serving to modify the NK cell activation state (see chapter by Carrington and Martin, this volume) (Parham 2005). This is illustrated in the finding that preeclampsia, a complication associated with insufficient remodeling of the uterine spiral arteries that provide a blood supply for the fetus during pregnancy, is associated with HLA-C group 2 molecules that could theoretically provide strong inhibitory signals to decidual NK cells (Hiby et al. 2004). It is also known that NK KIR-HLA interactions can be exploited during certain bone marrow transplantation procedures where incompatibility decreases the likelihood of graft-versus-host disease and leukemia relapse (Ruggeri et al. 2002). Of importance in each role is the repertoire of NK cell specificity. Almost all NK cell MHC class I receptors are expressed in a variegated fashion by the NK population, resulting in a broad range of MHC class I specificities within any individual's NK population (see chapter by Anderson, this volume).

3.2
Inhibitory Receptors for Non-MHC Ligands

A number of NK receptors whose ligands are non-MHC class I molecules also contain ITIMs and have the capacity to function as inhibitory receptors. These include glycoprotein 49 B1 (gp49B1) and certain NK cell receptor protein 1 (NKR-P1) family members found only in mice, along with carcinoembryonic antigen-related cell adhesion molecule 1 (CEACAM1) and sialic acid-binding immunoglobulin-like lectin (SIGLEC) family members found in both humans and mice. The roles of these receptors are currently obscure, but the broad expression of many of their ligands suggests that some may perform "missing-self" functions in a similar way to MHC class I receptors (see chapter by Plougastel and Yokoyama, this volume) (Kumar and McNerney 2005).

4
Activating Recognition and Signaling

4.1
Some ITAM-Based Receptors

In a similar way to the antigen receptors expressed by T and B cells, many of the NK receptors that induce strong activation of NK cells upon receptor cross-linking or ligation use immunoreceptor tyrosine-based activation motifs (ITAMs) to transduce these signals. In many cases these ITAMs are not present in the polypeptide conferring ligand binding capacity but are connected with it through noncovalent association of a transmembrane ITAM-bearing adaptor molecule. DNAX-activating protein of 12 kDa [DAP12, or KARAP (killer cell activating receptor-associated protein)], FcRγ, and CD3ζ are such signaling adaptors expressed by NK cells and involved in signal transduction from multiple distinct surface receptors. Two members of the NCRs, NKp46 and NKp30, along with the FcγRIIIA CD16 receptor responsible for NK cell antibody-dependent cellular cytotoxicity (ADCC) couple with FcRγ and CD3ζ. The other NCR, NKp44, couples with DAP12. As previously stated, NCRs are NK cell-specific receptors. Their name derives from their critical involvement in natural cytotoxicity against a broad panel of target cell types without prior NK cell sensitization, as demonstrated by antibody blocking of the cytolysis (see chapter by Bottino et al., this volume). Despite the reported NCR interaction with viral products (Arnon et al. 2005; Mandelboim et al. 2001), the identity of the NCR ligands expressed by tumor cells is still unknown, but it is tempting to speculate that these could either be normal self molecules or moieties upregulated on stress (Bloushtain et al. 2004).

4.2
NKG2D

NKG2D is an outlying member of the NKG2 family that forms homodimers and does not heterodimerize with CD94 (see chapters by González et al. and Jabri and Meresse, this volume). Many NKG2D ligands are class I MHC-related molecules that are expressed very selectively or at low levels by normal cells but are upregulated during stress and cellular transformation. In humans, NKG2D ligands include MICA, MICB, and various ULBP/RAET1 molecules, and murine H60, MULT1, and Rae1 molecules provide these roles in the mouse. The NKG2D ligands MICA, MICB, and Rae1 are all upregulated in tumor cells (Cerwenka et al. 2000; Diefenbach et al. 2000; Groh et al. 1996). NKG2D stimulation on NK cells leads to strong activation, and transfection-mediated NKG2D ligand expression on tumor cells leads to their rapid rejection in syngeneic mice (Cerwenka et al. 2001; Diefenbach et al. 2001). NKG2D is also expressed by $CD8^+$ T cells. However, NKG2D stimulation is not sufficient to induce effector functions of $CD8^+$ T cells without a primary activating signal coming from, for example, the TCR. The inability of NKG2D to directly stimulate $CD8^+$ T cells without additional signals is partially a consequence of its method of signal transduction. Human NKG2D and the long splice-variant form of mouse NKG2D (NKG2D-L) associate exclusively with the DAP10 (DNAX-activating protein of 10 kDa) signaling adaptor. Unlike the signaling adaptors used by the NCRs, DAP10 contains a YxxM motif that links to signaling pathways distinct from those of ITAM-bearing receptors. In the mouse, an additional short splice-variant form of NKG2D (NKG2D-S) is able to associate with both DAP10 and DAP12, but the lack of DAP12 expression in the majority of T cells restricts its association to the NK cell compartment (Diefenbach et al. 2002; Gilfillan et al. 2002).

4.3
Activating Homologs of Inhibitory MHC Class I Receptors

All the families of MHC class I receptors previously mentioned in the context of their inhibitory function also include activating molecules. Activating members of the Ly49, KIR, and NKG2 families (excepting NKG2D, which does not complex with CD94) are highly homologous to inhibitory receptors within these families but contain no ITIM and associate with DAP12. Where it has been possible to show direct binding to MHC class I molecules, the affinities of these activating interactions are much lower than those of activating counterparts (Vales-Gomez et al. 2000), questioning whether MHC class I molecules are their functional ligands. For the activating Ly49s, an astonishing role for Ly49H has been demonstrated in the control of murine cytomegalovirus (MCMV) infection. This receptor directly binds the MCMV *m157* gene product and is critical in control of infection by certain strains of mice (see chapters by Vidal and Lanier and Gumá et al., this volume). In addition, the activating receptor KIR2DS4 has been reported to bind a non-MHC class I ligand expressed by melanoma cells, suggesting a role in recognition of altered self (Katz et al. 2004).

It is not yet known whether such MHC class I-independent functions also apply to other activating members of these families. The high genetic polymorphism of activating receptors from the Ly49 and KIR families and a recent report supporting the continuous evolution of activating genes from inhibitory genes suggest that strong positive and negative evolutionary pressures are acting on them (Abi-Rached and Parham 2005). These pressures could be due to host-pathogen interactions in which pathogen "decoy" molecules for inhibitory receptors become detectable by a newly evolved activating receptor, giving a host with this receptor the upper hand (Arase and Lanier 2002). Alternatively, the selection pressures may be entirely due to interactions with self MHC molecules. Support for this comes from disease association studies in which both KIR and HLA have been studied in parallel. The genetic combination of an activating KIR and its known or potential (based on inhibitory KIR homology) HLA ligand is beneficial during HIV or hepatitis C virus (HCV) infection but increases the risk of developing certain autoimmune diseases including type I diabetes and psoriasis vulgaris (see chapters by Carrington and Martin and Johansson et al., this volume). Activating KIRs are also reported as beneficial during pregnancy, where their genetic presence reduces the risk of preeclampsia (Hiby et al. 2004). These findings point to a MHC-based role for activating KIR in regulation of immune responses and/or homeostasis of the NK and T cells that bear them.

Unlike activating *KIR* and *Ly49*, the *NKG2C* and *E* genes are highly conserved, suggesting a long-running evolutionary pressure for their maintenance. Along with changes in CD94/NKG2C expression observed on NK and T cells during infection, this argues for a role in modifying the activation capacity of these lymphocytes (see chapter by Gumá et al.).

5
The NK Cell Activation Cascade: From Surface Triggers to Effector Function

Engagement of NK-activating receptors induces tyrosine phosphorylation of their associated adaptor proteins. After phosphorylation by Src family kinases, ITAM-containing adaptors recruit the protein tyrosine kinases Syk and ZAP70, ultimately triggering NK cell effector functions. Alternatively, the YINM motif of DAP10, which signals for the receptor NKG2D (Wu et al. 1999), binds the p85 regulatory subunit of phosphatidylinositol 3-kinase (PI3K) (Chang et al. 1999; Wu et al. 1999) and the adaptor Grb2 (Chang et al. 1999) upon tyrosine phosphorylation.

Researchers are now actively exploring membrane-distal signaling molecules that mediate NK cell effector functions, particularly cytotoxicity. This process involves several steps including (a) rearrangement of actin cytoskeleton and formation of an immune synapse (IS) between NK cells and target cells, (b) reorientation of the Golgi complex and microtubule organizing center (MTOC) to polarize the lytic granules toward the IS, and (c) release of lytic granule contents (perforin and granzymes). The Vav guanine nucleotide exchange factors are implicated in all three of these processes as they play a central role in the activation of GTP-binding proteins (Billadeau et al. 1998; Chan et al. 2001; Colucci et al. 2001; Galandrini et al. 1999). Specifically, Vav1 is required for DAP10-mediated cytotoxicity, whereas Vav2 and Vav3 are essential for ITAM-mediated cytotoxicity (Cella et al. 2004). The Rho family of GTP-binding proteins (Rac1, RhoA, and Cdc42) and the Wiskott–Aldrich syndrome protein (WASP) regulate cytoskeleton rearrangements required for IS formation and MTOC-directed granule polarization (Gismondi et al. 2004; Khurana and Leibson 2003). Ras-related GTPase Arf6 promotes the release of cytolytic granule contents (Galandrini et al. 2005). Specifically, Arf6 activates the phosphatidylinositol 4-phosphate 5-kinase type Iα (PI5KIα), contributing to the generation of a phosphatidylinositol 4,5-bisphosphate (PIP$_2$) plasma membrane pool required for granule secretion.

Exocytosis of lytic granules also involves phospholipases Cγ1 and -2 (PLCγ1, PLCγ2) and intracellular Ca^{2+} mobilization (Azzoni et al. 1992; Billadeau et al. 2003; Liao et al. 1993; McVicar et al. 1998; Ting et al. 1992). Analysis of PLCγ2$-/-$ mice has demonstrated that PLCγ2 is essential for all activating NK cell receptors to trigger granule exocytosis (Wang et al. 2000; Tassi et al. 2005). Studies with pharmacological inhibitors have strongly implicated the MAP kinase (MAPK) MAPK ERK1/2 and p38 in granule exocytosis (Chini et al. 2000; Trotta et al. 2000, 1998). Although multiple signaling pathways that lead to MAPK activation have been identified (Perussia 2000), how ERK1/2 and p38 elicit release of lytic granules remains to be determined. PI3K activates the NK cytolytic machinery by inducing sequential activation of the GTP-binding protein Rac1, followed by the kinases Pak1, MEK, and ERK1/2 (Jiang et al. 2000). In addition, PI3K generates phosphatidylinositol 3,4,5-trisphosphate (PIP$_3$), which mediates recruitment of PLCγ1 and PLCγ2 to the cell membrane and their activation (Deane and Fruman 2004; Koyasu 2003;

Okkenhaug and Vanhaesebroeck 2003). Surprisingly, mice lacking the p85α regulatory subunit of PI3K do not exhibit major NK cell cytolytic defects. As PI3K includes multiple regulatory and catalytic subunits, redundancy may be in place. Like T and B lymphocytes, NK cells express intracellular adaptors such as the linker for activation of T cells (LAT), SLP-76, Gads, Grb2-associated binder 2 (Gab2), and 3BP2, which bridge together various components of signal transduction pathways. Although several signaling pathways have been shown to involve these adapters (Billadeau et al. 2003; Bottino et al. 2000; Chuang et al. 2001; Jevremovic et al. 1999, 2001; Klem et al. 2002; Zompi et al. 2004), it is not yet known whether any of them is required for NK cell activation.

6
Complexities in NK Cell Activation

6.1
Consequences of ITIM Phosphorylation

ITIM-bearing inhibitory NK receptors have been shown to recruit the protein tyrosine phosphatases SHP-1 and SHP-2 after ITIM phosphorylation (Colucci et al. 2002; Lanier 2003; McVicar and Burshtyn 2001; Vivier et al. 2004). In general, SHP-1 and SHP-2 dephosphorylate and deactivate multiple substrates that mediate NK cell activation, such as ITAM adaptors, protein tyrosine kinases, and Vav. However, SHP-1 and SHP-2 have different preferences for both phosphorylated ITIMs and substrates. Furthermore, each of them can either negatively or positively regulate signaling pathways depending on the experimental system studied. It is therefore not always trivial to ascribe a downregulating function to an ITIM-bearing receptor (see chapter by MacFarlane and Campbell, this volume).

6.2
2B4 Inhibition and Activation

In addition to ITIM-bearing inhibitory receptors, NK cells also express an unusual receptor, called 2B4, which binds CD48 on other cells. 2B4-mediated recognition of CD48 on target cells inhibits NK cell cytotoxicity (Lee et al. 2004), but 2B4-CD48 interaction between T cells and T cells or NK cells and NK cells enhances their activation (Lee et al. 2003). This intriguing dichotomy may be explained by the complexity of 2B4 signaling. 2B4 is a member of the CD2-like family of receptors, which also includes CD2, CD150, CD58, CD48, CD84, CD229, NTB-A, and CRACC (Engel et al. 2003; Nichols et al. 2005).

Some of these receptors, including 2B4, contain cytoplasmic immunoreceptor tyrosine-based switch motifs (ITSMs), which are distinct from ITAMs and ITIMs. Through ITSMs, CD2-like receptors bind a SH2 domain-containing cytoplasmic protein called SH2D1A (or SAP). SH2D1A recruits the Src kinase FynT, which phosphorylates the cytoplasmic tyrosines of the receptors. After tyrosine phosphorylation, CD2-like receptors sequentially recruit the SH2 domain-containing inositol-5 phosphatase-1 (SHIP-1), Shc, Dok1/2, and Ras-GAP, ultimately modulating MAPK activation (Veillette and Latour 2003).

Recently, it has been shown that cytoplasmic ITSMs, including those of 2B4, can also recruit a homolog of SH2D1A, called EWS-activated transcript 2 (EAT-2) (Morra et al. 2001b; Veillette and Latour 2003). EAT-2 may mediate a signaling cascade similar to that of SH2D1A. Alternatively, it could compete with SH2D1A for binding ITSM, thereby blocking the signaling cascade mediated by SH2D1A. Moreover, EAT-2 may block binding of other SH2-containing proteins, such as SHP-2, to ITSMs (Morra et al. 2001b). In this way, one current hypothesis is that the balance of SH2D1A and EAT-2 associated with the cytoplasmic domains of 2B4 and other ITSM-containing NK cell receptors determines the inhibitory or activating outcome of signaling. Importantly, mutations in SH2D1A cause X-linked lymphoproliferative disorder (XLP), a progressive combined variable immunodeficiency in which symptoms appear on Epstein-Barr virus (EBV) infection (Morra et al. 2001a; Nichols et al. 2005). Therefore, altered signaling by 2B4 and other ITSM-containing proteins expressed on NK cells may contribute to the pathogenesis of XLP. Understanding the function of SH2D1A and EAT-2 in NK cell inhibition and activation represents an important goal for NK cell research.

6.3
Roles of Adhesion

Early on in NK cell research, adhesion molecules were recognized as central players in NK cell-target cell and NK cell-matrix interactions as well as in NK cell effector functions (Helander and Timonen 1998). Mature NK cells constitutively express both β_1 and β_2 integrins. Their ligation results in rapid phosphorylation and activation of proline-rich tyrosine kinase 2 (Pyk2) (Gismondi et al. 2000), which regulates rearrangement of actin cytoskeleton through its constitutive association with paxillin. Pyk2 also contributes to NK cell activation by promoting ERK1/2 phosphorylation. Moreover, integrins activate a signaling cascade involving Vav1, Rac1, Pak1, and MKK3, ultimately leading to the activation of the MAPK p38 (Mainiero et al. 2000).

Recent evidence indicates that NK cells express a novel family of receptors, including DNAM-1, Tactile, and CRTAM, which bind a group of adhesion molecules called nectins and nectin-like molecules (Necls) (Boles et al. 2005; Bottino et al. 2003; Fuchs et al. 2004). Nectins and Necls are expressed on epithelial cells and mediate cell-cell adhesion (Sakisaka and Takai 2004). In addition, they are expressed on antigen-presenting cells (Boles et al. 2005). DNAM-1 binds Necl-5 and Nectin-2, Tactile binds Necl-5, and CRTAM binds Necl-2 (Boles et al. 2005; Bottino et al. 2003; Fuchs et al. 2004). The function of these adhesion interactions is under investigation. DNAM-1 triggers NK cell-mediated cytotoxicity (Shibuya et al. 1996) and has been reported to be physically and functionally associated with the β_2 integrin LFA-1, which induces DNAM-1 phosphorylation through the Src kinase Fyn-T (Shibuya et al. 1999). Thus DNAM-1-Necl-5/Nectin-2 interactions may be crucial in regulating NK cell adhesion to and lysis of target cells (Bottino et al. 2003). Tactile and CRTAM mediate strong adhesion but stimulate cytotoxicity weakly (Boles et al. 2005; Fuchs et al. 2004). Therefore, they may be preferentially implicated in NK cell migration into lymph nodes and peripheral tissues and/or NK cell proliferation and differentiation. Interestingly, Necl-2 is poorly expressed in epithelial tumors and overexpression of Necl-2 suppresses tumorigenesis of human tumor cell lines injected into nude mice (Kuramochi et al. 2001). This suggests that Necl-2 could be a major determinant of tumor immunogenicity, promoting anti-tumor NK cell responses through CRTAM (Boles et al. 2005).

6.4
Cytotoxicity and Cytokine Responses

Many NK cell ITAM-based receptors are capable of inducing full NK cell activation with intracellular Ca^{2+} mobilization, cytotoxic responses, and cytokine production (Moretta et al. 2001). However, signaling through certain NK cell receptors leads to more restricted effector function (see chapter by MacFarlane and Campbell, this volume). For example, stimulation of DAP10-linked NKG2D on NK cells leads to cytotoxicity but not IFN-γ secretion (Billadeau et al. 2003; Zompi et al. 2003). Alternatively, triggering of the unusual KIR family member KIR2DL4 has been found to result in IFN-γ secretion but not cytotoxicity (Rajagopalan et al. 2001). These findings illustrate how effector functions can be differentially triggered depending on the signaling pathway used and fit with their diverse roles in regulating and conducting immune responses.

7
A Challenge for the Future: Understanding the Integration of Signals by NK Cells

Although the reductionist analysis of NK cell signaling is rapidly leading to a detailed knowledge of individual pathways, it is essential to reconstruct the complexity of NK cell signaling and establish how these different components are integrated. In one experimental system, NK cell cytotoxicity has been tested against individual ligands expressed on a *Drosophila* insect cell line or directly coupled to beads (Barber et al. 2004). Remarkably, this approach has shown that expression of ICAM-1 on insect cells is sufficient not only to induce adhesion of NK cells to *Drosophila* cells through the β_2 integrin LFA-1 but also to induce activation signals that trigger lysis by NK cells. Coexpression of multiple activating and inhibitory ligands on *Drosophila* cells or beads will allow analysis of the relative contribution of the many different activating and inhibitory NK cell receptors (Barber and Long 2003).

Another powerful approach to reconstruct the complexity of NK cell signaling is three-dimensional immunofluorescence imaging (Davis 2002; Vyas et al. 2002). Interaction of NK cells with target cells leads to formation of an immunological synapse (IS) at the contact site. Molecules accumulating at the IS segregate in distinct domains. Segregated molecules are driven into specific arrangements depending on differences in cumulative activating and inhibitory signals. When inhibitory signals prevail over activating signals, SHP-1 clusters in the center of the cytolytic synapse, the Src kinase Lck has a multifocal distribution, and LFA-1 and LFA-1-associated talin form a ring that encloses SHP-1 and Lck. This inhibitory synapse is short-lived, the contact surface area shrinks rapidly, and deconjugation occurs within 2 or 3 min. In contrast, when activating signals overcome inhibitory signals, many activating molecules, such as protein kinase C-θ, WASP, Nck, SLP76, and LAT, as well as lytic granules, are recruited to the center of the IS. LFA-1 and talin form a peripheral ring, Lck maintains a multifocal distribution, and SHP-1 clusters in the periphery of the IS. This cytolytic IS is sustained and can last more than 15 min.

The complexity of NK cell signaling may go well beyond the integration of activating and inhibitory signals. Recent studies demonstrate that NK cells express multiple chemokine receptors, which trigger $G\alpha_i$ protein-mediated signals when engaged by constitutive or inflammatory chemokines (Maghazachi 2003). Moreover, NK cells express Toll-like receptors, which can sense pathogen components and trigger cytokine secretion (Chalifour et al. 2004; Hornung et al. 2002; Sivori et al. 2004). Finally, there is abundant evidence that IL-2, which is commonly used to culture NK cells, has profound effects on NK cell signaling, potentiating alternative cytotoxicity pathways that may not operate in freshly isolated NK cells. For example, WASP deficiency affects cytotoxicity of fresh but not IL-2-cultured NK cells (Gismondi et al. 2004). Additional cytokines, such as IFN-α, IL-12, IL-23, IL-15, and IL-21, influence NK cell maturation and/or acquisition of effector functions (Bonnema et al. 1994; Nguyen et al. 2002; Nutt et al. 2004; Vosshenrich et al. 2005). Understanding how these signaling pathways are integrated in vivo during NK cell-mediated immunosurveillance against viruses and tumors represents a challenging goal for NK cell research in the near future.

Acknowledgements We thank Elena Tomasello and Mathieu Bléry for useful discussion and review of the manuscript. Thanks to Corinne Beziers for artwork. EV is supported by specific grants from European Union ("ALLOSTEM"), Ligue Nationale contre le Cancer ('Equipe labellisée La Ligue'), and institutional grants from INSERM, CNRS, and Ministère de l'Enseignement Supérieur et de la Recherche. CAS is supported by the Fondation pour la Recherche Médicale. MC is supported by NIH grant 5R01AI056139-03.

References

Abi-Rached L, and Parham P (2005). Natural selection drives recurrent formation of activating KIR and Ly49 from inhibitory homologues. J Exp Med 201:1319–1332

Arase H, and Lanier LL (2002). Virus-driven evolution of natural killer cell receptors. Microbes Infect 4:1505–12

Arnon TI, Achdout H, Levi O, Markel G, Saleh N, Katz G, Gazit R, Gonen-Gross T, Hanna J, Nahari E, Porgador A, Honigman A, Plachter B, Mevorach D, Wolf DG, and Mandelboim O (2005). Inhibition of the NKp30 activating receptor by pp65 of human cytomegalovirus. Nat Immunol 6:515–23

Azzoni L, Kamoun M, Salcedo TW, Kanakaraj P, and Perussia B (1992). Stimulation of Fcγ RIIIA results in phospholipase C-γ1 tyrosine phosphorylation and p56lck activation. J Exp Med 176:1745–50

Barber DF, Faure M, and Long EO (2004). LFA-1 contributes an early signal for NK cell cytotoxicity. J Immunol 173:3653–9

Barber DF, and Long EO (2003). Coexpression of CD58 or CD48 with intercellular adhesion molecule 1 on target cells enhances adhesion of resting NK cells. J Immunol 170:294–9

Billadeau DD, Brumbaugh KM, Dick CJ, Schoon RA, Bustelo XR, and Leibson PJ (1998). The Vav-Rac1 pathway in cytotoxic lymphocytes regulates the generation of cell-mediated killing. J Exp Med 188:549–59

Billadeau DD, Upshaw JL, Schoon RA, Dick CJ, and Leibson PJ (2003). NKG2D-DAP10 triggers human NK cell-mediated killing via a Syk-independent regulatory pathway. Nat Immunol 4:557–64

Bloushtain N, Qimron U, Bar-Ilan A, Hershkovitz O, Gazit R, Fima E, Korc M, Vlodavsky I, Bovin NV, and Porgador A (2004). Membrane-associated heparan sulfate proteoglycans are involved in the recognition of cellular targets by NKp30 and NKp46. J Immunol 173:2392–401

Boles KS, Barchet W, Diacovo T, Cella M, and Colonna M (2005). The tumor suppressor TSLC1/NECL-2 triggers NK cell and CD8+ T cell responses through the cell surface receptor CRTAM. Blood 106:779–786

Bonnema JD, Rivlin KA, Ting AT, Schoon RA, Abraham RT, and Leibson PJ (1994). Cytokine-enhanced NK cell-mediated cytotoxicity. Positive modulatory effects of IL-2 and IL-12 on stimulus-dependent granule exocytosis. J Immunol 152:2098–104

Borrego F, Ulbrecht M, Weiss EH, Coligan JE, and Brooks AG (1998). Recognition of human histocompatibility leukocyte antigen (HLA)-E complexed with HLA class I signal sequence-derived peptides by CD94/NKG2 confers protection from natural killer cell-mediated lysis. J Exp Med 187:813–8

Bottino C, Augugliaro R, Castriconi R, Nanni M, Biassoni R, Moretta L, and Moretta A (2000). Analysis of the molecular mechanism involved in 2B4-mediated NK cell activation: evidence that human 2B4 is physically and functionally associated with the linker for activation of T cells. Eur J Immunol 30:3718–22

Bottino C, Castriconi R, Pende D, Rivera P, Nanni M, Carnemolla B, Cantoni C, Grassi J, Marcenaro S, Reymond N, Vitale M, Moretta L, Lopez M, and Moretta A (2003). Identification of PVR (CD155) and Nectin-2 (CD112) as cell surface ligands for the human DNAM-1 (CD226) activating molecule. J Exp Med 198:557–67

Braud V, Jones EY, and McMichael M (1997). The human major histocompatibility complex class Ib molecule HLA-E binds signal sequence-derived peptides with primary anchor residues at positions 2 and 9. Eur J Immunol 27:1164–9

Braud VM, Allan DS, O'Callaghan CA, Soderstrom K, D'Andrea A, Ogg GS, Lazetic S, Young NT, Bell JI, Phillips JH, Lanier LL, and McMichael AJ (1998). HLA-E binds to natural killer cell receptors CD94/NKG2A, B and C. Nature 391:795–9

Cella M, Fujikawa K, Tassi I, Kim S, Latinis K, Nishi S, Yokoyama W, Colonna M, and Swat W (2004). Differential requirements for Vav proteins in DAP10- and ITAM-mediated NK cell cytotoxicity. J Exp Med 200:817–23

Cerwenka A, Bakker ABH, McClanahan T, Wagner J, Wu J, Phillips JH, and Lanier LL (2000). Retinoic acid early inducible genes define a ligand family for the activating NKG2D receptor in Mice. Immunity 12:721–7

Cerwenka A, Baron JL, and Lanier LL (2001). Ectopic expression of retinoic acid early inducible-1 gene (RAE-1) permits natural killer cell-mediated rejection of a MHC class I-bearing tumor in vivo. Proc Natl Acad Sci USA 98:11521–6.

Cerwenka A, and Lanier L (2001). Natural killer cells, viruses and cancer. Nat Rev Immunol 1:41–9

Chalifour A, Jeannin P, Gauchat JF, Blaecke A, Malissard M, N'Guyen T, Thieblemont N, and Delneste Y (2004). Direct bacterial protein PAMP recognition by human NK cells involves TLRs and triggers α-defensin production. Blood 104:1778–83

Chan G, Hanke T, and Fischer KD (2001). Vav-1 regulates NK T cell development and NK cell cytotoxicity. Eur J Immunol 31:2403–10

Chang C, Dietrich J, Harpur AG, Lindquist JA, Haude A, Loke YW, King A, Colonna M, Trowsdale J, and Wilson MJ (1999). Cutting edge: KAP10, a novel transmembrane adapter protein genetically linked to DAP12 but with unique signaling properties. J Immunol 163:4651–4

Chapman TL, Heikeman AP, and Bjorkman PJ (1999). The inhibitory receptor LIR-1 uses a common binding interaction to recognize class I MHC molecules and the viral homolog UL18. Immunity 11:603–13

Chini CC, Boos MD, Dick CJ, Schoon RA, and Leibson PJ (2000). Regulation of p38 mitogen-activated protein kinase during NK cell activation. Eur J Immunol 30:2791–8

Chuang SS, Kumaresan PR, and Mathew PA (2001). 2B4 (CD244)-mediated activation of cytotoxicity and IFN-γ release in human NK cells involves distinct pathways. J Immunol 167:6210–6

Colonna M, Navarro F, Bellon T, Liano M, Garcia P, Samaridis J, Angman L, Cella M, and Lopez-Botet M (1997). A common inhibitory receptor for major histocompatibility complex class I molecules on human lymphoid and myelomonocytic cells. J Exp Med 186:1809–18

Colucci F, Di Santo JP, and Leibson PJ (2002). Natural killer cell activation in mice and men: different triggers for similar weapons? Nat Immunol 3:807–13

Colucci F, Rosmaraki E, Bregenholt S, Samson SI, Di Bartolo V, Turner M, Vanes L, Tybulewicz V, and Di Santo JP (2001). Functional dichotomy in natural killer cell signaling: Vav1-dependent and -independent mechanisms. J Exp Med 193:1413–24

Cooper MA, Fehniger TA, Fuchs A, Colonna M, and Caligiuri MA (2004). NK cell and DC interactions. Trends Immunol 25:47–52

Davis DM (2002). Assembly of the immunological synapse for T cells and NK cells. Trends Immunol 23:356–63

Deane JA, and Fruman DA (2004). Phosphoinositide 3-kinase: diverse roles in immune cell activation. Annu Rev Immunol 22:563–98

Diefenbach A, Jamieson AM, Liu SD, Shastri N, and Raulet DH (2000). Ligands for the murine NKG2D receptor: expression by tumor cells and activation of NK cells and macrophages. Nat Immunol 1:119–26.

Diefenbach A, Jensen ER, Jamieson AM, and Raulet DH (2001). Rae1 and H60 ligands of the NKG2D receptor stimulate tumour immunity. Nature 413:165–71.

Diefenbach A, Tomasello E, Lucas M, Jamieson AM, Hsia JK, Vivier E, and Raulet DH (2002). Selective associations with signaling proteins determine stimulatory versus costimulatory activity of NKG2D. Nat Immunol 3:1142–9.

Engel P, Eck MJ, and Terhorst C (2003). The SAP and SLAM families in immune responses and X-linked lymphoproliferative disease. Nat Rev Immunol 3:813–21

Ferlazzo G, and Munz C (2004). NK cell compartments and their activation by dendritic cells. J Immunol 172:1333–9

Franksson L, Sundback J, Achour A, Bernlind J, Glas R, and Karre K (1999). Peptide dependency and selectivity of the NK cell inhibitory receptor Ly-49C. Eur J Immunol 29:2748–58

Fuchs A, Cella M, Giurisato E, Shaw AS, and Colonna M (2004). Cutting edge: CD96 (tactile) promotes NK cell-target cell adhesion by interacting with the poliovirus receptor (CD155). J Immunol 172:3994–8

Galandrini R, Micucci F, Tassi I, Cifone MG, Cinque B, Piccoli M, Frati L, and Santoni A (2005). ARF6: A new player in the FcγRIIIA lymphocyte-mediated cytotoxicity. Blood 106:577–583

Galandrini R, Palmieri G, Piccoli M, Frati L, and Santoni A (1999). Role for the Rac1 exchange factor Vav in the signaling pathways leading to NK cell cytotoxicity. J Immunol 162:3148–52

Garcia-Lora A, Algarra I, Collado A, and Garrido F (2003). Tumour immunology, vaccination and escape strategies. Eur J Immunogenet 30:177–83.

Gilfillan S, Ho EL, Cella M, Yokoyama WM, and Colonna M (2002). NKG2D recruits two distinct adapters to trigger NK cell activation and costimulation. Nat Immunol 3:1150–5.

Gismondi A, Cifaldi L, Mazza C, Giliani S, Parolini S, Morrone S, Jacobelli J, Bandiera E, Notarangelo L, and Santoni A (2004). Impaired natural and CD16-mediated NK cell cytotoxicity in patients with WAS and XLT: ability of IL-2 to correct NK cell functional defect. Blood 104:436–43

Gismondi A, Jacobelli J, Mainiero F, Paolini R, Piccoli M, Frati L, and Santoni A (2000). Cutting edge: functional role for proline-rich tyrosine kinase 2 in NK cell-mediated natural cytotoxicity. J Immunol 164:2272–6

Groh V, Bahram S, Bauer S, Herman A, Beauchamp M, and Spies T (1996). Cell stress-regulated human major histocompatibility complex class I gene expressed in gastrointestinal epithelium. Proc Natl Acad Sci USA 93:12445–50.

Hanke T, Takizawa H, McMahon CW, Busch DH, Pamer EG, Miller JD, Altman JD, Liu Y, Cado D, Lemonnier FA, Bjorkman PJ, and Raulet DH (1999). Direct assessment of MHC class I binding by seven Ly49 inhibitory NK cell receptors. Immunity 11:67–77

Hansasuta P, Dong T, Thananchai H, Weekes M, Willberg C, Aldemir H, Rowland-Jones S, and Braud VM (2004). Recognition of HLA-A3 and HLA-A11 by KIR3DL2 is peptide-specific. Eur J Immunol 34:1673–9

Helander TS, and Timonen T (1998). Adhesion in NK cell function. Curr Top Microbiol Immunol 230:89–99

Hiby SE, Walker JJ, O'Shaughnessy K M, Redman CW, Carrington M, Trowsdale J, and Moffett A (2004). Combinations of maternal KIR and fetal HLA-C genes influence the risk of preeclampsia and reproductive success. J Exp Med 200:957–65

Hornung V, Rothenfusser S, Britsch S, Krug A, Jahrsdorfer B, Giese T, Endres S, and Hartmann G (2002). Quantitative expression of toll-like receptor 1–10 mRNA in cellular subsets of human peripheral blood mononuclear cells and sensitivity to CpG oligodeoxynucleotides. J Immunol 168:4531–7

Jevremovic D, Billadeau DD, Schoon RA, Dick CJ, Irvin BJ, Zhang W, Samelson LE, Abraham RT, and Leibson PJ (1999). Cutting edge: a role for the adaptor protein LAT in human NK cell-mediated cytotoxicity. J Immunol 162:2453–6

Jevremovic D, Billadeau DD, Schoon RA, Dick CJ, and Leibson PJ (2001). Regulation of NK cell-mediated cytotoxicity by the adaptor protein 3BP2. J Immunol 166:7219–28

Jiang K, Zhong B, Gilvary DL, Corliss BC, Hong-Geller E, Wei S, and Djeu JY (2000). Pivotal role of phosphoinositide-3 kinase in regulation of cytotoxicity in natural killer cells. Nat Immunol 1:419–25

Karre K, Ljunggren HG, Piontek G, and Kiessling R (1986). Selective rejection of H-2-deficient lymphoma variants suggests alternative immune defence strategy. Nature 319:675–8

Katz G, Gazit R, Arnon TI, Gonen-Gross T, Tarcic G, Markel G, Gruda R, Achdout H, Drize O, Merims S, and Mandelboim O (2004). MHC class I-independent recognition of NK-activating receptor KIR2DS4. J Immunol 173:1819–25

Khurana D, and Leibson PJ (2003). Regulation of lymphocyte-mediated killing by GTP-binding proteins. J Leukoc Biol 73:333–8

Klem J, Verrett PC, Kumar V, and Schatzle JD (2002). 2B4 is constitutively associated with linker for the activation of T cells in glycolipid-enriched microdomains: properties required for 2B4 lytic function. J Immunol 169:55–62

Koyasu S (2003). The role of PI3K in immune cells. Nat Immunol 4:313–9

Kraft JR, Vance RE, Pohl J, Martin AM, Raulet DH, and Jensen PE (2000). Analysis of Qa-1(b) peptide binding specificity and the capacity of CD94/NKG2A to discriminate between Qa-1-peptide complexes. J Exp Med 192:613–24

Kumar V, and McNerney ME (2005). A new self: MHC-class-I-independent Natural-killer-cell self-tolerance. Nat Rev Immunol 5:363–74

Kuramochi M, Fukuhara H, Nobukuni T, Kanbe T, Maruyama T, Ghosh HP, Pletcher M, Isomura M, Onizuka M, Kitamura T, Sekiya T, Reeves RH, and Murakami Y (2001). TSLC1 is a tumor-suppressor gene in human non-small-cell lung cancer. Nat Genet 27:427–30

Lanier LL (2003). Natural killer cell receptor signaling. Curr Opin Immunol 15:308–14

Lee KM, Bhawan S, Majima T, Wei H, Nishimura MI, Yagita H, and Kumar V (2003). Cutting edge: the NK cell receptor 2B4 augments antigen-specific T cell cytotoxicity through CD48 ligation on neighboring T cells. J Immunol 170:4881–5

Lee KM, McNerney ME, Stepp SE, Mathew PA, Schatzle JD, Bennett M, and Kumar V (2004). 2B4 acts as a non-major histocompatibility complex binding inhibitory receptor on mouse natural killer cells. J Exp Med 199:1245–54

Lee N, Llano M, Carretero M, Ishitani A, Navarro F, Lopez-Botet M, and Geraghty DE (1998). HLA-E is a major ligand for the natural killer inhibitory receptor CD94/NKG2A. Proc Natl Acad Sci USA 95:5199–204

Liao F, Shin HS, and Rhee SG (1993). Cross-linking of Fcγ RIIIA on natural killer cells results in tyrosine phosphorylation of PLC-γ1 and PLC-γ2. J Immunol 150:2668–74

Long EO (1999). Regulation of immune responses through inhibitory receptors. Annu Rev Immunol 17:875–904

Maenaka K, Juji T, Nakayama T, Wyer JR, Gao GF, Maenaka T, Zaccai NR, Kikuchi A, Yabe T, Tokunaga K, Tadokoro K, Stuart DI, Jones EY, and Van Der Merwe PA (1999). Killer cell immunoglobulin receptors and T cell receptors bind peptide-major histocompatibility complex class i with distinct thermodynamic and kinetic properties. J Biol Chem 274:28329–34

Maghazachi AA (2003). G protein-coupled receptors in natural killer cells. J Leukoc Biol 74:16–24

Mainiero F, Soriani A, Strippoli R, Jacobelli J, Gismondi A, Piccoli M, Frati L, and Santoni A (2000). RAC1/P38 MAPK signaling pathway controls β1 integrin-induced interleukin-8 production in human natural killer cells. Immunity 12:7–16

Mandelboim O, Lieberman N, Lev M, Paul L, Arnon TI, Bushkin Y, Davis DM, Strominger JL, Yewdell JW, and Porgador A (2001). Recognition of haemagglutinins on virus-infected cells by NKp46 activates lysis by human NK cells. Nature 409:1055–60.

Martin-Fontecha A, Thomsen LL, Brett S, Gerard C, Lipp M, Lanzavecchia A, and Sallusto F (2004). Induced recruitment of NK cells to lymph nodes provides IFN-γ for T_H1 priming. Nat Immunol 5:1260–5

McVicar DW, and Burshtyn DN (2001). Intracellular signaling by the killer immunoglobulin-like receptors and Ly49. Sci. STKE 2001:RE1

McVicar DW, Taylor LS, Gosselin P, Willette-Brown J, Mikhael AI, Geahlen RL, Nakamura MC, Linnemeyer P, Seaman WE, Anderson SK, Ortaldo JR, and Mason LH (1998). DAP12-mediated signal transduction in natural killer cells. A dominant role for the Syk protein-tyrosine kinase. J Biol Chem 273:32934–42

Moretta A, Bottino C, Vitale M, Pende D, Cantoni C, Mingari MC, Biassoni R, and Moretta L (2001). Activating receptors and coreceptors involved in human natural killer cell-mediated cytolysis. Ann Rev Immunol 19:197–223.

Moretta L, Bottino C, Pende D, Mingari MC, Biassoni R, and Moretta A (2002). Human natural killer cells: their origin, receptors and function. Eur J Immunol 32:1205–11.

Morra M, Howie D, Grande MS, Sayos J, Wang N, Wu C, Engel P, and Terhorst C (2001a). X-linked lymphoproliferative disease: a progressive immunodeficiency. Annu Rev Immunol 19:657–82

Morra M, Lu J, Poy F, Martin M, Sayos J, Calpe S, Gullo C, Howie D, Rietdijk S, Thompson A, Coyle AJ, Denny C, Yaffe MB, Engel P, Eck MJ, and Terhorst C (2001b). Structural basis for the interaction of the free SH2 domain EAT-2 with SLAM receptors in hematopoietic cells. EMBO J 20:5840–52

Nguyen KB, Salazar-Mather TP, Dalod MY, Van Deusen JB, Wei XQ, Liew FY, Caligiuri MA, Durbin JE, and Biron CA (2002). Coordinated and distinct roles for IFN-αβ, IL-12, and IL-15 regulation of NK cell responses to viral infection. J Immunol 169:4279–87

Nichols KE, Ma CS, Cannons JL, Schwartzberg PL, and Tangye SG (2005). Molecular and cellular pathogenesis of X-linked lymphoproliferative disease. Immunol Rev 203:180–99

Nutt SL, Brady J, Hayakawa Y, and Smyth MJ (2004). Interleukin 21:a key player in lymphocyte maturation. Crit Rev Immunol 24:239–50

Okkenhaug K, and Vanhaesebroeck B (2003). PI3K in lymphocyte development, differentiation and activation. Nat Rev Immunol 3:317–30

Parham P (2005). MHC class I molecules and KIRs in human history, health and survival. Nat Rev Immunol 5: 201–14

Perussia B (2000). Signaling for cytotoxicity. Nat Immunol 1:372–4

Peruzzi M, Wagtmann N, and Long EO (1996). A p70 killer inhibitory receptor specific for several HLA-B allotypes discriminates among peptides bound to HLA-B*2705. J Exp Med 184:1585–90

Rajagopalan S, Fu J, and Long EO (2001). Cutting edge: induction of IFN-γ production but not cytotoxicity by the killer cell Ig-like receptor KIR2DL4 (CD158d) in resting NK cells. J Immunol 167:1877–81

Rajagopalan S, and Long EO (1997). The direct binding of a p58 killer cell inhibitory receptor to human histocompatibility leukocyte antigen (HLA)-Cw4 exhibits peptide selectivity. J Exp Med 185:1523–8

Raulet DH (2004). Interplay of natural killer cells and their receptors with the adaptive immune response. Nat Immunol 5:996–1002

Ruggeri L, Capanni M, Urbani E, Perruccio K, Shlomchik WD, Tosti A, Posati S, Rogaia D, Frassoni F, Aversa F, Martelli MF, and Velardi A (2002). Effectiveness of donor natural killer cell alloreactivity in mismatched hematopoietic transplants. Science 295:2097–100.

Sakisaka T, and Takai Y (2004). Biology and pathology of nectins and nectin-like molecules. Curr Opin Cell Biol 16:513–21

Shibuya A, Campbell D, Hannum C, Yssel H, Franz-Bacon K, McClanahan T, Kitamura T, Nicholl J, Sutherland GR, Lanier LL, and Phillips JH (1996). DNAM-1, a novel adhesion molecule involved in the cytolytic function of T lymphocytes. Immunity 4:573–81

Shibuya K, Lanier LL, Phillips JH, Ochs HD, Shimizu K, Nakayama E, Nakauchi H, and Shibuya A (1999). Physical and functional association of LFA-1 with DNAM-1 adhesion molecule. Immunity 11:615–23

Sivori S, Falco M, Della Chiesa M, Carlomagno S, Vitale M, Moretta L, and Moretta A (2004). CpG and double-stranded RNA trigger human NK cells by Toll-like receptors: induction of cytokine release and cytotoxicity against tumors and dendritic cells. Proc Natl Acad Sci USA 101:10116–21

Tassi I, Presti R, Kim S, Yokoyama WM, Giltillan S, and Colonna M (2005). Phospholipase C-gamma2 is a critical signaling mediator for murine NK cell activating receptors. J Immunol 175:749–754

Ting AT, Karnitz LM, Schoon RA, Abraham RT, and Leibson PJ (1992). Fc γ receptor activation induces the tyrosine phosphorylation of both phospholipase C (PLC)-γ1 and PLC-γ2 in natural killer cells. J Exp Med 176:1751–5

Trotta R, Fettucciari K, Azzoni L, Abebe B, Puorro KA, Eisenlohr LC, and Perussia B (2000). Differential role of p38 and c-Jun N-terminal kinase 1 mitogen-activated protein kinases in NK cell cytotoxicity. J Immunol 165:1782–9

Trotta R, Puorro KA, Paroli M, Azzoni L, Abebe B, Eisenlohr LC, and Perussia B (1998). Dependence of both spontaneous and antibody-dependent, granule exocytosis-mediated NK cell cytotoxicity on extracellular signal-regulated kinases. J Immunol 161:6648–56

Vales-Gomez M, Reyburn H, and Strominger J (2000). Interaction between the human NK receptors and their ligands. Crit Rev Immunol 20:223–44

Vales-Gomez M, Reyburn HT, Mandelboim M, and Strominger JL (1998). Kinetics of interaction of HLA-C ligands with natural killer cell inhibitory receptors. Immunity 9:892

Vance RE, Kraft JR, Altman JD, Jensen PE, and Raulet DH (1998). Mouse CD94/NKG2A Is a natural killer cell receptor for the nonclassical major histocompatibility complex (MHC) class i molecule Qa-1(b). J Exp Med 188:1841–8

Veillette A, and Latour S (2003). The SLAM family of immune-cell receptors. Curr Opin Immunol 15:277–85

Vilches C, and Parham P (2002). KIR: diverse, rapidly evolving receptors of innate and adaptive immunity. Annu Rev Immunol 20:217–51

Vivier E, and Biron CA (2002). A pathogen receptor on natural killer cells. Science 296:1248–9

Vivier E, and Daëron M (1997). Immunoreceptor tyrosine-based inhibition motifs (ITIMs). Immunol Today 18:286–91

Vivier E, and Malissen B (2005). Innate and adaptive immunity: specificities and signaling hierarchies revisited. Nat Immunol 6:17–21

Vivier E, Nunes JA, and Vely F (2004). Natural killer cell signaling pathways. Science 306:1517–9

Vosshenrich CA, Ranson T, Samson SI, Corcuff E, Colucci F, Rosmaraki EE, and Di Santo JP (2005). Roles for common cytokine receptor gamma-chain-dependent cytokines in the generation, differentiation, and maturation of NK cell precursors and peripheral NK cells in vivo. J Immunol 174:1213–21

Vyas YM, Maniar H, and Dupont B (2002). Visualization of signaling pathways and cortical cytoskeleton in cytolytic and noncytolytic natural killer cell immune synapses. Immunol Rev 189:161–78

Wang D, Feng J, Wen R, Marine JC, Sangster MY, Parganas E, Hoffmeyer A, Jackson CW, Cleveland JL, Murray PJ, and Ihle JN (2000). Phospholipase Cγ2 is essential in the functions of B cell and several Fc receptors. Immunity 13:25–35

Wu J, Song Y, Bakker AB, Bauer S, Spies T, Lanier LL, and Phillips JH (1999). An activating immunoreceptor complex formed by NKG2D and DAP10. Science 285:730–2

Wu LC, Tuot DS, Lyons DS, Garcia KC, and Davis MM (2002). Two-step binding mechanism for T-cell receptor recognition of peptide MHC. Nature 418:552–6

Yokoyama WM (1998). Natural killer cell receptors. Curr Opin Immunol 10:298–305

Zappacosta F, Borrego F, Brooks AG, Parker KC, and Coligan JE (1997). Peptides isolated from HLA-CW 0304 confer different degrees of protection from natural killer cell-mediated lysis. Proc. Natl Acad Sci USA 94:6313–8

Zompi S, Gu H, and Colucci F (2004). The absence of Grb2-associated binder 2 (Gab2) does not disrupt NK cell development and functions. J Leukoc Biol 76:896–903

Zompi S, Hamerman JA, Ogasawara K, Schweighoffer E, Tybulewicz VL, Di Santo JP, Lanier LL, and Colucci F (2003). NKG2D triggers cytotoxicity in mouse NK cells lacking DAP12 or Syk family kinases. Nat Immunol 4:565–72

Signal Transduction in Natural Killer Cells

A. W. MacFarlane IV · K. S. Campbell (✉)

Fox Chase Cancer Center, Division of Basic Science, Institute for Cancer Research, 333 Cottman Ave., Philadelphia, PA 19111, USA
kerry.campbell@fccc.edu

1	Introduction	24
2	Physical Parameters of NK Cell Activation: The Cytolytic NK Cell Immune Synapse	25
3	Activation Signaling Through Receptor-Associated Transmembrane Accessory Proteins	27
4	Signals Downstream of ITAMs	28
5	Signaling Through DAP10	31
6	Vav, Rho Family GTPases, and MAP Kinases	32
7	Negative Signaling by Inhibitory Receptors	35
8	2B4	39
9	KIR2DL4	42
10	Considerations and Summary	43
	References	44

Abstract Tolerance of natural killer (NK) cells toward normal cells is mediated through their expression of inhibitory receptors that detect the normal expression of self in the form of class I major histocompatibility complex (MHC-I) molecules on target cells. These MHC-I-binding inhibitory receptors recruit tyrosine phosphatases, which are believed to counteract activating receptor-stimulated tyrosine kinases. The perpetual balance between signals derived from inhibitory and activating receptors controls NK cell responsiveness and provides an interesting paradigm of signaling cross talk. This review summarizes our knowledge of the intracellular mechanisms by which cell surface receptors influence biological responses by NK cells. Special emphasis focuses on the dynamic signaling events at the NK immune synapse and the unique signaling characteristics of specific receptors, such as NKG2D, 2B4, and KIR2DL4.

1
Introduction

The observation that natural killer (NK) cells selectively attack abnormal cells lacking proper display of self molecules of the class I major histocompatibility complex (MHC-I) spawned the "missing self" hypothesis [101]. By attacking cells that do not properly express MHC-I, NK cells can destroy mutant cells that cytolytic T cells would miss. Many pathogenic conditions are marked by MHC-I downregulation, including cells infected with varicella-zoster virus [3] or cytomegalovirus [118] and numerous tumor cells [63, 64].

The strategy of "missing self recognition" differs from that governing T- and B cell activation, which is triggered by the specific recognition of antigen (nonself) through expression of a wide repertoire of polymorphic receptors. It has come to light that a complex interplay of signals initiates upon engagement of numerous diverse NK cell receptors during interactions with other cells in the body. Some of these receptors are activating, whereas others are inhibitory. Activating receptors can initiate adhesion, cytotoxicity, and cytokine release. The key regulators of NK cell activation, however, are inhibitory receptors that recognize MHC-I and are responsible for limiting the activating signals. In this way, recognition of normal MHC-I expression dominantly suppresses NK attack of normal cells, whereas a lack of self MHC-I recognition shifts the balance toward target cell killing.

Contemporary NK signaling theory holds that "positive signals" derived from activating receptors are transduced through protein tyrosine kinase (PTK)-dependent pathways to phosphorylate signaling intermediates that polarize the cell toward its target, causing focused release of cytolytic granules and cytokine production. The granules contain perforin and granzymes that perforate the target and induce apoptosis, respectively. Cytokines, especially IFNγ, TNFα, and GM-CSF activate other immune cells, promote viral clearance, and elicit antitumor effects. In contrast, tolerance toward normal cells is mediated by "negative" signals derived from engagement of the MHC-I-binding receptors that recruit protein tyrosine phosphatases (PTP), which are believed to dephosphorylate the activation signaling intermediates. Specific details of how the activating and inhibitory signals propagate and interact within the cell are the subject of this review. After introducing major general concepts of NK cell signaling, we will highlight details relevant to some specific receptors of interest.

2
Physical Parameters of NK Cell Activation: The Cytolytic NK Cell Immune Synapse

The surface of contact between NK cell and target cell has been termed the NK immune synapse (NKIS). Contact with a susceptible target cell has been named the cytolytic NKIS (cNKIS), and a noncytolytic interaction with a normal cell is defined as an inhibitory NKIS (iNKIS), which will be discussed later. Numerous activating receptor-ligand pairs and effector signaling molecules accumulate at the cNKIS, forming an aggregate called the central supramolecular activation cluster (c-SMAC) (see Fig. 1). The peripheral region (p) of the SMAC rings the c-SMAC. The p-SMAC characteristically contains NK cell adhesion molecules, including LFA-1 (CD11a) and Mac-1 (CD11b), which both tether to their ICAM-1 ligand on the target cell. CD2 is an NK cell adhesion molecule in the p-SMAC that interacts with CD58 on target cells in humans and CD48 in rodents. Accordingly, coexpression of ICAM-1 in combination with either CD48 or CD58 on target cells has been shown to initiate strong adhesion by resting NK cells [9]. The actin-binding protein talin characteristically accumulates beneath these adhesion molecules in the p-SMAC, providing a link to the cytoskeleton during cNKIS establishment [126, 139, 169].

During cNKIS formation, focused talin recruitment and actin polymerization in the NK cell organize the assembly of signaling molecules at the target interface. This stabilizes NK cell adhesion to the target cell and initiates subsequent actin-directed reorientation of the microtubule-organizing center (MTOC) toward the target cell [181]. Perforin-containing cytolytic granules are then shuttled to the cNKIS by microtubule-associated kinesin motors, resulting in the focused release of their contents at the target interface [90]. A ring of F-actin surrounding the site of granule release [126] is believed to localize the release of cytolytic effectors and thereby prevent killing of normal "bystander" cells. Interestingly, multiple cNKIS can simultaneously occur toward susceptible target cells on opposite poles of an NK cell, but one report suggests that c-SMAC formation can only occur at one of the multiple interfaces at a given time [169]. Wülfing and colleagues have provided evidence that actin polarization is a key element in a series of sequential cytoskeletal polarization events that are required to trigger NK cell cytotoxicity [181]. Furthermore, they found that cytotoxicity by NK cells was more sensitive than that of CTL to a pharmacological inhibitor of actin dynamics [181]. Separately, Orange et al. found sequential cytoskeletal reorganization requirements, in which actin function was necessary for adhesion molecule redistribution within the cNKIS, whereas tubulin assembly was not obligatory until subsequent perforin polarization toward the target [126].

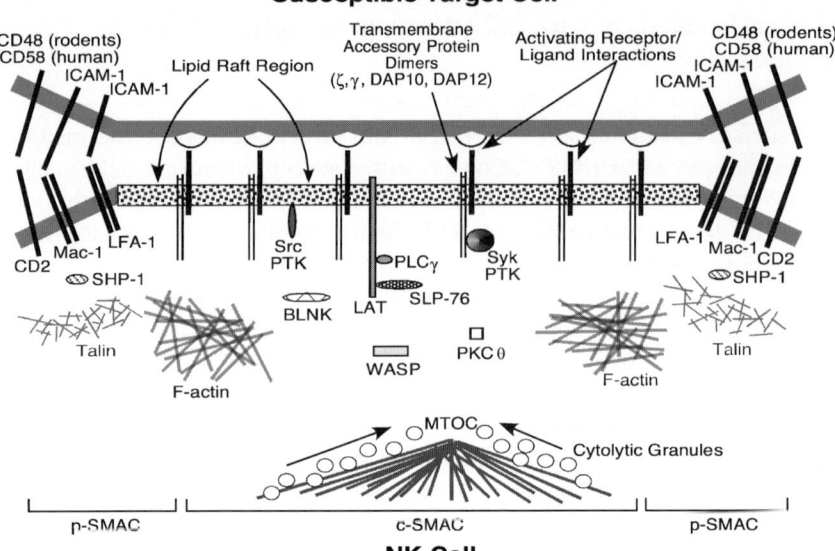

Fig. 1 The cytolytic NK immune synapse (cNKIS). A wide array of molecular interactions between receptor-ligand pairs, signaling effectors, signaling adaptors, lipid rafts, and cytoskeletal components occur at the contact interface between an NK cell (*bottom*) and a susceptible target cell (*top*). The lipid raft subdomain is designated as a speckled region of the overall plasma membrane (*gray bar*). The diagram is a simplified model to visualize the general physical localization of some of these molecules within the c-SMAC and p-SMAC regions of the developing cNKIS. Their locations are based on numerous immunofluorescence studies as described in the text

Lipid rafts are glycosphingolipid-enriched membrane microdomains that rapidly accumulate at the c-SMAC in a cytoskeleton-dependent manner [54, 104, 126, 168]. A number of important signaling markers are anchored in rafts, including the Src family PTK Lck and the linker for activation of T cells (LAT), which is a transmembrane adaptor [77, 194]. The c-SMAC becomes the focal point of intense positive signaling that is initiated by recruitment of a wide array of signaling effector proteins. The functions of these effectors will be discussed below in greater detail, but they include the membrane-active enzyme phospholipase Cγ (PLCγ)$_1$, the cytosolic adaptors SLP-76, BLNK, and Wiskott-Aldrich syndrome protein (WASP), and the protein kinases Itk, Fyn, Lck, Syk, ZAP-70, and protein kinase C (PKC)-θ [127, 169]. Recruitment of lipid rafts to the c-SMAC requires the Src family PTKs (Fyn and Lck), Syk family PTKs (Syk and ZAP-70), and the serine/threonine kinase, PKC-θ [13, 104]. Src homology 2 (SH2) domain-containing PTP-1 (SHP-1) is also recruited to the p-SMAC within 1 min of target cell conjugation [167, 168]. This may provide a mechanism for limiting the spread of activation beyond the c-SMAC. After 10 min of conjugation, SHP-1 enriches at the c-SMAC, possibly indicating a negative feedback role in limiting the duration of the activation response.

Many signaling events at the cNKIS lead to actin polymerization, which is crucial for cytotoxicity responses. The c-SMAC component WASP interacts with Cdc42 and the ARP2/3 complex to drive actin polymerization [128]. Patients with Wiskott-Aldrich syndrome exhibit defects in WASP and notably display impaired NK cell cytotoxicity that correlates with decreased frequency of F-actin and perforin at the cNKIS [66, 127].

The above discussion has outlined the known physical parameters that occur at the cNKIS to trigger cytoskeletal polarization and the cytolytic response. The following sections will examine specific signaling pathways that are triggered downstream from activating receptors engaged with ligands at the cNKIS.

3
Activation Signaling Through Receptor-Associated Transmembrane Accessory Proteins

Most NK cell-activating receptors communicate external stimuli to the cellular interior through noncovalent association with disulfide-linked dimers of transmembrane (TM) accessory proteins. The four TM accessory proteins known to exist in NK cells are TCRζ (ζ), FcεRIγ (γ), and DNAX activating proteins of 10 kDa (DAP10, also known as KAP10) and 12 kDa (DAP12, also known as KARAP). All four TM accessory proteins exist as disulfide-linked homodimers, whereas γ and ζ can also disulfide-link as heterodimers. For details about pairing between specific receptors and accessory proteins, see Table 1. Association of activating receptors with TM accessory proteins is generally promoted by electrostatic interactions between a TM arginine or lysine residue in the receptor that pairs with a corresponding aspartic or glutamic acid residue on the accessory protein. One notable exception is the receptor for antibody-dependent cytotoxicity (ADCC), FcγRIII (CD16), which associates with γ and ζ, despite the presence of a TM glutamic acid residue [92]. The cytoplasmic domains of DAP12, γ, and ζ all contain one or more immunoreceptor tyrosine-based activation motif (ITAM), whereas DAP10 has a YINM sequence. The following discussion will examine ITAM-mediated signaling and a subsequent section will detail events downstream from DAP10.

Table 1 Transmembrane accessory proteins associated with various NK cell-activating receptors from mouse and human

Receptor	Species	Accessory protein
CD16 (FcεRIII)	Mouse	γ
CD16 (FcεRIII)	Human	γ and ζ
KIR2DS	Human	DAP12
KIR3DS	Human	N.D. (probably DAP12)
KIR2DL4	Human	γ (some ζ)
Ly49D, H	Mouse	DAP12
CD94/NKG2C, E	Mouse and human	DAP12
NKG2D	Mouse	DAP10 and DAP12
NKG2D	Human	DAP10
NKp30	Human	γ and ζ
NKp44	Human	DAP12
NKp46	Human	γ and ζ
NKR-P1C	Mouse	γ

N.D., not determined

4
Signals Downstream of ITAMs

The ITAM is characterized by an amino acid sequence of $Yxx(L/I/V)x_{(6-8)}Yxx(L/I/V)$ [71]. When a receptor associated with an ITAM containing accessory protein binds to its ligand, the tyrosine residues in the ITAM become phosphorylated by a Src family kinase (e.g., Lyn, Lck, or Fyn). It is believed that this important phosphorylation event is primarily initiated by ligand interaction-mediated recruitment of these receptor-associated domains into lipid rafts at the c-SMAC, where Src family PTKs are resident. The bisphosphorylated ITAM establishes a highly specific binding site for the tandem SH2 domains of the Syk family PTKs: spleen tyrosine kinase (Syk) and ζ-associated protein of 70 kDa (ZAP-70). Membrane recruitment of these PTKs and their subsequent activation by Src family kinases represent significant signal-initiating events that are analogous to those of numerous antigen and Fc receptors on lymphocytes [159]. Although either Syk or ZAP-70 is capable of binding to all three ITAM-containing TM accessory proteins, several reports have described preferential association of Syk with DAP12 and γ, whereas ZAP-70 reportedly binds most tightly to ζ, as the name would imply [88, 114, 156].

Syk and ZAP-70 are critical PTKs for the function of ITAM-containing receptor complexes, and Syk has been shown to be required for human NK cell cytotoxicity [22, 80]. It was surprising, however, that NK cells from mice deficient in both of these PTKs still exhibited cytotoxicity toward a number of target cells [43]. At least part of the residual activation signaling in Syk-/ZAP-70-deficient NK cells is likely mediated through integrins, a receptor associated with DAP10, and the 2B4 receptor, all of which function independently of ITAMs, as will be discussed in subsequent sections [6, 8, 16, 146].

Phosphorylation of Syk or ZAP-70 initiates a cascade of downstream events that are fundamental to our understanding of general lymphocyte activation and important for initiating cytotoxicity and cytokine release by NK cells. Some of the major activating signal pathways emanating from ITAMs are outlined in Fig. 2. Initial substrates of Syk and ZAP-70 include phosphatidylinositol 3-kinase (PI3K) and PLCγ [79, 80, 160]. PLCγ activation also requires phosphorylation by a Tec family PTK, such as Itk, which is activated by Syk family PTKs in T cells [105]. PLCγ cleaves phosphatidylinositol 4,5-bisphosphate (PIP_2) in the plasma membrane to release inositol 1,4,5-trisphosphate (IP_3) and diacylglycerol (DAG). IP_3 migrates to the endoplasmic reticulum to release stored calcium, and DAG activates PKC at the plasma membrane [82, 97]. Alternately, PI3K phosphorylates the 3′-inositol hydroxyl group of PIP_2 to generate phosphatidylinositol 3,4,5-trisphosphate (PIP_3). PIP_3 production creates a specific plasma membrane binding site for recruitment of certain signaling proteins containing pleckstrin homology (PH) domains, which include PLCγ, Vav, Itk, and 3BP2. 3BP2 is an adaptor protein that brings PLCγ and Vav together at the assembling signalosome [78, 107]. Syk-phosphorylated Vav activates GTPases of the Rhofamily [60], which will be covered in Sect. 6 below. Activation of PLCγ, PKC, Vav, and PI3K as well as elevation of cytosolic calcium concentrations are important events for initiation of the cytolytic hit by NK cells [19, 34, 42, 60, 79, 82, 158–160, 181].

Another substrate of Syk and ZAP-70 kinases is growth factor receptor-bound protein 2 (Grb2), which is an adaptor that recruits son of sevenless (SOS). SOS is a guanine nucleotide exchange factor (GEF) that activates the Ras family GTPases, which trigger the Ras→RAF→MEK→ERK cascade [59]. Extracellular signal-regulated kinase (ERK) is a mitogen-activated protein kinase (MAPK) involved in regulating growth, proliferation, and cytotoxicity. ERK is activated by ITAM-coupled receptors and integrins in NK cells and important for granule-mediated cytotoxicity and IFNγ production [27, 29, 108, 115, 163, 174]. One report, however, showed that ERK does not contribute to conjugation with target cells or reorganization of actin or tubulin cytoskeleton in NK cells [163]. It was recently reported that abnormal NK

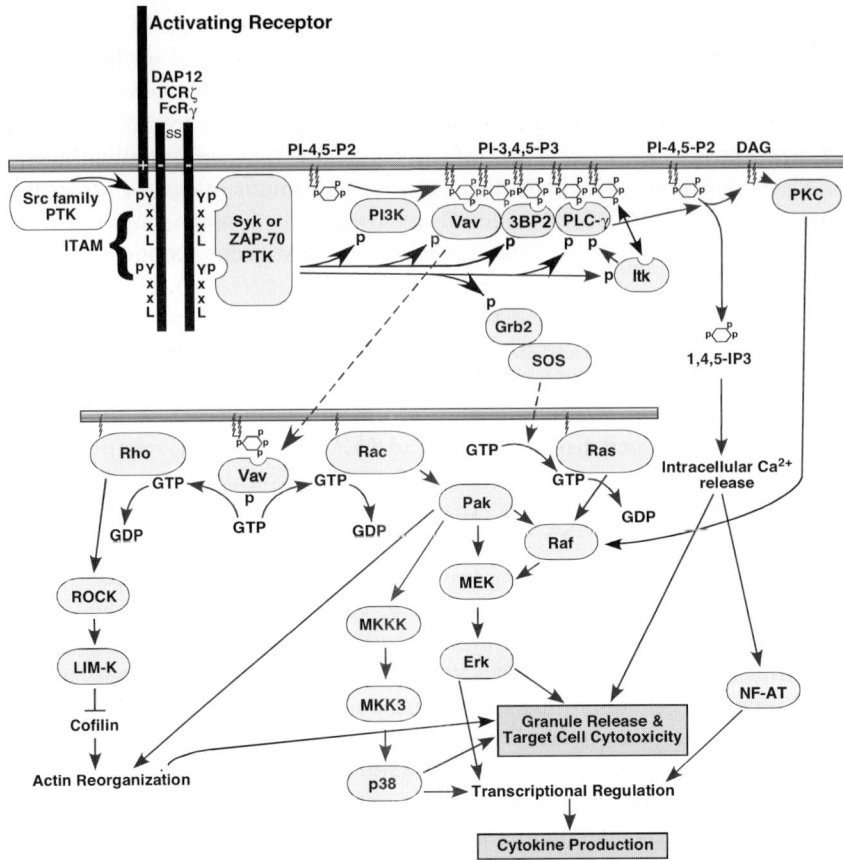

Fig. 2 Signaling cascades downstream from ITAM-coupled receptors. This model diagrams the major downstream intracellular events emanating from an engaged NK cell-activating receptor that is noncovalently associated with a disulfide-linked (*SS*) dimer of ITAM-containing TM accessory proteins. *Single arrows* label activation impacts or motility of molecules, *double-headed arrow* designates physical interaction, *dash-lined arrows* specify links to effector functions in another portion of the cell surface plasma membrane (*gray bar*) for clarity, *p* signifies a phosphorylation event, and *gray boxes* highlight ultimate biological responses. *Rounded notches* in individual effector modules represent SH2 or PH domains that interact with tyrosine phosphorylated proteins or PIP_3, respectively. Abbreviations correspond with the text

cells from patients with lymphoproliferative disease of granular lymphocytes (NK-LDGL) exhibit constitutive Ras and ERK activation that contributes to their accumulation [52].

5
Signaling Through DAP10

DAP10 is only associated with one activating receptor, which is NKG2D. Human NKG2D only associates with homodimers of DAP10, and murine NK cells possess a similar version, NKG2D-L, which also associates only with DAP10 dimers [50, 65, 140]. Murine NK cells, however, also express a shorter version, NKG2D-S, which lacks 13 amino-terminal amino acids in the cytoplasmic domain and can uniquely associate with homodimers of both DAP10 and DAP12 [50, 65, 140]. In contrast to ITAM-signaling receptors, the previously mentioned YINM motif on DAP10 becomes phosphorylated on ligation of NKG2D [10], thereby establishing a membrane-proximal binding site for SH2 domains of the Grb2 adaptor and the p85 subunit of PI3K [35, 180]. Grb2 and PI3K recruitment are also part of the ITAM-initiated activating pathway, and it has been shown that DAP10 signaling plays a costimulatory role that amplifies ITAM signaling [65, 69, 141, 178]. Similar costimulatory functions by CD28 and CD19 that enhance antigen receptor signaling in T- and B-cells, respectively, are also thought to be derived mainly from recruitment of PI3K [4, 30]. Numerous reports, however, indicate that NKG2D/DAP10 can also directly stimulate cytotoxicity [6, 16, 75, 196]. One of these studies even utilized NK cells from mice lacking Syk, ZAP-70, and DAP12 [196].

Significant differences have emerged that distinguish DAP10-initiated signals from those downstream of ITAMs. First, Billadeau et al. have shown in human NK cells that DAP10 signaling through the YINM motif is independent of Syk but involves Src kinases, SLP-76, PLCγ, Vav-1, and Rho family GTPases, whereas ITAM signaling involves all of these, including Syk [16]. Their evidence also indicates that DAP10-mediated phosphorylation of PLCγ and Vav requires the YINM tyrosine, but is independent of PI3K [16]. This suggests important roles for other effector proteins that might be recruited to the phosphorylated YINM. In line with this possibility, one study has found that NKG2D ligation stimulates Janus kinase 2 (Jak2) and STAT5, which are not characteristic effectors in ITAM signaling [153]. Several reports indicate that DAP10 can stimulate cytotoxicity, but not IFNγ production by NK cells, whereas DAP12 can trigger both responses [50, 69, 178, 196]. Although the basis of this is not entirely clear, the activation of Syk/ZAP-70 through ITAMs, which represents a major distinction from DAP10 signaling, may be critical for the cytokine response [80]. Second, evidence has been provided that NKG2D/DAP10-mediated activation is apparently less sensitive to attenuation by MHC class I-binding inhibitory receptors, such as KIR, whereas ITAM-containing receptor signaling is readily blocked by these inhibitory receptors [10, 32, 44, 49]. The molecular basis for this insensitivity to inhibition is currently unclear, but it allows NK cells to attack tumors that upregulate NKG2D ligands yet still express MHC-I. A third difference in downstream signaling is the activation of different Vav subtypes by ITAM- and YINM-coupled receptors [31]. These differences in Vav activation will be detailed in the next section.

6
Vav, Rho Family GTPases, and MAP Kinases

Vav proteins are major players in numerous downstream NK cell activation events and have been the subject of intense research in recent years. The Vav proteins are GEFs that activate certain Rho family GTPases by promoting the exchange of enzyme-bound GDP for GTP [45]. Rho family GTPases serve as molecular switches that are "on" when bound with GTP, but "off" when the nucleotide is hydrolyzed to GDP. The best-characterized subgroups of the Rho family are Rho (three members), Rac (four members), and Cdc42 (five members) [148]. By stimulating Rho family GTPases, Vav activation impacts upon a wide range of NK cell processes, including adhesion, cytoskeletal polarization toward the target cell, cytolytic granule release, transcriptional regulation, and cytokine production [45, 60, 164].

Vav-mediated activation of Rho family GTPases ultimately leads to the activation of members of the MAPK family, namely ERK, p38, and c-Jun N-terminal kinase (JNK). Evidence indicates that the p38 and ERK subgroups are important for IFNγ production and cytotoxicity, whereas JNK is dispensable for the cytolytic response [38, 108, 115, 162, 174, 175]. Importantly, the effector phase of the NK cell cytotoxicity response has been shown to require ERK activation that is mediated through Rac1 instead of its typical upstream effector, Ras [14, 79, 175]. This Rac1→Pak→MEK→ERK pathway was shown to be critical for polarization of cytolytic granules toward target cells [14, 60, 79, 175]. In line with these studies, activation of Rac GTPases in NK cells with a pharmacological agent was recently shown to dramatically reorganize actin dynamics, increase target cell adhesion, and enhance cytotoxicity [109]. In addition to their roles in the cytolytic response, activated MAPKs can be transported to the nucleus to regulate transcription [36, 177]. A growing body of evidence demonstrates selective transcriptional regulation events resulting from the activation of specific MAPKs [138, 177].

The Vav family GEFs are believed to be recruited to the plasma membrane by the binding of their PH domain to PIP_3, where they become activated [68], but evidence also exists for PI3K-independent Vav activation [16, 51, 73]. In addition to stimulation through ITAM and YINM signaling,

Vav proteins can also be activated by adhesion-related integrins [137]. In a quiescent cell, Vav exists in an inactive state where it is folded back upon itself in a hairpinlike conformation by an interaction between regulatory tyrosine residues and other amino acids within the Dbl homology domain. When the regulatory tyrosines become phosphorylated, these interactions are broken and Vav unfolds into its active conformation [5, 15]. (For an excellent review of the structure and function of Vav domains, see [164].) Three members of the Vav family have been identified and to a certain extent characterized. Vav-1 is restricted to hematopoietic cells, but Vav-2 and Vav-3 are ubiquitously expressed [26]. Vav-1 is sometimes referred to simply as Vav, but here we will specify Vav-1 in reference to the first member discovered and use Vav when referring to all three family members collectively.

Recent experiments with mice deficient in one or more Vav family members have demonstrated specific functional linkage to distinct TM accessory proteins. These experiments showed Vav-1 to be essential for NKG2D/DAP10 (YINM)-mediated signaling, whereas DAP12 (ITAM)-mediated signals are transduced by Vav-2 and Vav-3 [31]. The fact that loss of both Vav-2 and Vav-3 was required to abolish signals through DAP12 suggests that these two GEFs function in a redundant fashion in ITAM-dependent NK cell signaling pathways. This correlates well with the observations that DAP12- but not DAP10-derived signals induce IFNγ secretion [196] and that IFNγ secretion by NK cells is independent of VAV-1 [42]. Further evidence for alternative methods of Vav activation was provided by Riteau et al., who showed that Vav-2 can become activated in NK cells by a signal originating from the β_2 integrin LFA-1 [137]. Although clear distinctions that account for functional differences between Vav family members are not yet well established, many of the downstream impacts mediated through Rho family GTPases are outlined in the following discussion and schematized in Figs. 2 and 3.

Vav-1 has been shown to function as a GEF for Rac members [Rac-1 [46], Rac-2 [145], RhoG [145]], Cdc42 [191], and possibly RhoA [129]. Vav-2 and Vav-3 have been shown to activate Rac members (Rac-1, RhoG) and RhoA [121, 122]. There are numerous conflicting reports as to whether Vav-2 is also a GEF for Cdc42 [2, 99, 122, 145, 176]. The Rac, Rho, and Cdc42 subgroups of GTPases impart distinct effects on the actin cytoskeleton as described below. Rac-1, Cdc42, and RhoA can also stimulate transcription through NF-κB [132]. Furthermore, Vav-1 itself has been shown to migrate directly to the nucleus to associate with and facilitate transcription by nuclear factor for activation of T cells (NF-AT) and NF-κB family members [72].

As previously mentioned, Rac-1 initiates a signaling cascade that is important during NK cell cytolytic responses by directly stimulating p21-activated

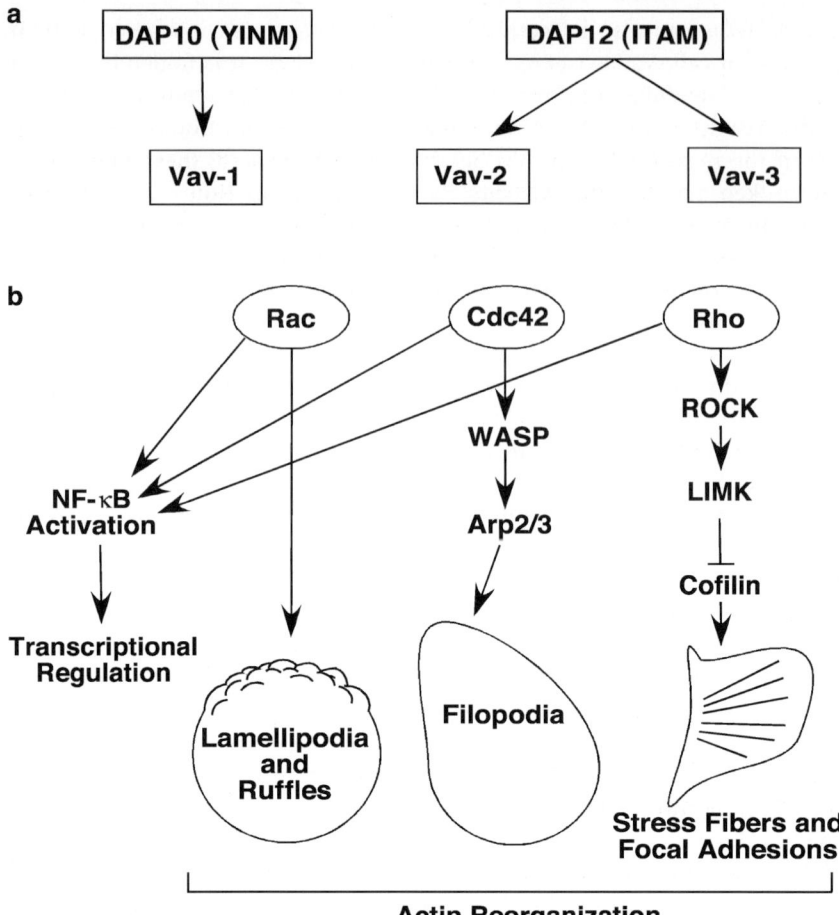

Fig. 3a, b Selective impacts of receptors coupled to YINM- or ITAM-containing receptor complexes on subtypes of Vav and downstream impacts of the major subgroups of Rho family GTPases that are stimulated by Vav. **a** Receptors coupled to DAP10 (containing a YINM motif) and DAP12 (containing an ITAM) activate distinct subsets of Vav subtypes as designated by the *arrows*. **b** Three major Rho family subgroups (Rac, Cdc42, and Rho) can be activated by Vav subtypes to stimulate distinct downstream cascades that lead to radically different impacts on the actin cytoskeleton. In addition, all three Rho subgroups can impact upon NF-κB to regulate transcription. Major effectors in downstream signaling cascades are designated with *arrows*

kinase (Pak), which activates MEK1 to stimulate ERK [79, 175]. Activation of Rac-1 brings about morphological changes in the actin cytoskeleton that produce lamellipodia and ruffles [136]. Lamellipodia are the actin-rich leading edges of motile cells, and ruffles are dorsal circular structures. Rac-2 is also known to act through ERK and p38 and to promote actin polymerization in T cells [186] and granule exocytosis in neutrophils [1]. Rho-G also generates lamellipodia and ruffles, but in a more site-specific manner than Rac-1 [176].

RhoA has been shown in NK cells to activate Rho-associated kinase (ROCK), which subsequently phosphorylates and activates LIM-kinase (LIMK) [103]. Active LIMK inhibits the actin-depolymerizing protein cofilin. Disruption of cofilin function leads to the formation of focal adhesions and stress fibers that are involved in cell adhesion and motility [103]. Integrity of the RhoA→ROCK→LIMK pathway has been shown to be essential for recruitment of lipid rafts and actin polymerization at the cNKIS and for target cytotoxicity [103].

Members of the Cdc42 subgroup of the Rho family recruit WASP. WASP facilitates Arp2/3-mediated actin nucleation, which promotes growth of elongated cytoskeletal protrusions called filopodia [128]. Although a clear role for Cdc42 in NK cell function has not been defined, WASP is important in cytotoxicity responses [66, 127], as mentioned above. Like Rac, Cdc42 can also activate Pak and its downstream signaling events [148].

7
Negative Signaling by Inhibitory Receptors

NK cell tolerance toward normal cells is derived from "negative signaling" that originates through cell surface inhibitory receptors, which detect MHC-I molecules on the surface of normal cells. The MHC-I-binding inhibitory receptors expressed on NK cells include killer cell Ig-like receptors (KIR; human), Ly49 (mouse), NKG2A/CD94 (human and mouse), and ILT2/LIR1 (CD85j; human). The engagement of NK cell inhibitory receptors with MHC-I molecules on normal target cells causes them to coaggregate with activating receptors that are simultaneously interacting with ligands at the target cell interface. The magnitude of inhibition is proportional to the degree of MHC-I engagement. If sufficiently engaged, the inhibitory receptors efficiently and dominantly block downstream signals that are initiated by the activating receptors. Accumulated evidence indicates that this inhibition is primarily mediated through recruitment of two PTPs, named SH2 domain-containing protein tyrosine phosphatase-1 (SHP-1) and SHP-2, to the cytoplasmic domains of the inhibitory receptors. Numerous early activation signaling events are abolished upon inhibitory receptor engagement with MHC-I, most notably intracellular calcium mobilization [28, 82].

As mentioned above, the physical contact interface between an NK cell and a normal MHC-I-expressing cell that is resistant to attack has been termed the inhibitory NKIS (iNKIS). The accumulation of receptors and signaling molecules at the iNKIS is referred to as the supramolecular inhibition cluster (SMIC). Target cell contact at the iNKIS still initiates transient LFA-1-mediated adhesion and the rapid polarization of talin toward the target cell [167]. The accumulation of talin and Lck quickly dissipates from the iNKIS, however, and adhesion is disrupted within minutes, in sharp contrast with the stable adhesion and accumulation of these molecules at the cNKIS [25, 167]. Furthermore, raft polarization, actin polymerization, and MTOC reorientation are lacking in the iNKIS, whereas these events can last more than 15 min in the cNKIS [54, 104, 142, 167, 169]. PKC-θ, PLCγ, Itk, ZAP-70, SLP-76, and BLNK do not accumulate at the iNKIS [169]. In fact, the only signaling molecules known to be recruited to the c-SMIC within 1 min of target cell conjugation are Lck and SHP-1 [167]. A major distinguishing feature of the iNKIS is early SHP-1 accumulation at the c-SMIC, which is also the site at which inhibitory KIR or Ly49 interacts with MHC-I [47, 53, 167]. One report noted that CD45, CD43, and ezrin are lacking at the iNKIS, whereas all three are evenly distributed within the cNKIS [112]. Further analysis in that report revealed that the narrow gap between human NK cell and target cell surfaces within the iNKIS (about 15 nm) corresponds to the height of interacting KIR/HLA-C extracellular domains, whereas CD45 and CD43 are taller, which may explain their physical exclusion from this narrow interface at the c-SMIC [112].

NK cell inhibitory receptors function through immunoreceptor tyrosine-based inhibitory motifs (ITIMs) in their cytoplasmic domains. ITIMs are (I/V)xYxx(L/V) sequences that, when phosphorylated on NK cell inhibitory receptors, become specific binding sites for SHP-1 and SHP-2 [21, 24, 28, 101, 102, 113, 188]. SHP-1 and SHP-2 contain tandem SH2 domains that interact with the tyrosine-phosphorylated ITIMs. Inhibitory Ly49, KIR, ILT2/LIR1, and NKG2A have been shown to recruit SHP-1 and/or SHP-2 to varying degrees via phosphorylated ITIMs [48, 81, 94, 113]. KIR enrichment at the iNKIS is delayed on truncation of the cytoplasmic domain or in the presence of high doses of an inhibitor of actin polymerization, indicating roles for the cytoplasmic domain and actin in the efficiency of KIR clustering toward a resistant target cell [149]. KIR with mutant ITIM tyrosines can still accumulate at the iNKIS but are unable to inhibit lipid raft polarization [54], and dominant-negative SHP-1 can block KIR-mediated inhibition of raft polarization [104].

The following discussion will focus primarily on studies with KIR, which are the best-characterized MHC-I-binding inhibitory receptors. SHP-1 binding to the cytoplasmic domain of KIR occurs only when both ITIMs become tyrosine-phosphorylated. SHP-2, however, can bind when only one ITIM is phosphorylated [21, 58, 188, 189]. Mutational analysis has shown that SHP-2 binds with higher avidity to the phosphorylated amino-terminal ITIM on KIR, and SHP-2 binding avidity correlates well with inhibitory capacity of various mutant receptors [21, 188, 189]. The PTP recruitment patterns from these studies form the basis of the model shown in Fig. 4. Surprisingly, mutation of both KIR ITIM tyrosines to phenylalanine has been shown to result in a receptor that weakly associates with SHP-2 and is still slightly inhibitory [188, 189]. Furthermore, an unphosphorylated peptide encompassing the amino-terminal ITIM readily binds SHP-2, suggesting that SHP-2 may constitutively interact with KIR in the unphosphorylated, resting state [189]. One KIR, named KIR2DL5, uniquely possesses an altered carboxy-terminal ITIM (TxYxxL), which results in a receptor that inhibits NK cell cytotoxicity in a SHP-2-dependent manner [190]. In addition to direct recruitment of SHP-1 and SHP-2 to the iNKIS by inhibitory receptors, binding of these PTPs to phosphorylated ITIMs releases them from a self-inhibiting conformation in the cytosol where the amino-terminal SH2 domain blocks the catalytic domain [70, 161]. This autoinhibition has been shown to be abrogated in vitro by binding of the SH2 domains to tyrosine-phosphorylated KIR ITIM peptides [24, 28, 131].

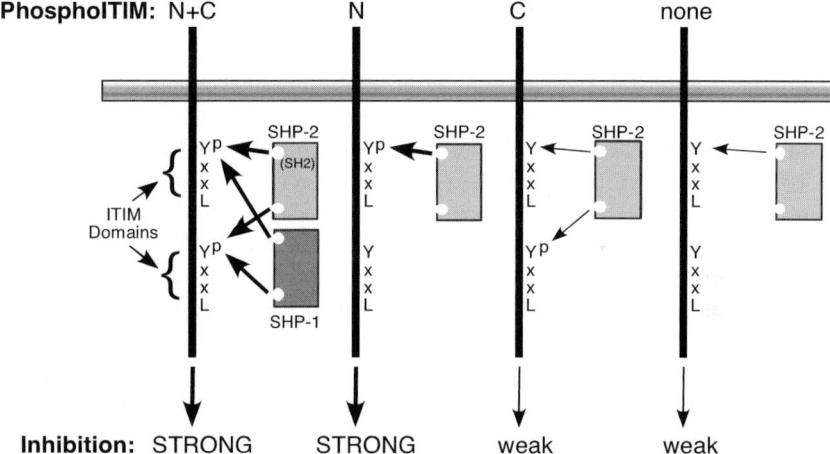

Fig. 4 A model of the patterns of recruitment of SHP-1 and SHP-2 to phosphorylated amino (N)- and carboxy (C)-terminal ITIMs of KIR and their inhibitory consequences. This model is based on biochemical and functional studies described in the text that examined mutant KIR in which the cytoplasmic ITIM tyrosines were selectively changed to phenylalanine, which cannot be phosphorylated

SHP-1 and SHP-2 share 60% sequence identity and very high homology in secondary and tertiary structures. Despite the high homology, they generally play very different roles in vivo, with SHP-1 acting as a negative regulator for many inhibitory receptors (including CD22, CD72, PIR-B, and CD5) [147, 192], whereas SHP-2 is primarily a positive regulator (PDGFR, EGFR, ICAM-1, PAR-2, and leptin receptor) [11, 18, 56, 57, 134, 166, 187, 192]. Nonetheless, examples of positive effects on signaling by SHP-1 [117, 182] and negative influences mediated by SHP-2 [41, 86, 95, 110, 185] have also been reported. It is important to note that electrostatic charge differences surrounding the catalytic clefts influence substrate recognition by the two PTPs, with SHP-2 expected to prefer phosphotyrosines flanked by more acidic residues [184]. Accordingly, numerous examples of differential substrate specificities between SHP-1 and SHP-2 catalytic domains have been reported [116, 125, 157, 172, 183]. Therefore, it is tempting to speculate that these two PTPs may play different functional roles at the iNKIS as a consequence of both recruitment differences dependent on phosphoITIM status of inhibitory receptors and their distinct substrate recognition capacities.

Recruitment and activation of SHP-1 and SHP-2 by phosphorylated inhibitory receptors is believed to prevent NK cell activation by dephosphorylating numerous signaling intermediates at the iNKIS. When human NK cells engage with MHC-I-expressing target cells, tyrosine phosphorylation has been shown to be abrogated in a number of substrates, including Src family PTKs, PLCγ, ZAP-70, Vav, SLP-76, LAT, Grb2, PI3K, and the ITAMS of ζ [17, 150, 165]. It is unclear which of these are direct substrates of SHP-1 or SHP-2 or whether the reduced phosphorylation of some is a consequence of upstream dephosphorylation events. The inhibitory impact, however, appears to be at the level of and downstream from Syk family PTKs [17].

Two studies have provided evidence for direct SHP-1 substrates in human NK cells using substrate-trapping forms of SHP-1. First, Binstadt et al. specifically isolated tyrosine-phosphorylated SLP-76 from NK cell lysates in vitro [17]. Second, Stebbins et al. specifically isolated Vav-1 as a substrate on engaging a chimeric KIR/SHP-1 receptor during conjugation of an NK cell line with MHC-I-expressing target cells [150]. Although both of these studies offer important mechanistic insight, alternative evidence suggests that other relevant substrates exist. For instance, NK cells from SLP-76-deficient mice exhibit normal natural cytotoxicity and ADCC [133], suggesting that SLP-76 is not the key substrate that blocks activation. Futhermore, SHP-1 was shown previously to physically associate with Vav-1 via SH2/SH3 domain interactions [87], suggesting that this interaction might have enhanced capture in the substrate trapping experiments of Stebbins et al. Nonetheless, Vav activation is clearly an important early event in development of the cNKIS, and reversal of its activation by SHP-1-mediated dephosphorylation would indeed abrogate key activation events within the iNKIS.

SH2 domain-containing inositol 5'-phosphatase-1 (SHIP-1) is another negative effector enzyme that can be recruited to ITIMs on several inhibitory receptors, including the B cell receptor, FcγRIIb [67]. By cleaving the 5'-phosphate on PIP_2 and PIP_3 in the plasma membrane, SHIP-1 has the capacity to deplete the substrate for PLCγ and eliminate PI3K-generated binding sites for certain proteins containing PH domains. Gupta et al. have provided convincing evidence that SHIP-1 is not involved in inhibitory KIR function [67]. Wang and colleagues, however, have shown that SHIP-1 can associate with certain inhibitory Ly49 receptors, notably Ly49A and Ly49C, which have broad capacity to bind most MHC-I ligands in mice [48, 171]. Interestingly, a substantially greater number of the NK cells that develop in SHIP-1-deficient mice express Ly49A and Ly49C and survive longer, presumably because of enhanced Akt recruitment to elevated PIP3 in their plasma membranes [171]. SHIP-1 can also transiently localize within lipid rafts at the plasma membrane of NK cells during ADCC responses, apparently through associations with ζ and an adaptor named Shc [61, 62]. Overexpression of SHIP-1 was also shown to suppress ADCC responses, indicating that it can negatively impact upon CD16 function [61]. Therefore, a growing body of evidence suggests that SHIP-1 also plays important negative regulatory roles in NK cell functions.

8
2B4

2B4 (CD244) is a receptor with divergent functional properties that is present on all murine NK cells as well as a subset of T cells [111, 124]. In humans, 2B4 has been detected on NK cells, T cells, basophils, and macrophages [124]. Murine 2B4 receptors are predominantly inhibitory in nature, because mouse NK cells lacking 2B4 show enhanced cytotoxicity [96, 119]. On the other hand, human 2B4 appears to be predominantly an activating receptor, because human NK cells are more cytotoxic toward target cells transfected with the 2B4 ligand CD48 [89]. The murine 2B4 gene alternately expresses two distinct cytoplasmic domains that are either longer (2B4L) or shorter (2B4S) [151]. 2B4S enhances cytolytic activity in murine NK cells, whereas 2B4L is inhibitory [144]. The inhibitory nature of 2B4 in mice is believed to be due to the predominant expression of 2B4L [96, 119]. Downstream signaling events generated from 2B4 ligation are outlined below and diagrammed in Fig. 5.

The cytoplasmic domains of murine 2B4L and human 2B4 contain three and four immunoreceptor tyrosine-based switch motifs (ITSM; TxYxxV/L/I),

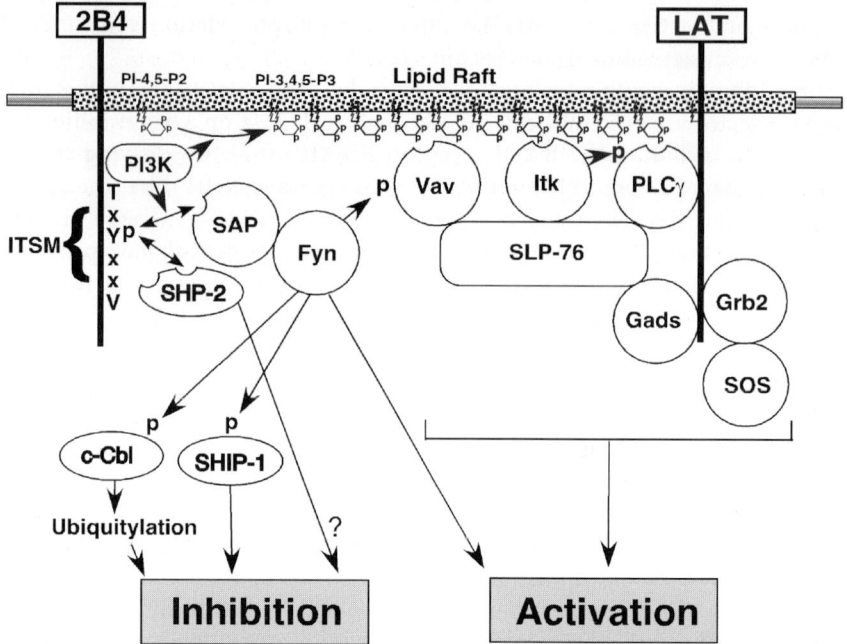

Fig. 5 Downstream signaling from 2B4 and LAT. A schematized model shows protein interactions (*physically attached modules* or *double-headed arrows*) and downstream functional impacts (*single-headed arrows*; p signifies phosphorylation). The lipid raft subdomain is designated as a *speckled region* of the overall plasma membrane (*gray bar*). *Rounded notches* in effector modules represent SH2 or PH domains that interact with tyrosine-phosphorylated proteins or PIP_3, respectively. Ultimate biological impacts on NK cell activation or inhibition are signified in the *gray boxes*. This is a simplified model based on current evidence from a number of studies that are described in the text

respectively, whereas 2B4S has only one [85]. Upon engagement, the receptor is recruited to lipid rafts at the target cell interface in an actin-dependent manner, and tyrosine residues in the ITSM sequences are phosphorylated [173]. Phosphorylation of the ITSM sequences creates specific binding sites for SH2 domain-containing proteins, most notably signaling lymphocyte activation molecule (SLAM)-associated protein (SAP, also known as SH2D1A) [98, 143, 154]. SAP is an SH2 domain-containing adaptor that links 2B4 to the Src family PTK Fyn [33, 93]. One report claims that PI3K is also recruited to 2B4 on ligation and that the recruitment of SAP to 2B4 requires PI3K function [7]. Recruitment of SAP and Fyn was shown in one report to be essential for 2B4-mediated tyrosine phosphorylation of Vav-1, c-Cbl, and SHIP [37].

While Vav-1 initiates activation signaling, both c-Cbl and SHIP may be part of a negative feedback mechanism to dampen activation responses through 2B4. c-Cbl is an ubiquitin ligase that can promote the degradation of PTKs [106] and receptors [170]. It is important to note that another report demonstrated that 2B4 ligation alone did not induce tyrosine phosphorylation of Vav-1, but coligation with the integrin LFA-1 synergistically enhanced phosphorylation and raft recruitment of Vav-1 [137].

A genetic mutation that renders the SH2 domain of SAP inoperative causes X-linked proliferative disease (XLP) in humans [152]. NK cells from humans with XLP have attenuated cytotoxic capability [33, 93, 130] that correlates with a lack of activation capacity through 2B4 [12, 123, 155]. Only one report has found 2B4 to act as an inhibitory receptor in NK cells from XLP patients [130]. EWS/FLI1-activated transcript 2 (EAT-2) is an SH2-containing adaptor that is related to SAP but lacks the PxxP motif necessary to bind Fyn [120]. Therefore, it could potentially competitively inhibit SAP-mediated activation through 2B4, but little data exist on the function of EAT-2 in NK cells. Even if EAT-2 can be recruited to 2B4, the evidence indicates that it cannot substitute for the activating function of SAP.

SHP-2 has also been shown to be recruited to murine 2B4L and is presumed to mediate the inhibitory function of that receptor [144]. Tangye et al. reported that SHP-2 was recruited to phosphorylated human 2B4 and competed for SAP recruitment when these proteins were transfected into the murine B cell line BaF3 [155]. Others, however, have failed to demonstrate SHP-2 recruitment to tyrosine-phosphorylated human 2B4 in NK cells [123, 130, 190], although one of these reports alternatively found SHP-1 recruitment [130].

2B4 is also widely believed to interact with the TM adaptor LAT in lipid rafts, and this association was proposed to contribute significantly to activating function by the receptor [20, 39, 40, 85]. It is possible that this interaction may not be direct, but a consequence of colocalization of the two proteins in lipid rafts on 2B4 ligation [139, 173]. LAT is a transmembrane adaptor protein that serves as a major linker for nucleating numerous signaling molecules at the c-SMAC during NK cell activation. LAT is localized to lipid rafts by means of palmitoylation at a CxxC motif [194]. Ligation of 2B4 (CD244) [20], CD2 [74], and FcγRIII (CD16) [76] in NK cells leads to phosphorylation of LAT that recruits PLCγ [195], Grb2 [193], and Gads [100]. Gads (Grb2-related adaptor protein) further links LAT to another adaptor, SLP-76 (signaling lymphocyte protein of 76 kDa) [100], which binds Vav [179]. Itk can also associate with SLP-76 and subsequently phosphorylate PLCγ [23, 91]. In a cNKIS with target cells expressing the 2B4 ligand, CD48, Roda-Navarro et al. reported that the c-SMAC is enriched with 2B4, SAP, and partial colocalization of LAT, which are surrounded by a ring of talin in the p-SMACw [139]. Although 2B4 ligation can stimulate both cytotoxicity and IFNγ release by NK cells, studies with pharmacological inhibitors indicate that downstream signals required for cytotoxicity responses (PKC, Ras, Raf, ERK, and p38) differ substantially from those required to initiate IFNγ production (p38 and the AP-1 transcription factor) [39, 40].

9
KIR2DL4

KIR2DL4 (CD158d) is an intriguing NK cell-activating receptor that is upregulated on IL-2-stimulated NK cells and contains both a transmembrane arginine and a cytoplasmic ITIM [55, 84, 135]. In contrast to most other NK cell-activating receptors, KIR2DL4 is very effective at stimulating IFNγ secretion but induces only weak cytotoxicity in resting NK cells [84, 135]. The ITIM sequence in KIR2DL4 was found to be strongly inhibitory in isolation, as assessed in a chimeric receptor construct in which the cytoplasmic domain selectively recruited SHP-2 [189]. The ITIM does not seem to dampen activating function in the intact receptor, however [55, 84]. Perhaps SHP-2 recruitment may contribute to activation signaling in this context.

Mutation of the transmembrane arginine in KIR2DL4 resulted in a receptor with weak inhibitory capacity, suggesting that the arginine links the receptor to a TM accessory protein [55]. In stark contrast to the other activating members of the KIR family (KIR2DS1–5 and KIR3DS1) that associate with DAP12, KIR2DL4 was recently found to associate strongly with γ and only very weakly with ζ [83]. Association with γ was shown to increase the surface expression of KIR2DL4 and promote its capacity to stimulate cytotoxicity [83]. KIR2DL4 stimulates only weak activation of cytotoxicity in resting NK cells, and this has been proposed to be the result of low stoichiometric association with γ [83]. Alternatively, selective association with γ may directly contribute to the unique functional capacity of KIR2DL4 to stimulate strong IFNγ responses in resting NK cells and the upregulation of KIR2DL4 by IL-2 stimulation. Although there is no definitive evidence that KIR2DL4 can act as an inhibitory receptor in NK cells (unless the transmembrane arginine is mutated [55]), the receptor can reach the cell surface in the absence of associated accessory protein [83]. This suggests that KIR2DL4 might exhibit some inhibitory function when expressed under conditions in which γ expression is limiting.

10
Considerations and Summary

It is important to note that several factors must be considered when interpreting the NK cell signal transduction literature. First, although they mediate the same general biological responses, human and mouse NK cell receptors and signaling pathways can differ substantially because of species differences that are sometimes highly divergent. Second, NK cells share many signal transduction effector proteins that are otherwise uniquely found only in B cells or T cells. Therefore, functionality of NK cells from mice with deficiencies in some of these effectors is sometimes only modestly affected as compared to T- or B cell defects. This appears to be due to greater redundancy from other related effector proteins or alternative signaling pathways that are found in NK cells. Third, signaling mechanisms may be substantially different in resting vs. IL-2-activated NK cells, because of different levels of or activity of certain effector proteins and/or receptors. Fourth, studies in NK-like cell lines should be confirmed in primary NK cells or at least multiple NK-like cell lines. Fifth, the signaling events in NK cells that occur during target cell conjugation are the consequence of simultaneous engagement of numerous cell surface receptors, and therefore it is difficult to ascribe particular events to just one receptor. Furthermore, different NK cell lines or primary clones express varied receptor repertoires and different targets exhibit unique arrays of ligands (some of which have not yet been discovered), which further complicates interpretations between different target cell conjugation experiments. Finally, many NK cell signal transduction studies have used overexpression of wild-type or dominant-negative forms of certain effector proteins with vaccinia virus or pharmacological inhibitors. These methods have limitations and potential side effects, however, and conclusions based solely upon the biological impacts of one of these should be interpreted with caution.

Although our understanding of the signaling mechanisms that control NK cell activation has improved substantially in recent years, there are still enormous opportunities for future discovery. The predominant mechanism controlling NK cell function is negative signaling that commences when inhibitory receptors engage with MHC-I on normal cells of the body. The dynamic balance between negative and positive signals in NK cells makes them an ideal and unique cellular model system for studying signaling cross talk between activating and inhibitory receptors. Better understanding of the molecular basis of NK cell activation should eventually lead to therapeutic methods to manipulate the function of NK cells for facilitating bone marrow transplantation or improving the treatment of cancer or viral infection.

Acknowledgements The authors thank Drs. Erica Golemis, Jonathan Chernoff, and Diana Alvarez Arias for constructive comments on the manuscript. This work was supported by NIH R01 Grants CA-083859 and CA-100226 to K.S.C. A.W.F. was supported by NRSA training grant T32-AI07492; support was also provided in part by NIH CORE Grant CA-06927 and an appropriation from the Commonwealth of Pennsylvania. Its contents are solely the responsibility of the authors and do not necessarily represent the official views of the National Cancer Institute.

References

1. Abdel-Latif D, Steward M, Macdonald DL, Francis GA, Dinauer MC, Lacy P (2004) Rac2 is critical for neutrophil primary granule exocytosis. Blood 104:832–839
2. Abe K, Rossman KL, Liu B, Ritola KD, Chiang D, Campbell SL, Burridge K, Der CJ (2000) Vav2 is an activator of Cdc42, Rac1, and RhoA. J Biol Chem 275:10141–10149
3. Abendroth A, Lin I, Slobedman B, Ploegh H, Arvin AM (2001) Varicella-zoster virus retains major histocompatibility complex class I proteins in the Golgi compartment of infected cells. J Virol 75:4878–4888
4. Acuto O, Michel F (2003) CD28-mediated co-stimulation: a quantitative support for TCR signalling. Nat Rev Immunol 3:939–951
5. Aghazadeh B, Lowry WE, Huang XY, Rosen MK (2000) Structural basis for relief of autoinhibition of the Dbl homology domain of proto-oncogene Vav by tyrosine phosphorylation. Cell 102:625–633
6. Andre P, Castriconi R, Espeli M, Anfossi N, Juarez T, Hue S, Conway H, Romagne F, Dondero A, Nanni M, Caillat-Zucman S, Raulet DH, Bottino C, Vivier E, Moretta A, Paul P (2004) Comparative analysis of human NK cell activation induced by NKG2D and natural cytotoxicity receptors. Eur J Immunol 34:961–971
7. Aoukaty A, Tan R (2002) Association of the X-linked lymphoproliferative disease gene product SAP/SH2D1A with 2B4, a natural killer cell-activating molecule, is dependent on phosphoinositide 3-kinase. J Biol Chem 277:13331–13337
8. Barber DF, Faure M, Long EO (2004) LFA-1 contributes an early signal for NK cell cytotoxicity. J Immunol 173:3653–3659
9. Barber DF, Long EO (2003) Coexpression of CD58 or CD48 with intercellular adhesion molecule 1 on target cells enhances adhesion of resting NK cells. J Immunol 170:294–299
10. Bauer S, Groh V, Wu J, Steinle A, Phillips JH, Lanier LL, Spies T (1999) Activation of NK cells and T cells by NKG2D, a receptor for stress-inducible MICA. Science 285:727–729
11. Bennett AM, Tang TL, Sugimoto S, Walsh CT (1994) Protein-tyrosine-phosphatase SHPTP2 couples platelet-derived growth factor receptor β to Ras. Proc Natl Acad Sci USA 91:7335–7339
12. Benoit L, Wang X, Pabst HF, Dutz J, Tan R (2000) Defective NK cell activation in X-linked lymphoproliferative disease. J Immunol 165:3549–3553
13. Bi K, Tanaka Y, Coudronniere N, Sugie K, Hong S, van Stipdonk MJ, Altman A (2001) Antigen-induced translocation of PKC-θ to membrane rafts is required for T cell activation. Nat Immunol 2:556–563

14. Billadeau DD, Brumbaugh KM, Dick CJ, Schoon RA, Bustelo XR, Leibson PJ (1998) The Vav-Rac1 pathway in cytotoxic lymphocytes regulates the generation of cell-mediated killing. J Exp Med 188:549–559
15. Billadeau DD, Mackie SM, Schoon RA, Leibson PJ (2000) Specific subdomains of Vav differentially affect T cell and NK cell activation. J Immunol 164:3971–3981
16. Billadeau DD, Upshaw JL, Schoon RA, Dick CJ, Leibson PJ (2003) NKG2D-DAP10 triggers human NK cell-mediated killing via a Syk-independent regulatory pathway. Nat Immunol 4:557–564
17. Binstadt BA, Billadeau DD, Jevremovic D, Williams BL, Fang N, Yi T, Koretzky GA, Abraham RT, Leibson PJ (1998) SLP-76 is a direct substrate of SHP-1 recruited to killer cell inhibitory receptors. J Biol Chem 273:27518–27523
18. Bjørbaek C, Buchholz RM, Davis SM, Bates SH, Pierroz DD, Gu H, Neel BG, Myers J, M.G., Flier JS (2001) Divergent roles of SHP-2 in ERK activation by leptin receptors. J Biol Chem 276:4747–4755
19. Bonnema JD, Karnitz LM, Schoon RA, Abraham RT, Leibson PJ (1994) Fc receptor stimulation of phosphatidylinositol 3-kinase in natural killer cells is associated with protein kinase C-independent granule release and cell-mediated cytotoxicity. J Exp Med 180:1427–1435
20. Bottino C, Augugliaro R, Castriconi R, Nanni M, Biassoni R, Moretta L, Moretta A (2000) Analysis of the molecular mechanism involved in 2B4-mediated NK cell activation: evidence that human 2B4 is physically and functionally associated with the linker for activation of T cells. Eur J Immunol 30:3718–3722
21. Bruhns P, Marchetti P, Fridman WH, Vivier E, Daëron M (1999) Differential roles of N- and C-terminal immunoreceptor tyrosine-based inhibition motifs during inhibition of cell activation by killer cell inhibitory receptors. J Immunol 162:3168–3175
22. Brumbaugh KM, Binstadt BA, Billadeau DD, Schoon RA, Dick CJ, Ten RM, Leibson PJ (1997) Functional role for Syk tyrosine kinase in natural killer cell-mediated natural cytotoxicity. J Exp Med 186:1965–1974
23. Bunnell SC, Diehn M, Yaffe MB, Findell PR, Cantley LC, Berg LJ (2000) Biochemical interactions integrating Itk with the T cell receptor-initiated signaling cascade. J Biol Chem 275:2219–2230
24. Burshtyn DN, Scharenberg AM, Wagtmann N, Rajogopalan S, Berrada K, Yi T, Kinet J-P, Long EO (1996) Recruitment of tyrosine phosphatase HCP by the killer cell inhibitory receptor. Immunity 4:77–85
25. Burshtyn DN, Shin J, Stebbins C, Long EO (2000) Adhesion to target cells is disrupted by the killer cell inhibitory receptor. Curr Biol 10:777–780
26. Bustelo XR (2001) Vav proteins, adaptors, and cell signaling. Oncogene 20:6372–6381
27. Campbell KS, Cella M, Carretero M, Lopez-Botet M, Colonna M (1998) Signaling through human killer cell activating receptors triggers tyrosine phosphorylation of an associated protein complex. Eur J Immunol 28:599–609
28. Campbell KS, Dessing M, Lopez-Botet M, Cella M, Colonna M (1996) Tyrosine phosphorylation of a human killer inhibitory receptor recruits protein tyrosine phosphatase 1C. J Exp Med 184:93–100

29. Carretero M, Llano M, Navarro F, Bellon T, Lopez-Botet M (2000) Mitogen-activated protein kinase activity is involved in effector functions triggered by the CD94/NKG2-C NK receptor specific for HLA-E. Eur J Immunol 30:2842–2848
30. Carter RH, Wang Y, Brooks S (2002) Role of CD19 signal transduction in B cell biology. Immunol Res 26:45–54
31. Cella M, Fujikawa K, Tassi I, Kim S, Latinis K, Nishi S, Yokoyama W, Colonna M, Swat W (2004) Differential requirements for Vav proteins in DAP10- and ITAM-mediated NK cell cytotoxicity. J Exp Med 200:817–823
32. Cerwenka A, Baron JL, Lanier LL (2001) Ectopic expression of retinoic acid early inducible-1 gene (RAE-1) permits natural killer cell-mediated rejection of a MHC class I-bearing tumor in vivo. Proc Natl Acad Sci USA 98:11521–11526
33. Chan B, Lanyi A, Song HK, Griesbach J, Simarro-Grande M, Poy F, Howie D, Sumegi J, Terhorst C, Eck MJ (2003) SAP couples Fyn to SLAM immune receptors. Nat Cell Biol 5:155–160
34. Chan G, Hanke T, Fischer KD (2001) Vav-1 regulates NK T cell development and NK cell cytotoxicity. Eur J Immunol 31:2403–2410
35. Chang C, Dietrich J, Harpur AG, Lindquist JA, Haude A, Loke YW, King A, Colonna M, Trowsdale J, Wilson MJ (1999) Cutting edge: KAP10, a novel transmembrane adapter protein genetically linked to DAP12 but with unique signaling properties. J Immunol 163:4651–4654
36. Chang L, Karin M (2001) Mammalian MAP kinase signaling cascades. Nature 410:37–40
37. Chen R, Relouzat F, Roncagalli R, Aoukaty A, Tan R, Latour S, Veillette A (2004) Molecular dissection of 2B4 signaling: implications for signal transduction by SLAM-related receptors. Mol Cell Biol 24:5144–5156
38. Chini CCS, Boos MD, Dick CJ, Schoon RA, Leibson PJ (2000) Regulation of p38 mitogen-activated protein kinase during NK cell activation. Eur J Immunol 30:2791–2798
39. Chuang SS, Kumaresan PR, Mathew PA (2001) 2B4 (CD244)-mediated activation of cytotoxicity and IFN-γ release in human NK cells involves distinct pathways. J Immunol 167:6210–6216
40. Chuang SS, Lee JK, Mathew PA (2003) Protein kinase C is involved in 2B4 (CD244)-mediated cytotoxicity and AP-1 activation in natural killer cells. Immunology 109:432–439
41. Cilio CM, Daws MR, Malashicheva A, Sentman CL, Holmberg D (1998) Cytotoxic T lymphocyte antigen 4 is induced in the thymus upon in vivo activation and its blockade prevents anti-CD3-mediated depletion of thymocytes. J Exp Med 188:1239–1246
42. Colucci F, Rosmaraki E, Bregenholt S, Samson SI, Di Bartolo V, Turner M, Vanes L, Tybulewicz V, Di Santo JP (2001) Functional dichotomy in natural killer cell signaling: Vav1-dependent and -independent mechanisms. J Exp Med 193:1413–1424
43. Colucci F, Scweighoffer E, Tomasello E, Turner M, Ortaldo JR, Vivier E, Tybulewicz VLJ, DiSanto JP (2002) Natural cytotoxicity uncoupled from the Syk and ZAP-70 intracellular kinases. Nat Immunol 3:288–294

44. Cosman D, Mullberg J, Sutherland CL, Chin W, Armitage R, Fanslow W, Kubin M, Chalupny NJ (2001) ULBPs, novel MHC class I-related molecules, bind to CMV glycoprotein UL16 and stimulate NK cytotoxicity through the NKG2D receptor. Immunity 14:123–133
45. Costello PS, Walters AE, Mee PJ, Turner M, Reynolds LF, Prisco A, Sarner N, Zamoyska R, Tybulewicz VL (1999) The Rho-family GTP exchange factor Vav is a critical transducer of T cell receptor signals to the calcium, ERK, and NF-κB pathways. Proc Natl Acad Sci USA 96:3035–3040
46. Crespo P, Schuebel KE, Ostrom AA, Gutkind JS, Bustelo XR (1997) Phosphotyrosine-dependent activation of Rac-1 GDP/GTP exchange by the vav proto-oncogene product. Nature 385:169–172
47. Davis DM, Chiu I, Fassett M, Cohen GB, Mandelboim O, Strominger JL (1999) The human natural killer cell immune synapse. Proc Natl Acad Sci USA 96:15062–15067
48. Daws MR, Eriksson M, Oberg L, Ullen A, Sentman CL (1999) H-2D^d engagement of Ly49A leads directly to Ly49A phosphorylation and recruitment of SHP1. Immunology 97:656–664
49. Diefenbach A, Jamieson AM, Liu SD, Shastri N, Raulet DH (2000) Ligands for the murine NKG2D receptor: expression by tumor cells and activation of NK cells and macrophages. Nat Immunol 1:119–126
50. Diefenbach A, Tomasello E, Lucas M, Jamieson AM, Hsia JK, Vivier E, Raulet DH (2002) Selective associations with signaling proteins determine stimulatory versus costimulatory activity of NKG2D. Nat Immunol 3:1142–1149.
51. Djouder N, Schmidt G, Frings M, Cavalie A, Thelen M, Aktories K (2001) Rac and phosphatidylinositol 3-kinase regulate the protein kinase B in FcεRI signaling in RBL 2H3 mast cells. J Immunol 166:1627–1634
52. Epling-Burnette PK, Bai F, Wei S, Chaurasia P, Painter JS, Olashaw N, Hamilton A, Sebti S, Djeu JY, Loughran TP (2004) ERK couples chronic survival of NK cells to constitutively activated Ras in lymphoproliferative disease of granular lymphocytes (LDGL). Oncogene 23:9220–9229
53. Eriksson M, Ryan JC, Nakamura MC, Sentman CL (1999) Ly49A inhibitory receptors redistribute on natural killer cells during target cell interaction. Immunology 97:341–347
54. Fassett MS, Davis DM, Valter MM, Cohen GB, Strominger JL (2001) Signaling at the inhibitory natural killer cell immune synapse regulates lipid raft polarization but not class I MHC clustering. Proc Natl Acad Sci USA 98:14547–14552
55. Faure M, Long EO (2002) KIR2DL4 (CD158d), an NK cell-activating receptor with inhibitory potential. J Immunol 168:6208–6214
56. Feng G-S (1999) Shp-2 tyrosine phosphatase: signaling one cell or many. Exp Cell Res 253:47–54
57. Feng G-S, Hiui C-C, Pawson T (1993) SH2-containing phosphotyrosine phosphatase as a target of protein-tyrosine kinases. Science 259:1607–1611
58. Fry AM, Lanier LL, Weiss A (1996) Phosphotyrosines in the killer cell inhibitory receptor motif of NKB1 are required for negative signaling and for association with protein tyrosine phosphatase 1C. J Exp Med 184:295–300

59. Galandrini R, Palmieri G, Piccoli M, Frati L, Santoni A (1996) CD16-mediated p21ras activation is associated with Shc and p36 tyrosine phosphorylation and their binding with Grb2 in human natural killer cells. J Exp Med 183:179–186
60. Galandrini R, Palmieri G, Piccoli M, Frati L, Santoni A (1999) Role for the Rac1 exchange factor Vav in the signaling pathways leading to NK cell cytotoxicity. J Immunol 162:3148–3152
61. Galandrini R, Tassi I, Mattia G, Lenti L, Piccoli M, Frati L, Santoni A (2002) SH2-containing inositol phosphatase (SHIP-1) transiently translocates to raft domains and modulates CD16-mediated cytotoxicity in human NK cells. Blood 100:4581–4589
62. Galandrini R, Tassi I, Morrone S, Lanfrancone L, Pelicci P, Piccoli M, Frati L, Santoni A (2001) The adaptor protein shc is involved in the negative regulation of NK cell-mediated cytotoxicity. Eur J Immunol 31:2016–2025
63. Garrido F, Cabrera T, Concha A, Glew S, Ruiz-Cabello F, Stern PL (1993) Natural history of HLA expression during tumor development. Immunol Today 14:491–499
64. Garrido F, Cabrera T, Lopez-Nevot MA, Ruiz-Cabello F (1995) HLA class I antigens in human tumors. Adv Cancer Res 67:155–194
65. Gilfillan S, Ho EL, Cella M, Yokoyama WM, Colonna M (2002) NKG2D recruits two distinct adapters to trigger NK cell activation and costimulation. Nat Immunol 3:1150–1155.
66. Gismondi A, Cifaldi L, Mazza C, Giliani S, Parolini S, Morrone S, Jacobelli J, Bandiera E, Notarangelo L, Santoni A (2004) Impaired natural and CD16-mediated NK cell cytotoxicity in patients with WAS and XLT: ability of IL-2 to correct NK cell functional defect. Blood 104:436–443
67. Gupta N, Scharenberg AM, Burshtyn DN, Wagtmann N, Lioubin MN, Rohrschneider LR, Kinet JP, Long EO (1997) Negative signaling pathways of the killer cell inhibitory receptor and Fcγ RIIb1 require distinct phosphatases. J Exp Med 186:473–478
68. Han J, Luby-Phelps K, Das B, Shu X, Xia Y, Mosteller RD, Krishna UM, Falck JR, White MA, Broek D (1998) Role of substrates and products of PI 3-kinase in regulating activation of Rac-related guanosine triphosphatases by Vav. Science 279:558–560
69. Ho EL, Carayannopoulos LN, Poursine-Laurent J, Kinder J, Plougastel B, Smith HR, Yokoyama WM (2002) Costimulation of multiple NK cell activation receptors by NKG2D. J Immunol 169:3667–3675
70. Hof P, Pluskey S, Dhe-Paganon S, Eck MJ, Shoelson SE (1998) Crystal structure of the tyrosine phosphatase SHP-2. Cell 92:441–450
71. Horejsi V, Zhang W, Schraven B (2004) Transmembrane adaptor proteins: organizers of immunoreceptor signalling. Nat Rev Immunol 4:603–614
72. Houlard M, Arudchandran R, Regnier-Ricard F, Germani A, Gisselbrecht, S, Blank U. Rivera J, Varin-Blank N (2002) Vav1 is a component of transcriptionally active complexes. J Exp Med 195:1115–1127
73. Inabe K, Ishiai M, Sharenberg AM, Freshney N, Downward J, Kurosaki T (2002) Vav3 modulates B cell receptor responses by regulating phosphoinositide 3-kinase activation. J Exp Med 195:189–200

74. Inoue H, Miyaji M, Kosugi A, Nagafuku M, Okazaki T, Mimori T, Amakawa R, Fukuhara S, Domae N, Bloom ET, Umehara H (2002) Lipid rafts as the signaling scaffold for NK cell activation: tyrosine phosphorylation and association of LAT with phosphatidylinositol 3-kinase and phospholipase C-γ following CD2 stimulation. Eur J Immunol 32:2188–2198
75. Jamieson AM, Diefenbach A, McMahon CW, Xiong N, Carlyle JR, Raulet DH (2004) The role of the NKG2D immunoreceptor in immune cell activation and natural killing. Immunity 20:799
76. Jevremovic D, Billadeau DD, Schoon RA, Dick CJ, Irvin BJ, Zhang W, Samelson LE, Abraham RT, Leibson PJ (1999) Cutting edge: a role for the adaptor protein LAT in human NK cell-mediated cytotoxicity. J Immunol 162:2453–2456
77. Jevremovic D, Billadeau DD, Schoon RA, Dick CJ, Irvin BJ, Zhang W, Samelson LE, Abraham RT, Leibson PJ (1999) Cutting edge: a role for the adaptor protein LAT in human NK cell-mediated cytotoxicity. J Immunol 162:2453–2456
78. Jevremovic D, Billadeau DD, Schoon RA, Dick CJ, Leibson PJ (2001) Regulation of NK cell-mediated cytotoxicity by the adaptor protein 3BP2. J Immunol 166:7219–7228
79. Jiang K, Zhong B, Gilvary DL, Corliss BC, Hong-Geller E, Wei S, Djeu JY (2000) Pivotal role of phosphoinositide-3 kinase in regulation of cytotoxicity in natural killer cells. Nat Immunol 1:419–425
80. Jiang K, Zhong B, Gilvary DL, Corliss BC, Vivier E, Hong-Geller E, Wei S, Djeu JY (2002) Syk regulation of phosphoinositide 3-kinase-dependent NK cell function. J Immunol 168:3155–3164
81. Kabat J, Borrego F, Brooks A, Coligan JE (2002) Role that each NKG2A immunoreceptor tyrosine-based inhibitory motif plays in mediating the human CD94/NKG2A inhibitory signal. J Immunol 169:1948–1958
82. Kaufman DS, Schoon RA, Robertson MJ, Leibson PJ (1995) Inhibition of selective signaling events in natural killer cells recognizing major histocompatibility complex class I. Proc Natl Acad Sci USA 92:6484–6488
83. Kikuchi-Maki A, Catina TL, Campbell KS (2005) Cutting edge: KIR2DL4 transduces signals into human NK cells through association with the Fc receptor gamma protein. J Immunol 174:3859–3863
84. Kikuchi-Maki A, Yusa S, Catina TL, Campbell KS (2003) KIR2DL4 is an IL-2 regulated NK cell receptor that exhibits limited expression in humans but triggers strong IFNγ production. J Immunol 171:3415–3425
85. Klem J, Verrett PC, Kumar V, Schatzle JD (2002) 2B4 is constitutively associated with linker for the activation of T cells in glycolipid-enriched microdomains: properties required for 2B4 lytic function. J Immunol 169:55–62
86. Klinghoffer RA, Kazlauskas A (1995) Identification of a putative Syp substrate, the PDGF receptor. J Biol Chem 270:22208–22217
87. Kon-Kozlowski M, Pani G, Pawson T, Siminovitch KA (1996) The tyrosine phosphatase PTP1C associates with Vav, Grb2, and mSos1 in hematopoietic cells. J Biol Chem 271:3856–3862
88. Krishnan S, Warke VG, Nambiar MP, Tsokos GC, Farber DL (2003) The FcR gamma subunit and Syk kinase replace the CD3 ζ-chain and ZAP-70 kinase in the TCR signaling complex of human effector CD4 T cells. J Immunol 170:4189–4195

89. Kubin MZ, Parshley DL, Din W, Waugh JY, Davis-Smith T, Smith CA, Macduff BM, Armitage RJ, Chin W, Cassiano L, Borges L, Petersen M, Trinchieri G, Goodwin RG (1999) Molecular cloning and biological characterization of NK cell activation-inducing ligand, a counterstructure for CD48. Eur J Immunol 29:3466–3477
90. Kuhn JR, Poenie M (2002) Dynamic polarization of the microtubule cytoskeleton during CTL-mediated killing. Immunity 16:111–121
91. Labno CM, Lewis CM, You D, Leung DW, Takesono A, Kamberos N, Seth A, Finkelstein LD, Rosen MK, Schwartzberg PL, Burkhardt JK (2003) Itk functions to control actin polymerization at the immune synapse through localized activation of Cdc42 and WASP. Curr Biol 13:1619–1624
92. Lanier LL, Yu G, Phillips JH (1989) Co-association of CD3ζ with a receptor (CD16) for IgG Fc on human natural killer cells. Nature 342:803–805.
93. Latour S, Roncagalli R, Chen R, Bakinowski M, Shi X, Schwartzberg PL, Davidson D, Veillette A (2003) Binding of SAP SH2 domain to FynT SH3 domain reveals a novel mechanism of receptor signalling in immune regulation. Nat Cell Biol 5:149–154
94. Le Drean E, Vely F, Olcese L, Cambiaggi A, Guia S, Krystal G, Gervois N, Moretta A, Jotereau F, Vivier E (1998) Inhibition of antigen-induced T cell response and antibody-induced NK cell cytotoxicity by NKG2A: association of NKG2A with SHP-1 and SHP-2 protein-tyrosine phosphatases. Eur J Immunol 28:264–276
95. Lee K-M, Chuang E, Griffin M, Khattri R, Hong DK, Zhang W, Straus D, Samelson LE, Thompson CB, Bluestone JA (1998) Molecular basis of T cell inactivation by CTLA-4. Science 282:2263–2266
96. Lee KM, McNerney ME, Stepp SE, Mathew PA, Schatzle JD, Bennett M, Kumar V (2004) 2B4 acts as a non-major histocompatibility complex binding inhibitory receptor on mouse natural killer cells. J Exp Med 199:1245–1254
97. Leibson PJ, Midthun DE, Windebank KP, Abraham RT (1990) Transmembrane signaling during natural killer cell-mediated cytotoxicity. Regulation by protein kinase C activation. J Immunol 145:1498–1504
98. Lewis J, Eiben LJ, Nelson DL, Cohen JI, Nichols KE, Ochs HD, Notarangelo LD, Duckett CS (2001) Distinct interactions of the X-linked lymphoproliferative syndrome gene product SAP with cytoplasmic domains of members of the CD2 receptor family. Clin Immunol 100:15–23
99. Liu BP, Burridge K (2000) Vav2 activates Rac1, Cdc42, and RhoA downstream from growth factor receptors but not β1 integrins. Mol Cell Biol 20:7160–7169
100. Liu SK, Fang N, Koretzky GA, McGlade CJ (1999) The hematopoietic-specific adaptor protein Gads functions in T-cell signaling via interactions with the SLP-76 and LAT adaptors. Curr Biol 9:67–75
101. Ljunggren H-G, Kärre K (1990) In search of the "missing self": MHC molecules and NK cell recognition. Immunol Today 11:237–244
102. Long EO (1999) Regulation of immune responses through inhibitory receptors. Annu Rev Immunol 17:875–904
103. Lou Z, Billadeau DD, Savoy DN, Schoon RA, Leibson PJ (2001) A role for a RhoA/ROCK/LIM-kinase pathway in the regulation of cytotoxic lymphocytes. J Immunol 167:5749–5757

104. Lou Z, Jevremovic D, Billadeau DD, Leibson PJ (2000) A balance between positive and negative signals in cytotoxic lymphocytes regulates the polarization of lipid rafts during the development of cell-mediated killing. J Exp Med 191:347–354
105. Lucas JA, Miller AT, Atherly LO, Berg LJ (2003) The role of Tec family kinases in T cell development and function. Immunol Rev 191:119–138
106. Lupher ML, Jr., Rao N, Lill NL, Andoniou CE, Miyake S, Clark EA, Druker B, Band H (1998) Cbl-mediated negative regulation of the Syk tyrosine kinase. A critical role for Cbl phosphotyrosine-binding domain binding to Syk phosphotyrosine 323. J Biol Chem 273:35273–35281
107. Maeno K, Sada K, Kyo S, Miah SM, Kawauchi-Kamata K, Qu X, Shi Y, Yamamura H (2003) Adaptor protein 3BP2 is a potential ligand of Src homology 2 and 3 domains of Lyn protein-tyrosine kinase. J Biol Chem 278:24912–24920
108. Mainiero F, Gismondi A, Soriani A, Cippitelli M, Palmieri G, Jacobelli J, Piccoli M, Frati L, Santoni A (1998) Integrin-mediated ras-extracellular regulated kinase (ERK) signaling regulates interferon γ production in human natural killer cells. J Exp Med 188:1267–1275
109. Malorni W, Quaranta MG, Straface E, Falzano L, Fabbri A, Viora M, Fiorentini C (2003) The Rac-activating toxin cytotoxic necrotizing factor 1 oversees NK cell-mediated activity by regulating the actin/microtubule interplay. J Immunol 171:4195–4202
110. Marengere LE, Waterhouse P, Duncan GS, Mittrucker HW, Feng GS, Mak TW (1996) Regulation of T cell receptor signaling by tyrosine phosphatase SYP association with CTLA-4. Science 272:1170–1173
111. Mathew PA, Garni-Wagner BA, Land K, Takashima A, Stoneman E, Bennett M, Kumar V (1993) Cloning and characterization of the 2B4 gene encoding a molecule associated with non-MHC-restricted killing mediated by activated natural killer cells and T cells. J Immunol 151:5328–5337
112. McCann FE, Vanherberghen B, Eleme K, Carlin LM, Newsam RJ, Goulding D, Davis DM (2003) The size of the synaptic cleft and distinct distributions of filamentous actin, ezrin, CD43, and CD45 at activating and inhibitory human NK cell immune synapses. J Immunol 170:2862–2870
113. McVicar DW, Burshtyn DN (2001) Intracellular signaling by the killer immunoglobulin-like receptors and Ly49. Sci STKE 2001:RE1
114. McVicar DW, Taylor LS, Gosselin P, Willette-Brown J, Mikhael AI, Geahlen RL, Nakamura MC, Linnemeyer P, Seaman WE, Anderson SK, Ortaldo JR, Mason LH (1998) DAP12-mediated signal transduction in natural killer cells. A dominant role for the Syk protein-tyrosine kinase. J Biol Chem 273:32934–32942
115. Milella M, Gismondi A, Roncaioli P, Bisogno L, Palmieri G, Frati L, Cifone MG, Santoni A (1997) CD16 cross-linking induces both secretory and extracellular signal-regulated kinase (ERK)-dependent cytosolic phospholipase A2 (PLA2) activity in human natural killer cells: involvement of ERK, but not PLA2, in CD16-triggered granule exocytosis. J Immunol 158:3148–3154
116. Mishra AK, Zhang A, Niu T, Yang J, Liang X, Zhao ZJ, Zhou GW (2002) Substrate specificity of protein tyrosine phosphatase: differential behavior of SHP-1 and SHP-2 towards signal regulation protein SIRPα1. J Cell Biochem 84:840–846

117. Mizuno K, Tagawa Y, Mitomo K, Watanabe N, Katagiri T, Ogimoto M, Yakura H (2002) Src homology region 2 domain-containing phosphatase 1 positively regulates B cell receptor-induced apoptosis by modulating association of B cell linker protein with Nck and activation of c-Jun NH_2-terminal kinase. J Immunol 169:778–786
118. Mocarski ES, Jr. (2004) Immune escape and exploitation strategies of cytomegaloviruses: impact on and imitation of the major histocompatibility system. Cell Microbiol 6:707–717
119. Mooney JM, Klem J, Wulfing C, Mijares LA, Schwartzberg PL, Bennett M, Schatzle JD (2004) The murine NK receptor 2B4 (CD244) exhibits inhibitory function independent of signaling lymphocytic activation molecule-associated protein expression. J Immunol 173:3953–3961
120. Morra M, Lu J, Poy F, Martin M, Sayos J, Calpe S, Gullo C, Howie D, Rietdijk S, Thompson A, Coyle AJ, Denny C, Yaffe MB, Engel P, Eck MJ, Terhorst C (2001) Structural basis for the interaction of the free SH2 domain EAT-2 with SLAM receptors in hematopoietic cells. EMBO J 20:5840–5852
121. Movilla N, Bustelo XR (1999) Biological and regulatory properties of Vav-3, a new member of the Vav family of oncoproteins. Mol Cell Biol 19:7870–7885
122. Movilla N, Dosil M, Zheng Y, Bustelo XR (2001) How Vav proteins discriminate the GTPases Rac1 and RhoA from Cdc42. Oncogene 20:8057–8065
123. Nakajima H, Cella M, Bouchon A, Grierson HL, Lewis J, Duckett CS, Cohen JI, Colonna M (2000) Patients with X-linked lymphoproliferative disease have a defect in 2B4 receptor-mediated NK cell cytotoxicity. Eur J Immunol 30:3309–3318
124. Nakajima H, Cella M, Langen H, Friedlein A, Colonna M (1999) Activating interactions in human NK cell recognition: the role of 2B4-CD48. Eur J Immunol 29:1676–1683
125. O'Reilly AM, Neel BG (1998) Structural determinants of SHP-2 function and specificity in *Xenopus* mesoderm induction. Mol Cell Biol 18:161–177
126. Orange JS, Harris KE, Andzelm MM, Valter MM, Geha RS, Strominger JL (2003) The mature activating natural killer cell immunologic synapse is formed in distinct stages. Proc Natl Acad Sci USA 100:14151–14156
127. Orange JS, Ramesh N, Remold-O'Donnell E, Sasahara Y, Koopman L, Byrne M, Bonilla FA, Rosen FS, Geha RS, Strominger JL (2002) Wiskott-Aldrich syndrome protein is required for NK cell cytotoxicity and colocalizes with actin to NK cell-activating immunological synapses. Proc Natl Acad Sci USA 99:11351–11356
128. Paavilainen VO, Bertling E, Falck S, Lappalainen P (2004) Regulation of cytoskeletal dynamics by actin-monomer-binding proteins. Trends Cell Biol 14:386–394
129. Palmby TR, Abe K, Karnoub AE, Der CJ (2004) Vav transformation requires activation of multiple GTPases and regulation of gene expression. Mol Cancer Res 2:702–711
130. Parolini S, Bottino C, Falco M, Augugliaro R, Giliani S, Franceschini R, Ochs HD, Wolf H, Bonnefoy JY, Biassoni R, Moretta L, Notarangelo LD, Moretta A (2000) X-linked lymphoproliferative disease. 2B4 molecules displaying inhibitory rather than activating function are responsible for the inability of natural killer cells to kill Epstein-Barr virus-infected cells. J Exp Med 192:337–346

131. Pei D, Wang J, Walsh CT (1996) Differential functions of the two Src homology 2 domains in protein tyrosine phosphatase SH-PTP1. Proc Natl Acad Sci USA 93:1141–1145
132. Perona R, Montaner S, Saniger L, Sanchez-Perez I, Bravo R, Lacal J (1997) Activation of the nuclear factor-κB by Rho, CDC42, and Rac-1 proteins. Genes Dev 11:463–475
133. Peterson EJ, Clements JL, Ballas ZK, Koretzky GA (1999) NK cytokine secretion and cytotoxicity occur independently of the SLP-76 adaptor protein. Eur J Immunol 29:2223–2232
134. Pluskota E, Chen Y, D'Souza SE (2000) Src homology domain 2-containing tyrosine phosphatase 2 associates with intercellular adhesion molecule 1 to regulate cell survival. J Biol Chem 275:30029–30036
135. Rajagopalan S, Fu J, Long EO (2001) Cutting Edge: Induction of IFN-γ production but not cytotoxicity by the killer cell Ig-like receptor KIR2DL4 (CD158d) in resting NK cells. J Immunol 167:1877–1881
136. Ridley AJ, Paterson CL, Johnston CL, Dickmann D, Hall A (1992) The small GTP-binding protein Rac regulates growth factor-induced membrane ruffling. Cell 70:401–410
137. Riteau B, Barber DF, Long EO (2003) Vav1 phosphorylation is induced by β2 integrin engagement on natural killer cells upstream of actin cytoskeleton and lipid raft reorganization. J Exp Med 198:469–474
138. Roberts CJ, Nelson B, Marton MJ, Stoghton R, Meyer MR, Bennett HA, He YD, Dai H, Walker WL, Hughes TR, Tyers M, Boone C, Friend SH (2000) Signaling and circuitry of multiple MAPK pathways revealed by a matrix of global gene expression profiles. Science 287:873–880
139. Roda-Navarro P, Mittelbrunn M, Ortega M, Howie D, Terhorst C, Sånchez-Madrid F, Fernåndez-Ruiz E (2004) Dynamic redistribution of the activating 2B4/SAP complex at the cytotoxic NK cell immune synapse. J Immunol 173:3640–3646
140. Rosen D, Araki M, Hamerman J, Chen T, Yamamura T, Lanier L (2004) A structural basis for the association of DAP12 with mouse, but not human, NKG2D. J Immunol 173:2470–2478
141. Rudd CR, M. (2003) Independent CD28 signaling via VAV and SLP-76: a model for in trans costimulation. Immunol Rev 192:32–41
142. Sanni TB, Masilamani M, Kabat J, Coligan JE, Borrego F (2004) Exclusion of lipid rafts and decreased mobility of CD94/NKG2A receptors at the inhibitory NK cell synapse. Mol Biol Cell 15:3210–3223
143. Sayos J, Martin M, Chen A, Simarro M, Howie D, Morra M, Engel P, Terhorst C (2001) Cell surface receptors Ly-9 and CD84 recruit the X-linked lymphoproliferative disease gene product SAP. Blood 97:3867–3874
144. Schatzle JD, Sheu S, Stepp SE, Mathew PA, Bennett M, Kumar V (1999) Characterization of inhibitory and stimulatory forms of the murine natural killer cell receptor 2B4. Proc Natl Acad Sci USA 96:3870–3875
145. Schuebel KE, Movilla N, Rosa JL, Bustelo XR (1998) Phosphorylation-dependent and constitutive activation of Rho proteins by wild-type and oncogenic Vav-2. EMBO J 17:6608–6621

146. Shibuya K, Lanier LL, Phillips JH, Ochs HD, Shimizu K, Nakayama E, Nakauchi H, Shibuya A (1999) Physical and functional association of LFA-1 with DNAM-1 adhesion molecule. Immunity 11:615–623
147. Siminovitch KA, Neel BG (1998) Regulation of B cell signal transduction by SH2-containing protein-tyrosine phosphatases. Semin Immunol 10:329–347
148. Sorokina EM, Chernoff J (2004) Rho-GTPases: New members, new pathways. J Cell Biochem 94:225–231
149. Standeven LJ, Carlin LM, Borszcz P, Davis DM, Burshtyn DN (2004) The actin cytoskeleton controls the efficiency of killer Ig-like receptor accumulation at inhibitory NK cell immune synapses. J Immunol 173:5617–5625
150. Stebbins CC, Watzl C, Billadeau DD, Leibson PJ, Burshtyn DN, Long EO (2003) Vav1 dephosphorylation by the tyrosine phosphatase SHP-1 as a mechanism for inhibition of cellular cytotoxicity. Mol Cell Biol 23:6291–6299
151. Stepp SE, Schatzle JD, Bennett M, Kumar V, Mathew PA (1999) Gene structure of the murine NK cell receptor 2B4: presence of two alternatively spliced isoforms with distinct cytoplasmic domains. Eur J Immunol 29:2392–2399
152. Sumegi J, Seemayer TA, Huang D, Davis JR, Morra M, Gross TG, Yin L, Romco G, Klein E, Terhorst C, Lanyi A (2002) A spectrum of mutations in SH2D1A that causes X-linked lymphoproliferative disease and other Epstein-Barr virus-associated illnesses. Leuk Lymphoma 43:1189–1201
153. Sutherland CL, Chalupny NJ, Schooley K, VandenBos T, Kubin M, Cosman D (2002) UL16-binding proteins, novel MHC class I-related proteins, bind to NKG2D and activate multiple signaling pathways in primary NK cells. J Immunol 168:671–679
154. Tangye SG, Lazetic S, Woollatt E, Sutherland GR, Lanier LL, Phillips JH (1999) Cutting edge: Human 2B4, an activating NK cell receptor, recruits the protein tyrosine phosphatase SHP-2 and the adaptor signaling protein SAP. J Immunol 162:6981–6985
155. Tangye SG, Phillips JH, Lanier LL, Nichols KE (2000) Functional requirement for SAP in 2B4-mediated activation of human natural killer cells as revealed by the X-linked lymphoproliferative syndrome. J Immunol 165:2932–2936
156. Taylor N, Jahn T, Smith S, Lamkin T, Uribe L, Liu Y, Durden DL, Weinberg K (1997) Differential activation of the tyrosine kinases ZAP-70 and Syk after FcγRI stimulation. Blood 89:388–396
157. Tenev T, Keilhack H, Tomic S, Stoyanov B, Stein-Gerlach M, Lammers R, Krivtsov AV, Ullrich A, Böhmer F-D (1997) Both SH2 domains are involved in interaction of SHP-1 with the epidermal growth factor receptor but cannot confer receptor-directed activity to SHP-1/SHP-2 chimera. J Biol Chem 272:5966–5973
158. Teng JMC, Liu X-R, Mills GB, Dupont B (1996) CD28-mediated cytotoxicity by the human leukemic NK cell line YT involves tyrosine phosphorylation, activation of phosphatidylinositol 3-kinase, and protein kinase C. J Immunol 156:3222–3232
159. Ting AT, Dick CJ, Schoon RA, Karnitz LM, Abraham RT, Leibson PJ (1995) Interaction between lck and syk family tyrosine kinases in Fcγ receptor-initiated activation of natural killer cells. J Biol Chem 270:16415–16421
160. Ting AT, Karnitz LM, Schoon RA, Abraham RT, Leibson PJ (1992) Fcγ receptor activation induces the tyrosine phosphorylation of both phospholipase C (PLC)-γ1 and PLC-γ2 in natural killer cells. J Exp Med 176:1751–1755

161. Tonks NK, Neel BG (1996) From form to function: signaling by protein tyrosine phosphatases. Cell 87:365–368
162. Trotta R, Fettucciari K, Azzoni L, Abebe B, Puorro KA, Eisenlohr LC, Perussia B (2000) Differential role of p38 and c-Jun N-terminal kinase 1 mitogen-activated protein kinases in NK cell cytotoxicity. J Immunol 165:1782–1789
163. Trotta R, Puorro KA, Paroli M, Azzoni L, Abebe B, Eisenlohr LC, Perussia B (1998) Dependence of both spontaneous and antibody-dependent, granule exocytosis-mediated NK cell cytotoxicity on extracellular signal-regulated kinases. J Immunol 152:6648–6656
164. Turner M, Billadeau DD (2002) VAV proteins as signal integrators for multisubunit immune-recognition receptors. Nat Rev Immunol 2:476–486
165. Valiante NM, Phillips JH, Lanier LL, Parham P (1996) Killer cell inhibitory receptor recognition of human leukocyte antigen (HLA) class I blocks formation of a pp36/PLC-γ signaling complex in human natural killer (NK) cells. J Exp Med 184:2243–2250
166. Vogel W, Lammers R, Huang J, Ullrich A (1993) Activation of a phosphotyrosine phosphatase by tyrosine phosphorylation. Science 259:1611–1614
167. Vyas YM, Maniar H, Dupont B (2002) Cutting edge: Differential segregation of the Src homology 2-containing protein tyrosine phosphatase-1 within the early NK cell immune synapse distinguishes noncytolytic from cytolytic interactions. J Immunol 168:3150–3154
168. Vyas YM, Maniar H, Lyddane CE, Sadelain M, Dupont B (2004) Ligand binding to inhibitory killer cell Ig-like receptors induce colocalization with Src homology domain 2-containing protein tyrosine phosphatase 1 and interruption of ongoing activation signals. J Immunol 173:1571–1578
169. Vyas YM, Mehta KM, Morgan M, Maniar H, Butros L, Jung S, Burkhardt JK, Dupont B (2001) Spatial organization of signal transduction molecules in the NK cell immune synapses during MHC class I-regulated noncytolytic and cytolytic interactions. J Immunol 167:4358–4367
170. Wang HY, Altman Y, Fang D, Elly C, Dai Y, Shao Y, Liu YC (2001) Cbl promotes ubiquitination of the T cell receptor ζ through an adaptor function of Zap-70. J Biol Chem 276:26004–26011
171. Wang JW, Howson JM, Ghansah T, Desponts C, Ninos JM, May SL, Nguyen KH, Toyama-Sorimachi N, Kerr WG (2002) Influence of SHIP on the NK repertoire and allogeneic bone marrow transplantation. Science 295:2094–2097
172. Wang P, Fu H, Snavley DF, Freitas MA, Pei D (2002) Screening combinatorial libraries by mass spectrometry. 2. Identification of optimal substrates of protein tyrosine phosphatase SHP-1. Biochemistry 41:6202–6210
173. Watzl C, Long EO (2003) Natural killer cell inhibitory receptors block actin cytoskeleton-dependent recruitment of 2B4 (CD244) to lipid rafts. J Exp Med 197:77–85
174. Wei S, Gamero AM, Liu JH, Daulton AA, Valkov NI, Trapani JA, Larner AC, Weber MJ, Djeu JY (1998) Control of lytic function by mitogen-activated protein kinase/extracellular regulatory kinase 2 (ERK2) in a human natural killer cell line: identification of perforin and granzyme B mobilization by functional ERK2. J Exp Med 187:1753–1765

175. Wei S, Gilvary DL, Corliss BC, Sebti S, Sun J, Straus DB, Leibson PJ, Trapani JA, Hamilton AD, Weber MJ, Djeu JY (2000) Direct tumor lysis by NK cells uses a Ras-independent mitogen-activated protein kinase signal pathway. J Immunol 165:3811–3819
176. Wennerberg K, Ellerbroek SM, Liu RY, Karnoub AE, Burridge K, Der CJ (2002) RhoG signals in parallel with Rac1 and Cdc42. J Biol Chem 277:47810–47817
177. Wilkinson MG, Millar JBA (1998) SAPKs and transcription factors do the nucleocytoplasmic tango. Genes Dev 12:1391–1397
178. Wu J, Cherwinski H, Spies T, Phillips JH, Lanier LL (2000) DAP10 and DAP12 form distinct, but functionally cooperative, receptor complexes in natural killer cells. J Exp Med 192:1059–1068
179. Wu J, Motto DG, Koretzky GA, Weiss A (1996) Vav and SLP-76 interact and functionally cooperate in IL-2 gene activation. Immunity 4:593–602
180. Wu J, Song Y, Bakker AB, Bauer S, Spies T, Lanier LL, Phillips JH (1999) An activating immunoreceptor complex formed by NKG2D and DAP10. Science 285:730–732
181. Wülfing C, Purtic B, Klem J, Schatzle JD (2003) Stepwise cytoskeletal polarization as a series of checkpoints in innate but not adaptive cytolytic killing. Proc Natl Acad Sci USA 100:7767–7772
182. Xie Z-H, Zhang J, Siraganian RP (2000) Positive regulation of c-Jun N-terminal kinase and TNF-α production but not histamine release by SHP-1 in RBL-2H3 mast cells. J Immunol 164:1521–1528
183. Yang J, Cheng Z, Niu T, Liang X, Zhao ZJ, Zhou GW (2001) Protein tyrosine phosphatase SHP-1 specifically recognizes C-terminal residues of its substrates via helix alpha0. J Cell Biochem 83:14–20
184. Yang J, X. L, Niu T, Meng W, Zhao Z, Zhou W (1998) Crystal structure of the catalytic domain of protein-tyrosine phosphatase SHP-1. J Biol Chem 273:28199–28207
185. You M, Yu D-H, Feng G-S (1999) Shp-2 tyrosine phosphatase functions as a negative regulator of the interferon-stimulated Jak/STAT pathway. Mol Cell Biol 19:2416–2424
186. Yu H, Leitenberg D, Li B, Flavell RA (2001) Deficiency of small GTPase Rac2 affects T cell activation. J Exp Med 194:915–926
187. Yu Z, Ahmad S, Schwartz J-L, Banville D, Shen S-H (1997) Protein-tyrosine phosphatase SHP2 is positively linked to proteinase-activated receptor 2-mediated mitogenic pathway. J Biol Chem 272:7519–7524
188. Yusa S, Campbell KS (2003) Src Homology 2-containing protein tyrosine phosphatase-2 (SHP-2) can play a direct role in the inhibitory function of killer cell Ig-like receptors in human NK cells. J Immmunol 170:4539–4547
189. Yusa S, Catina TL, Campbell KS (2002) SHP-1- and phosphotyrosine-independent inhibitory signaling by a killer cell Ig-like receptor cytoplasmic domain in human NK cells. J Immunol 168:5047–5057
190. Yusa S, Catina TL, Campbell KS (2004) KIR2DL5 can inhibit human NK cell activation via recruitment of Src homology region 2-containing protein tyrosine phosphatase-2 (SHP-2). J Immunol 172:7385–7392

191. Zeng R, Cannon JL, Abraham RT, Way M, Billadeau DD, Bubeck-Wardenberg J, Burkhardt JK (2003) SLP-76 coordinates Nck-dependent Wiskott-Aldrich Syndrome Protein recruitment with Vav-1/Cdc42-dependent Wiskott-Aldrich Syndrome Protein activation at the T cell-APC contact site. J Immunol 171:1360–1368
192. Zhang J, Somani A-K, Siminovitch KA (2000) Roles of the SHP-1 tyrosine phosphatase in the negative regulation of cell signalling. Semin Immunol 12:361–378
193. Zhang W, Sloan-Lancaster J, Kitchen J, Trible RP, Samelson LE (1998) LAT: The ZAP-70 tyrosine kinase substrate that links T cell receptor to cellular activation. Cell 92:83–92
194. Zhang W, Trible RP, Samelson LE (1998) LAT palmitoylation: its essential role in membrane microdomain targeting and tyrosine phosphorylation during T cell activation. Immunity 9:239–246
195. Zhang W, Trible RP, Zhu M, Liu SK, McGlade CJ, Samelson LE (2000) Association of Grb2, Gads, and phospholipase C-gamma 1 with phosphorylated LAT tyrosine residues. Effect of LAT tyrosine mutations on T cell antigen receptor-mediated signaling. J Biol Chem 275:23355–23361
196. Zompi S, Hamerman JA, Ogasawara K, Schweighoffer E, Tybulewicz VL, Di Santo JP, Lanier LL, Colucci F (2003) NKG2D triggers cytotoxicity in mouse NK cells lacking DAP12 or Syk family kinases. Nat Immunol 4:565–572

CTMI (2006) 298:59–75
© Springer-Verlag Berlin Heidelberg 2006

Transcriptional Regulation of NK Cell Receptors

S. K. Anderson (✉)

Basic Research Program, SAIC-Frederick, National Cancer Institute-Frederick, Bldg. 560, Rm. 31-93, Frederick, MD 21702-1201, USA
andersn@ncifcrf.gov

1	Introduction	60
2	*Ly49* Promoter Studies	61
2.1	Overview	61
2.2	The Role of TCF-1	62
2.3	Identification of Pro1, Pro2, and Pro3	63
2.4	Pro1 Is a Bidirectional Transcriptional Element	64
2.5	The Pro1 Probabilistic Switch	65
3	*NKR-P1* Promoters	67
4	*CD94* Promoter	67
5	*NKG2A* Promoter	68
6	*KIR* Promoters	69
7	Association of AP-1, SP-1, and Ets with NK Cell-Specific Promoters	71
8	Conclusion	72
	References	73

Abstract The stochastic expression of individual members of NK cell receptor gene families on subsets of NK cells has attracted considerable interest in the transcriptional regulation of these genes. Each receptor gene can contain up to three separate promoters with distinct properties. The recent discovery that an upstream promoter can function as a probabilistic switch element in the Ly49 gene family has revealed a novel mechanism of variegated gene expression. An important question to be answered is whether or not the other NK cell receptor gene families contain probabilistic switches. The promoter elements currently identified in the Ly49, NKR-P1, CD94, NKG2A, and KIR gene families are described.

The content of this publication does not necessarily reflect the views or policies of the Department of Health and Human Services, nor does mention of trade names, commercial products, or organizations imply endorsement by the U.S. Government.

1
Introduction

Although the NK cell receptor families have been known for over a decade, a detailed molecular characterization of promoter elements has only been performed for a small number of these genes. Current information indicates that each member of the lectin-related NK cell receptor families may contain up to three separate promoters that are active at distinct stages of NK or T cell development (Fig. 1). Information gained from the analysis of NK cell receptor promoters and the transcription factors required for their activity can provide important clues regarding the differentiation of NK cells and the T cell subsets that also express these receptors. The promoters of the Ly49 family of murine MHC class I receptors represent the most studied NK cell promoters, partly because of the large size of the gene family, and partly because of the interest generated by the demonstration that individual NK cells selectively express a subset of the available *Ly49* genes in a probabilistic fashion (Raulet

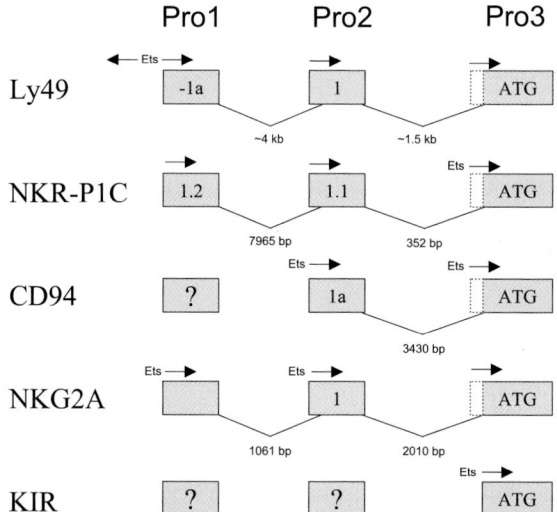

Fig. 1 Promoters of NK cell receptors. *Arrows* indicate known receptor transcripts. The genes have been aligned relative to the first coding exon, indicated by the *rectangle* labeled *ATG*. The upstream exons derived from additional promoters are labeled with the exon number used by the authors that have described them. *Rectangles* containing *a question mark* indicate the possibility that additional promoters exist for these genes. The splicing events observed in each gene are illustrated by the *lines underneath* each gene, and the sizes of the introns are indicated. The promoters that contain a consensus Ets-binding site are indicated by *Ets* preceding the transcript *arrow*

et al. 1997). Variegated expression has also been demonstrated for several other C-type lectin-related genes, including the *NKG2A/CD94* genes and the *NKR-P1B* gene (Takei et al. 2001; Carlyle et al. 1999; Kung et al. 1999; Liu et al. 2000). The major MHC class I receptor gene family in humans (*KIR*) is also expressed in a variegated fashion on NK cells (Valiante et al. 1997). Variegated expression is a common feature of sensory receptors, so that individual cells can be tuned to detect specific stimuli or combinations of stimuli. In the case of the MHC class I receptors found on NK cells, selective expression of inhibitory receptors ensures that there will be NK cells that are sensitive to the loss of a single class I allele. It has been suggested that the selective expression of individual members of these gene families may be due to competition of individual promoters for transcription factors available in limiting quantities (Ioannidis et al. 2003). The recent discovery of competing, overlapping promoters in the *Ly49* genes reveals a novel molecular mechanism responsible for generating variegated expression of receptor gene families (Saleh et al. 2004). The new model proposes that direct competition between opposing promoters generates a probabilistic switch that determines the frequency of gene activation for a given *Ly49* gene. There is a strong possibility that this type of switch element will be found in other variegated NK cell receptor gene families. This chapter reviews the current state of knowledge regarding NK receptor regulation and suggests future directions of research.

2
Ly49 Promoter Studies

2.1
Overview

The *Ly49a* promoter region was first identified in 1993 (Kubo et al. 1993); however, functional studies of this promoter were not reported until 1999 (Kubo et al. 1999; Held et al. 1999). The ATF-2 and TCF-1 transcription factors were shown to play a central role in *Ly49a* promoter activity assayed in a T cell line that expresses Ly49A protein (EL-4). Subsequent studies characterizing the *Ly49c, i,* and *j* promoters revealed a core promoter element that could generate EL-4 cell-specific activity (Gosselin et al. 2000; McQueen et al. 2001) However, in contrast to typical promoters, addition of sequence upstream of the *Ly49* core promoter element had a strong inhibitory effect on promoter activity. Comparative analysis of *Ly49* promoter sequences reveals that there are three distinct classes of *Ly49* promoters, the *Ly49a/g*-related family, the *Ly49e/c*-related family, and the activating *Ly49* gene family (Wilhelm et al.

2001). From an evolutionary standpoint, this supports the theory that the *Ly49e* and *Ly49a* genes located at either end of the *Ly49* gene cluster expressed by NK cells represent the original *Ly49* genes from which the remainder of the inhibitory genes were derived, and the activating genes are predicted to be evolved from a single ancestral activating gene.

2.2
The Role of TCF-1

A series of reports have investigated the role of TCF-1 in the expression of Ly49 proteins (Held et al. 1999, 2003; Kunz and Held 2001; Ioannidis et al. 2003). There are two TCF-1 sites in the *Ly49a* promoter, and TCF-1 binding to these sites was shown to regulate *Ly49a* promoter activity in EL-4 cells. TCF-1-null mice express Ly49A on only 1% of splenic NK cells as compared to the 20% of NK cells that express this receptor in wild-type C57BL/6 mice (Held et al. 1999). The effect of TCF-1 on the percentage of NK cells that express Ly49A is dose-dependent, because approximately 10% of NK cells from TCF-$1^{+/-}$ heterozygotes express Ly49A and the increased levels of TCF-1 protein expressed by TCF-1 transgenic mice correlate with increases in the percentage of NK cells expressing Ly49A (Ioannidis et al. 2003). This result was taken as evidence for limiting concentrations of TCF-1 controlling the probability of *Ly49* gene activation, but the presence or absence of TCF-1 sites in the *Ly49* promoters does not correlate with the effects of TCF-1 on receptor expression. The percentage of NK cells expressing the Ly49G protein in TCF-1-null mice are similar to wild-type levels, and the *Ly49g* gene contains TCF-1 sites that are identical to those found in the *Ly49a* gene. Conversely, the *Ly49d* promoter does not contain the TCF-1 sites, and the NK cell subset that expresses Ly49D is decreased in TCF-1-null mice. These contradictory observations may be resolved by recent observations with *Ly49a* transgenic mice, which indicate the crucial role of an upstream promoter element (Tanamachi et al. 2004) in the expression of Ly49A. The upstream promoter element is significantly different in the *Ly49a* and *Ly49g* genes, suggesting that this control region may be differentially affected by the loss of TCF-1. However, there are no consensus TCF-1 binding sites in the upstream element, and the possibility that the effects of TCF-1 on *Ly49a* gene activation are indirect must be entertained. $NK1.1^+$ $CD3^-$ cell numbers are significantly reduced in the bone marrow of TCF-null mice (Held et al. 1999), and this may be a reflection of decreased progenitor cell expansion in TCF-null mice (Schilham et al. 1998). If the activation of the *Ly49a* gene is strictly dependent on cell proliferation in the bone marrow, the expression of Ly49A would only be induced on cycling NK cells that have not received sufficient inhibitory receptor signaling to prevent the acquisition of additional receptors. It is noteworthy that SHIP-null mice have an unusually high percentage of splenic NK cells (>80%) that express Ly49A, and splenic NK cell numbers are increased in these mice (Wang et al. 2002). It would be of interest to examine whether there is increased proliferation of progenitor cells in the bone marrow of SHIP-null mice. If the *Ly49a* gene requires cell proliferation for activation and represents the last inhibitory *Ly49* gene to be activated during development, it could function as a fail-safe Ly49 that prevents the generation of overactive NK cells. Two studies have indicated that Ly49A is expressed later in development than the other inhibitory Ly49s (Williams et al. 2000; Stevenaert et al. 2003). Additional studies suggest that competence to express Ly49A is determined early in development (Dorfman and Raulet 1998; Roth et al. 2000). Perhaps activation of the *Ly49a* gene is possible at both early and late stages of NK cell development and the decision to express Ly49A may be related to NK cell proliferation as well as the balance of positive and negative signals present at a given point in development.

2.3
Identification of Pro1, Pro2, and Pro3

Recent studies have revealed the presence of two additional *Ly49* promoters, one upstream and one downstream of the previously defined promoter. The downstream promoter precedes the first *Ly49* coding exon (exon 2), and it has been shown to produce transcripts in the *Ly49j* and *Ly49g* genes (McQueen et al. 2001; Wilhelm et al. 2001). The upstream *Ly49* promoter was discovered as a result of the identification of a novel *Ly49g* transcript in 129J liver NK cells (Saleh et al. 2002). The novel promoter was named Pro1, and the downstream exon 1 and exon 2 promoters previously identified were labeled as Pro2 and Pro3, with Pro2 representing the first promoter to be defined and the most frequently studied. The Pro1 element was identified in all of the inhibitory *Ly49* family members, and it was shown to be active in immature NK cells but not mature cells. Although related elements are present in the activating *Ly49* genes, no transcripts originating from this region have been detected. If early transcripts of the activating *Ly49* genes do exist, they may only be present transiently during NK cell maturation, and the relative scarcity of these transcripts will require extensive screening of cDNA libraries from various tissues in order to detect them.

A major weakness of the *Ly49* promoter studies performed to date is that the majority of in vitro analyses of *Ly49* promoter activity have been performed in the EL-4 T cell line, and therefore may not be an accurate representation of the control of Ly49 expression in NK cells. Another weakness is revealed by the discovery that the majority of *Ly49g* transcripts detected in splenic NK cells originate from the exon 2 promoter (Pro3), indicating that the studies of the exon 1 promoter (Pro2) may only be relevant to the expression of Ly49 proteins in T cells (Wilhelm et al. 2001). It therefore appears that to fully understand the mechanisms controlling Ly49 expression in NK cells, additional studies should be performed with Pro2 and Pro3 in a cell line that corresponds to a mature murine NK cell. Unfortunately, no mature mouse NK cell lines are currently available.

2.4
Pro1 Is a Bidirectional Transcriptional Element

The in vitro characterization of the upstream Pro1 promoter element was possible because of the existence of a murine NK cell line (LNK) that represents an immature CD94-positive, Ly49-negative cell that produces transcripts from the *Ly49g* Pro1 promoter but no transcripts originating from the Pro2 or Pro3 promoters (Tsutsui et al. 1996; Saleh et al. 2002). A detailed analysis of the *Ly49g* Pro1 element led to the unexpected finding of bidirectional promoter activity (Saleh et al. 2004). The Pro1 element is therefore capable of producing a forward transcript containing the Ly49 coding region or a reverse transcript that extends into the intergenic region and contains no identifiable coding sequences. The presence of antisense intergenic *Ly49* transcripts in bone marrow NK1.1-positive cells was demonstrated by RT-PCR. Bidirectional promoters producing either a forward coding transcript or a reverse noncoding "sterile" transcript were previously observed in the immunoglobulin heavy chain variable genes (Nguyen et al. 1991; Sun and Kitchingman 1994), and at that time they were suggested to function in the opening of chromatin, because concurrent bidirectional transcription would be expected to have a dramatic effect on accessibility and potentially play a role in making a V_h gene available for recombination.

In the case of the bidirectional element discovered in the *Ly49* genes, the early activity of this promoter suggested that it might represent a switch controlling the variegated expression of members of this gene family. In vitro promoter studies indicated that the relative forward and reverse transcriptional activities of the Pro1 element varied among *Ly49* genes (Saleh et al. 2004). Pro1 elements with a dominant reverse promoter activity were found in *Ly49* genes coding for Ly49 proteins that were not expressed on a significant subset of splenic NK cells. Increased levels of forward Pro1 activity were associated with *Ly49* genes that are expressed on larger subsets of NK cells. Significant differences in the Pro1 structure and function in the *Ly49j* and *Ly49c* genes provided a possible explanation for the distinct expression patterns of these two highly related genes. Although the *Ly49j* and *Ly49c* genes possess greater than 96% nucleotide homology, Ly49J is only expressed on a small subset (<5%) of C57BL/6 adult NK cells whereas Ly49C is expressed on 50% (Kubota et al 1999). The Pro2 promoter activity of these genes had previously been shown to be functionally equivalent (McQueen et al, 2001); however, the Pro1 forward transcriptional activity of the *Ly49j* gene was severely decreased relative to *Ly49c* activity, and this correlates with a deletion of the transcript initiation region and disruption of the TATA box associated with forward transcription in the *Ly49j* Pro1 element. This result suggests that Pro1 is a key element controlling the activation of the inhibitory *Ly49* genes. Further evidence for the importance of the Pro1 element was provided by studies of Ly49A transgenic mice in which the entire *Ly49a* gene, including 8 kb 5′ of the Pro2 element was used to generate transgenic mice (Tanamachi et al. 2004). These mice showed normal variegated expression of the Ly49A protein in NK cells; however, the protein was also expressed by all B cells, suggesting that there may be an additional locus control region located elsewhere that is required for suppression of B cell expression. An upstream DNAse hypersensitive site was detected in the *Ly49a* gene. The region surrounding the hypersensitive site was deleted from the *Ly49a* gene, and this construct was used to generate additional transgenic mice. The hypersensitive site identified maps to the center of the Pro1 element. Ly49A transgenic mice lacking the Pro1 region no longer expressed Ly49A on NK cells or B cells, indicating an essential role of the Pro1 promoter in gene activation.

2.5
The Pro1 Probabilistic Switch

To test the possibility that Pro1 was functioning as a gene switch, the bidirectional element was cloned between two different fluorescent protein cDNAs, so that forward transcription could be detected by the expression of yellow fluorescent protein (YFP) and reverse transcription would result in cyan fluorescent protein (CFP) expression (Saleh et al. 2004). By isolating stable transfectants containing only a single copy of this two-color reporter vector, it was possible to monitor the transcriptional behavior of the Pro1 element in real time. The remarkable result of this experiment was that the Pro1 element did in fact represent a switch that could choose between two stable transcriptional states. A single-cell clone containing the two-color vector under the control of the *Ly49g* Pro1 element (Ly49G is expressed on 45% of adult splenic NK cells) produced a variegated cell population that contained nearly equivalent levels of blue (CFP) or yellow (YFP) cells. The stability of this switch was demonstrated by time-lapse imaging of the variegated cell population. In the absence of cell division, blue cells remained blue and yellow cells remained yellow—switching of cell color was associated with cell division. A subpopulation of dividing cells was detected that expressed both CFP and YFP simultaneously before cell division, and these cells gave rise to a CFP-expressing daughter and a YFP-expressing daughter. This result indicated that the new copy of the two-color construct produced by DNA replication could produce a transcript in the opposite direction relative to the transcript produced by the parental copy in the same cell. This result provides direct evidence that the transcriptional decision is not directed by the relative concentration of transcription factors present in the nucleus. The model of *Ly49* gene activation proposed does not require the existence of limiting concentrations of transcription factors, because the factors required to initiate forward transcription are identical to those needed for reverse transcription. The "decision" to produce a forward or reverse transcript should be based on the relative probability of transcription factor binding to the competing forward or reverse binding sites, and this was borne out by mutation studies showing that changing the relative affinity of binding sites could change the probability of forward or reverse transcription (Saleh et al. 2004).

The probabilistic switch identified in the *Ly49* genes provides a powerful new paradigm to explain cell fate decisions. Although chance events may not seem to be a desirable mechanism to produce defined cellular outcomes, if a single chance event is occurring in a large number of precursor cells, the cellular fates that are produced are based on probability, and therefore completely predictable and reproducible. Although one cannot know the eventual Ly49 fate of an individual NK cell precursor, the total Ly49 repertoire produced is constant, and each individual mouse of a given inbred strain produces an identical repertoire. The Ly49 repertoire is stable in mature NK cells because the switch promoter is only active in immature cells, and the unidirectional adult promoter takes over transcription of the *Ly49* gene in the mature NK cell. Presumably, it is the forward transcription from the switch promoter in the immature NK cell that prevents the adult promoter from assuming a closed chromatin state, resulting in promoter activation when the NK cell matures and the transcription factors required for adult promoter activity are expressed. Ligand interaction and signaling play an important role in the final repertoire, but the probabilistic switch provides the initial diversity of Ly49 expression that can be modified by the selection processes operating in NK cell development.

3
NKR-P1 Promoters

The *NKR-P1C* gene encodes the NK1.1 antigen expressed by all functional C57BL/6 NK cells and NKT cells (Ryan et al. 1992). This gene is also expressed early in development, because a CD117+, NK1.1+ progenitor cell in thymus was shown to produce both NK and T cells (Carlyle et al. 1997). There is a general conservation of exon structure among the lectin-related genes, and the *NKR-P1C* gene was recently shown to possess three distinct promoter elements in locations similar to the three promoters identified in the Ly49 genes (Ljutic et al. 2003). Furthermore, the 5'-most promoter in the *NKR-P1C* gene was shown to be active only in fetus-derived NK cells, analogous to the *Ly49* Pro1 promoter that was shown to be active in immature NK cells. The principal *NKR-P1C* promoter that is active in the adult precedes the first coding exon of the gene, and it is located in a position similar to the *Ly49* promoter (Pro3) that precedes the first Ly49 coding exon (exon 2). The *Ly49g* Pro3 promoter was shown to represent the major *Ly49g* promoter used by splenic NK cells in vivo (Wilhelm et al. 2001). The question that arises is whether the 5'-most promoter is required for the initial activation of the *NKR-P1C*, as has been shown for the *Ly49a* gene. Because the *NKR-P1C* gene is not selectively activated in a subset of NK cells, the complex system of gene activation used by the Ly49 genes may not be required. However, NKR-P1B is only expressed on approximately 60% of NK cells in the Sw, SJL, and FVB mouse strains (Carlyle et al. 1999; Kung et al. 1999; Liu et al. 2000), suggesting that this inhibitory receptor could be controlled by the same mechanism of gene activation discovered in the Ly49 inhibitory receptors. The C57BL/6 *NKR-P1D* gene may also be expressed in a variegated fashion, because it is highly related to the *NKR-P1B* gene. There is conservation of the region surrounding the *NKR-P1C* upstream promoter/enhancer in the *NKR-P1D* gene, suggesting that a fetus-specific promoter may also exist in this gene. A key question to be answered is whether or not this element has bidirectional transcriptional activity and potentially functions as a stochastic switch controlling the selective activation of the *NKR-P1B/D* genes.

4
CD94 Promoter

The CD94 protein interacts with NKG2 family members to form heterodimers that interact with the nonclassical MHC proteins Qa-1^b in mouse and HLA-E in humans. CD94/NKG2 proteins are selectively expressed on NK cells in a manner similar to that observed for Ly49s, however CD94 appears early in NK development and its expression decreases as Ly49 expression increases (Lohwasser et al. 2000; Takei et al. 2001). Another feature of CD94/NKG2 expression that is shared with Ly49 is their expression on some $CD8^+$ T cells (McMahon and Raulet 2001). *CD94* promoters have been studied extensively in both mouse and human. Two promoters have been shown to exist in both species. The human *CD94* proximal promoter is active in freshly isolated primary NK and $CD8^+$ $\alpha\beta$ T cells, whereas the distal promoter is only induced on culture of cells with IL-2 or IL-15 (Lieto et al. 2003). In the mouse *CD94* gene, the situation is reversed; the distal promoter is used almost exclusively in freshly isolated NK cells, and its use decreases on culture in IL-2 (Wilhelm et al. 2003). A comparison of the putative transcription factor binding sites in the human and mouse promoters demonstrates a high degree of conservation; however, there are some notable differences that might explain the differential activation properties of the two promoters. There are multiple Ikaros sites and a Myc site in the human proximal promoter, and none of these sites is present in the human distal promoter. The opposite situation exists in the mouse gene, with Ikaros and Myc sites found in the distal promoter but not the proximal promoter, suggesting that Myc and Ikaros are associated with constitutive expression in freshly isolated NK cells. CD94 may be expressed in a variegated fashion in immature NK cells (Takei et al. 2001); therefore it is possible that an additional upstream promoter with a function similar to that of Ly49 Pro1 is present in the *CD94* gene. Screening of bone marrow cDNA libraries with a *CD94* probe will be necessary to determine whether there are unique *CD94* transcripts present in immature NK cells.

5
NKG2A Promoter

The *NKG2* gene family is located centromeric of the *Ly49* gene family on mouse chromosome 6, and this family is conserved in the human NKC on chromosome 12 (Plougastel et al. 1997; Brostjian et al. 2000; Bull et al. 2000). There is only a single inhibitory *NKG2* family member, *NKG2A*, located at the beginning of the cluster in both humans and mice. The close proximity of *NKG2A* to the *Ly49* gene family and the observed variegated expression of this gene (Takei et al. 2001) suggest that the system of transcriptional control found in the Ly49 genes might also exist in the NKG2A gene. Two promoters have been reported in the human NKG2A gene (Plougastel et al. 1997), and cDNAs isolated from rhesus monkey decidua have been identified that indicate the existence of a third upstream promoter (Kravitz et al. 2001). An additional human *NKG2A* cDNA isolated from NK92 cells (GenBank accession BC053840) confirms the existence of this novel promoter in the human gene. The locations of the three promoters identified in the human *NKG2A* gene correspond to the positions of the three *Ly49* and *NKR-P1C* promoters, providing evidence for a similar system of gene regulation in the lectin-related NK cell receptor gene families (Fig. 1). The 3′-most promoter of *NKG2A* is adjacent to the first coding exon of the gene in a location analogous to the location of *Ly49* Pro3. This promoter contains typical TATA and CCAAT elements, and transcripts initiated from this promoter comprised 25% of the cDNAs isolated from normal circulating lymphocytes. The second promoter identified generates a noncoding exon (exon 1), and it is located approximately 2 kb upstream of exon 2 in a location similar to that of *Ly49* Pro2. Transcripts originating in this region comprised 75% of *NKG2A* cDNAs isolated from lymphocytes. No characterization of the 5′-most promoter has been performed. Further studies are required to determine whether this additional promoter is functionally related to the Ly49 Pro1 element.

6
KIR Promoters

To date, there are only a few reports that provide a detailed functional analysis of KIR promoters. The analysis of the promoter regions of the *2DL4* and *3DL1* genes revealed significant differences in promoter structure and function, consistent with the distinct expression patterns of these genes (Stewart et al. 2003). All NK cells transcribe the *2DL4* gene, whereas *3DL1* is expressed in a variegated fashion in NK cell subsets. DNAse I footprinting was used to identify several sites of protein interaction that correspond to predicted transcription factor binding sites. Consistent with the distinct regulation of the *2DL4* and *3DL1* genes, there were significant differences in the potential transcription factor binding sites identified. A *2DL4* core promoter fragment of 262 bp was sufficient to confer NK-specific activity in reporter gene assays, and DNAse I footprinting revealed potential involvement of GATA-3, TCF-2, MYC/MAX, AP-1, CREB/ATF, RUNX/AML, and c-Ets1 transcription factors. In contrast, the *3DL1* core promoter demonstrated weaker activity, and potential binding sites for TCF-2, STAT, c-Ets1, YY-1, CREB, RUNX/AML, and SP-1 were identified. The identification of a DNAse I footprint at the putative AML binding site of *3DL1* supports the proposed importance of this AML site suggested by a study that compared expressed versus nonexpressed variants of the *2DL5* gene (Vilches et al. 2000). This AML-binding site is conserved in the promoter region of all *KIR* genes (Trowsdale et al. 2001), and the nonexpressed

2DL5 variants contain a point mutation that disrupts this AML site, suggesting that AML binding is required for *KIR* gene transcription. In addition, there is a SP-1 site in close proximity to the transcriptional start site, suggesting that *KIR* transcription is SP-1 dependent. The SP-1 site is conserved in all *KIR* genes, with the exception of the *3DL3* gene. The observed deletion of the SP-1 site in the nontranscribed *3DL3* gene may represent the key mutation that has inactivated transcription of this gene. SP-1-driven promoters are generally associated with genes that are constitutively active, such as housekeeping genes, indicating that additional levels of control must exist to explain the variegated expression of *KIR* genes.

Two reports have demonstrated that DNA methylation is responsible for maintaining the variegated expression of the *KIR* genes (Santourlidis et al. 2002; Chan et al. 2003). The paper by Santourlidis et al. investigated the methylation status of the *2DL3*, *3DL2*, and *3DL1* genes in the NK3.3 and NKL cell lines as well as freshly isolated NK cells. A small CpG island surrounding the transcriptional start site of each *KIR* gene was consistently methylated in silent *KIR* genes and demethylated in active *KIR* genes. Treatment of polyclonal NK cells, an NK cell clone, and NK cell lines with the demethylating agent 5-aza-2'-deoxycytidine resulted in de novo expression of KIRs. Furthermore, in vitro methylation of a 2DL3 core promoter construct suppressed transcriptional activity in luciferase reporter assays, indicating that the methylation status of the core *KIR* promoter determines whether or not a particular *KIR* gene is transcriptionally active. The study by Chan et al. (Chan et al. 2003) demonstrated that human NK cell clones expressing the 3DL1 protein exhibit allele-specific demethylation of the *3DL1* gene. The broadly expressed *2DL4* gene was found to be demethylated on both alleles. Demethylation of the *3DL1* and *2DL4* genes also correlated with protein expression in freshly isolated NK cells. Furthermore, induction of hypomethylation by treatment of NK92 cells with 5-aza-2'-deoxycytidine leads to heterogeneous expression of multiple KIR proteins.

Together, these studies demonstrate that the promoter regions of silent *KIR* genes are methylated, and active *KIR* genes are associated with demethylation, indicating that methylation plays a key role in maintaining a stable KIR repertoire. The unanswered question is whether or not methylation plays a role in determining the variegated expression pattern of *KIR* genes. For methylation to determine the probabilistic expression of the *KIR* genes, the promoter regions of different *KIR* family members would have to possess intrinsically different susceptibilities to methylation or demethylation. To fully address this issue, it will be necessary to perform core promoter substitution experiments in *KIR* transgenic mice. Alternatively, the selective gene activation may be controlled by a distal element similar to the Pro1 element found in the *Ly49* genes. Although the *KIR* intergenic region is considerably smaller than the *Ly49* intergenic region (2 kb versus 15 kb average intergenic distance), it is still possible that an additional upstream promoter exists in the *KIR* genes. RT-PCR analyses of the *2DL4–3DL1–2DL5* region have revealed the presence of sense and antisense transcripts in the intergenic regions in several NK cell lines as well as polyclonal NK cell preparations (SK Anderson, unpublished observations). The potential role of upstream elements in KIR variegation could also be addressed by substitution of intergenic segments between *KIR* genes that are expressed in significantly different percentages of NK cells and testing these alterations in transgenic mice.

7
Association of AP-1, SP-1, and Ets with NK Cell-Specific Promoters

It is of interest to note that the core promoter regions of several NK cell-specific receptor genes contain potential Ets binding sites together with SP-1 or AP-1 binding sites. AP-1 plays a major role in the NK cell-specific transcription of the human 2B4 gene (Chuang et al. 2001), and AP-1 sites are found together with an Ets site in the *NKG2A* and *NKR-P1C* upstream promoters as well as the proximal *CD94* promoter and *Ly49g* Pro3. The major *NKR-P1C* promoter used by mature NK cells contains Ets and SP-1 sites, as does the distal *CD94* promoter. A detailed study of the NK cell-specific Pmed1 promoter of the human *FcγRIIIA* gene has shown that SP-1 binding is required for activity, and an Ets site is located between two SP-1 binding sites in this promoter (Heusohn et al. 2002). In addition, the core promoter region of the perforin gene contains SP-1 and Ets binding sites and the Ets-related MEF protein is required for expression of the mouse perforin gene (Lacorazza et al. 2002). MEF$^{-/-}$ mice displayed a severe reduction in NK1.1-positive lymphocytes, suggesting that MEF is also important for NKR-P1C expression. A comparison of the Ets-binding sites in NK-specific promoters reveals an expanded consensus of ACAGGAA(G/A)T that may represent a MEF-specific binding sequence. It is of interest to note that the Pro1 elements of the *Ly49* genes also contain this Ets-binding consensus, and specific binding of the Elf and MEF transcription factors but not other Ets family members was observed in EL4 nuclear lysates with this element (SK Anderson, unpublished observations). It therefore appears that the Elf/MEF subfamily of Ets transcription factors represent an important component of NK/T-specific expression of NK receptors.

8
Conclusion

Although significant progress has been made toward gaining a complete understanding of the mechanisms controlling NK receptor gene transcription, there are still many unanswered questions. The studies of NK cell receptor gene transcription performed to date have identified several transcription factors that play a role in the expression of the NK cell receptors. The analysis of mutant mice that lack specific transcription factors associated with NK receptor expression can provide data supporting the role of these transcription factors in NK-specific expression; however, results obtained from such experiments should be interpreted with caution because of the pleotrophic nature of transcription factors. The variegated expression of NK cell receptor gene families clearly requires a sophisticated system of control, and we are just beginning to understand the mechanisms underlying the selective activation of these genes. Because two of the lectin-related genes families have been found to contain additional promoters that are specifically active in immature NK cells, it is not unreasonable to expect that the other lectin-related gene families will contain similar promoters. Screening of cDNA libraries generated from immature NK cell populations with various NK receptor probes could identify novel NK receptor promoters that are only active in the early stages of NK cell development. It will also be important to examine the early-acting promoters of genes that are selectively activated for bidirectional transcriptional activity and the possibility that they behave as probabilistic switches. The NK cell-specificity of the receptor genes may also be controlled in part by locus control regions, and to date, no studies addressing this possibility have been performed. A complete understanding of the mechanisms underlying the selective expression of NK cell-specific receptors must await the identification of all genomic elements required for appropriate gene expression in vivo.

Acknowledgements This project has been funded in whole or in part with Federal funds from the National Cancer Institute, National Institutes of Health, under Contract No. NO1-CO-12400. The author is indebted to Drs. James Carlyle, Dixie Mager, Colin Brooks, Gareth Davies, and Veronique Pascal for critical reading of the manuscript.

By acceptance of this article, the publisher or recipient acknowledges the right of the U.S. Government to retain a non-exclusive, royalty-free license in and to any copyright covering the article.

References

Brostjan C, Sobanov Y, Glienke J, Hayer S, Lehrach H, Francis F, Hofer E (2000) The NKG2 natural killer cell receptor family: comparative analysis of promoter sequences. Genes Immun 1:504–508

Bull C, Sobanov Y, Rohrdanz B, O'Brien J, Lehrach H, Hofer E (2000) The centromeric part of the human NK gene complex: linkage of LOX-1 and LY49L with the CD94/NKG2 region. Genes Immun 1:280–287

Carlyle JR, Martin A, Mehra A, Attisano L, Tsui FW, Zúñiga-Pflücker JC (1999) Mouse NKR-P1B, a novel NK1.1 antigen with inhibitory function. J Immunol 162:5917–5923

Carlyle JR, Michie AM, Furlonger C, Nakano T, Lenardo MJ, Paige CJ, Zúñiga-Pflücker JC (1997) Identification of a novel developmental stage marking lineage commitment of progenitor thymocytes. J Exp Med 186:173–182

Chan HW, Kurago ZB, Stewart CA, Wilson MJ, Martin MP, Mace BE, Carrington M, Trowsdale J, Lutz CT (2003) DNA methylation maintains allele-specific KIR gene expression in human natural killer cells. J Exp Med 197:245–255

Chuang SS, Pham HT, Kumaresan PR, Mathew PA (2001) A prominent role for activator protein-1 in the transcription of the human 2B4 (CD244) gene in NK cells. J Immunol 166:6188–6195

Dorfman JR, Raulet DH (1998) Acquisition of Ly49 receptor expression by developing natural killer cells. J Exp Med 187:609–618

Gosselin P, Makrigiannis AP, Nalewaik R, Anderson SK (2000) Characterization of the Ly49I promoter. Immunogenetics 51:326–331

Held W, Kunz B, Lowin-Kropf B, van de Wetering M, Clevers H (1999) Clonal acquisition of the Ly49A NK cell receptor is dependent on the *trans*-acting factor TCF-1. Immunity 11:433–442

Held W, Clevers H, Grosschedl R (2003) Redundant functions of TCF-1 and LEF-1 during T and NK cell development, but unique role of TCF-1 for Ly49 NK cell receptor acquisition. Eur J Immunol 33:1393–1398

Heusohn F, Wirries G, Schmidt RE, Gessner JE (2002) The Pmed1 gene promoter of human FcγRIIIA can function as a NK/T cell-specific restriction element, which involves binding of Sp1 transcription factor. J Immunol 168:2857–2864

Ioannidis V, Kunz B, Tanamachi DM, Scarpellino L, Held W (2003) Initiation and limitation of Ly-49A NK cell receptor acquisition by T cell factor-1. J Immunol 171:769–775

Kravitz RH, Grendell RL, Slukvin II, Golos TG (2001) Selective expression of NKG2-A and NKG2-C mRNAs and novel alternative splicing of 5′ exons in rhesus monkey decidua. Immunogenetics 53:69–73

Kubo S, Itoh Y, Ishikawa N, Nagasawa R, Mitarai T, Maruyama N (1993) The gene encoding mouse lymphocyte antigen Ly-49: structural analysis and the 5′-flanking sequence. Gene 136:329–331

Kubo S, Nagasawa R, Nishimura H, Shigemoto K, Maruyama N (1999) ATF-2-binding regulatory element is responsible for the Ly49A expression in murine T lymphoid line, EL-4. Biochim Biophys Acta 1444:191–200

Kubota A, Kubota S, Lohwasser S, Mager DL, Takei F (1999) Diversity of NK cell receptor repertoire in adult and neonatal mice. J Immunol 163:212–216

Kung SKP, Su R-C, Shannon J, Miller RG (1999) The NKR-P1B gene product is an inhibitory receptor on SJL/J NK cells. J Immunol 162:5876–5887

Kunz B, Held W (2001) Positive and negative roles of the *trans*-acting T cell factor-1 for the acquisition of distinct Ly-49 MHC class I receptors by NK cells. J Immunol 166:6181–6187

Lacorazza HD, Miyazaki Y, Di Cristofano A, Deblasio A, Hedvat C, Zhang J, Cordon-Cardo C, Mao S, Pandolfi PP, and Nimer SD (2002) The ETS protein MEF plays a critical role in perforin gene expression and the development of natural killer and NK-T cells. Immunity 17:437–439

Lieto LD, Borrego F, You CH, Coligan JE (2003) Human CD94 gene expression: dual promoters differing in responsiveness to IL-2 or IL-15. J Immunol 171:5277–5286

Liu J, Morris MA, Nguyen P, George TC, Koulich E, Lai WC, Schatzle JD, Kumar V, Bennett M (2000) Ly49I NK cell receptor transgene inhibition of rejection of H2^b mouse bone marrow transplants. J Immunol 164:1793–1799

Ljutic B, Carlyle JR, Zuniga-Pflucker JC (2003) Identification of upstream *cis*-acting regulatory elements controlling lineage-specific expression of the mouse NK cell activation receptor, NKR-P1C. J Biol Chem 278:31909–31917

Lohwasser S, Wilhelm B, Mager DL, Takei F (2000) The genomic organization of the mouse CD94 C-type lectin gene. Eur J Immunogenet 27:149–151

McMahon CW, Raulet DH (2001) Expression and function of NK receptors in CD8$^+$ T cells. Curr Opin Immunol 13:465–470

McQueen KL, Wilhelm BT, Takei F, Mager DL (2001) Functional analysis of 5′ and 3′ regions of the closely related Ly49c and j genes. Immunogenetics 52:212–223

Nguyen QT, Doyen N, d'Andon MF, Rougeon F (1991). Demonstration of a divergent transcript from the bidirectional heavy chain immunoglobulin promoter V$_h$441 in B-cells. Nucleic Acids Res 19:5339–5344

Plougastel B, Trowsdale J (1998) Sequence analysis of a 62-kb region overlapping the human KLRC cluster of genes. Genomics 49:193–199

Raulet DH, Held W, Correa I, Dorfman J, Wu M-F, Corral L (1997) Specificity, tolerance and developmental regulation of natural killer cells defined by expression of class I specific Ly49 receptors. Immunol Rev 155:41–52

Roth C, Carlyle JR, Takizawa H, Raulet DH (2000) Clonal acquisition of inhibitory Ly49 receptors on developing NK cells is successively restricted and regulated by stromal class I MHC. Immunity 13:143–153

Ryan JC, Turck J, Niemi EC, Yokoyama WM, Seaman WE (1992) Molecular cloning of the NK1.1 antigen, a member of the NKR-P1 family of natural killer cell activation molecules. J Immunol 149:1631–1635

Saleh A, Makrigiannis AP, Hodge DL, Anderson SK (2002) Identification of a novel Ly49 promoter that is active in bone marrow and fetal thymus. J Immunol 168:5163–5169

Saleh A, Davies GE, Pascal V, Wright PW, Hodge DL, Cho EH, Lockett SJ, Abshari M, Anderson SK (2004) Identification of probabilistic transcriptional switches in the Ly49 gene cluster: a eukaryotic mechanism for selective gene activation. Immunity 21:55–66

Santourlidis S, Trompeter HI, Weinhold S, Eisermann B, Meyer KL, Wernet P, Uhrberg M (2002) Crucial role of DNA methylation in determination of clonally distributed killer cell Ig-like receptor expression patterns in NK cells. J Immunol 169:4253–4261

Schilham MW, Wilson A, Moerer P, Benaissa-Trouw BJ, Cumano A, Clevers HC (1998) Critical involvement of Tcf-1 in expansion of thymocytes. J Immunol 161:3984–3991

Stevenaert F, Van Beneden K, De Creus A, Debacker V, Plum J, Leclercq G (2003) Ly49E expression points toward overlapping, but distinct, natural killer (NK) cell differentiation kinetics and potential of fetal versus adult lymphoid progenitors. J Leukoc Biol 73:731–738

Stewart CA, Van Bergen J, Trowsdale J (2003) Different and divergent regulation of the KIR2DL4 and KIR3DL1 promoters. J Immunol 170:6073–6081

Sun G, Kitchingman GR (1994) Bidirectional transcription from the human immunoglobulin VH6 gene promoter. Nucleic Acids Res 22:861–868

Takei F, McQueen KL, Maeda M, Wilhelm BT, Lohwasser S, Lian RH, Mager DL (2001) Ly49 and CD94/NKG2: developmentally regulated expression and evolution. Immunol Rev 181:90–103

Tanamachi DM, Moniot DC, Cado D, Liu SD, Hsia JK, Raulet DH (2004) Genomic Ly49A transgenes: basis of variegated Ly49A gene expression and identification of a critical regulatory element. J Immunol 172:1074–1082

Trowsdale J, Barten R, Haude A, Stewart CA, Beck S, Wilson MJ (2001) The genomic context of natural killer receptor extended gene families. Immunol Rev 181:20–38

Tsutsui H, Nakanishi K, Matsui K, Higashino K, Okamura H, Miyazawa Y, Kaneda K. (1996). IFN-γ-inducing factor up-regulates Fas ligand-mediated cytotoxic activity of murine natural killer cell clones. J Immunol 157:3967–3973

Valiante NM, Uhrberg M, Shilling HG, Lienert-Weidenbach K, Arnett KL, D'Andrea A, Phillips JH, Lanier LL, Parham P (1997) Functionally and structurally distinct NK cell receptor repertoires in the peripheral blood of two human donors. Immunity 7:739–751

Vilches C, Gardiner CM, Parham P (2000) Gene structure and promoter variation of expressed and nonexpressed variants of the KIR2DL5 gene. J Immunol 165:6416–6421

Wang J-W, Howson JM, Ghansah T, Desponts C, Ninos JM, May SL, Nguyen KHT, Toyama-Sorimachi N, Kerr WG (2002) Influence of SHIP on the NK repertoire and allogeneic bone marrow transplantation. Science 295:2094–2097

Wilhelm BT, McQueen KL, Freeman JD, Takei F, Mager DL (2001) Comparative analysis of the promoter regions and transcriptional start sites of mouse Ly49 genes. Immunogenetics 53:215–224

Wilhelm BT, Landry JR, Takei F, Mager DL (2003) Transcriptional control of murine CD94 gene: differential usage of dual promoters by lymphoid cell types. J Immunol 171:4219–4226

Williams NS, Kubota A, Bennett M, Kumar V, Takei F (2000). Clonal analysis of NK cell development from bone marrow progenitors in vitro: orderly acquisition of receptor gene expression. Eur J Immunol 30:2074–2082

Extending Missing-Self? Functional Interactions Between Lectin-like Nkrp1 Receptors on NK Cells with Lectin-like Ligands

B. F. M. Plougastel · W. M. Yokoyama (✉)

Rheumatology Division, Department of Medicine, Howard Hughes Medical Institute, Washington University School of Medicine, St. Louis, MO 63110, USA
yokoyama@im.wustl.edu

1	Introduction	78
2	Nkrp1 and Clr Families	79
2.1	Nkrp1 and Clr Molecular Interactions	82
2.2	Nkrp1 and Clr Functions	83
2.3	Genetics of *Nkrp1* and *Clr*	85
3	Conclusions	86
	References	86

Abstract The functions of natural killer (NK) cells are clearly regulated by major histocompatibility complex (MHC) class I molecules on their cellular targets. In mice, this is due to the action of MHC-specific inhibitory receptors belonging to the Ly49 family of lectin-like molecules. The Ly49 receptors are encoded in the NK gene complex (NKC) that contains clusters of genes for other lectin-like receptors on NK cells and other hematopoietic cells. Interestingly, recent studies have shown that some of these lectin-like receptors, belonging to the Nkrp1 family, can recognize other lectin-like molecules, termed Clr, also encoded in the NKC. These genetically linked loci for receptor-ligand pairs suggest a genetic strategy to preserve this interaction and show several other contrasts with Ly49-MHC interactions. In this review, we discuss these issues and summarize recent developments concerning this non-MHC-dependent regulation of NK cell function.

Abbreviations
ITAM	Immunoreceptor tyrosine-based activation motif
ITIM	Immunoreceptor tyrosine-based inhibitory motif
KARAP	Killer activating receptor-associated protein
DAP12	DNAX-activation protein of 12 kDa
DAP10	DNAX-activation protein of 10 kDa
Clr	C-type lectin related
IFN-γ	Interferon-γ
NKC	NK gene complex

1
Introduction

The natural killer gene complex (NKC) contains gene clusters that encode mostly type II integral membrane proteins with extracellular domains that have structural features of the C-type lectins (Yokoyama and Plougastel 2003). These proteins can be classified into families (Ly49, NKRP1, NKG2, and CD94). Members within the same family may have opposing functions. For example, molecules belonging to the Ly49 family like Ly49D or Ly49H have been shown to activate NK cells (Mason et al. 1996; Smith et al. 2000), whereas the Ly49A receptor inhibits NK cell function after interaction with its major histocompatibility complex (MHC) class I-specific ligand (Karlhofer et al. 1992; Kim and Yokoyama 1998). Where functions have been described, cytoplasmic protein sequences known as immunoreceptor tyrosine-based activation motifs (ITAMs) and immunoreceptor tyrosine-based inhibitory motifs (ITIMs) (Vivier and Daeron 1997) are responsible for the activating or inhibitory signals, respectively. Whereas the inhibitory receptors contain ITIMs that recruit inhibitory phosphatases that influence intracellular signaling cascades, the activating receptors lack any known signaling domains of their own. Instead, they rely on association with adaptor proteins such as killer activating receptor-associated protein (KARAP), also known as DAP12 (DNAX-activation protein of 12 kDa), DAP10, or FcεRIγ that transmit signals through their intracellular ITAMs. Protein tyrosine kinases with Src homology 2 domains or phosphatidylinositol 3-kinase can then bind the phosphorylated tyrosine residues, leading to downstream signaling and gene modulation. NK receptors expressed on other cell types may recruit alternative protein kinases, or phosphatases, and therefore modulate a range of intracellular signaling pathways.

The integration of inhibitory and activation receptor signaling ultimately results in triggering (or not) of NK cells. In this regard, a guiding principle in NK cell biology is the "missing-self" hypothesis whereby target cells with defective MHC class I expression are eliminated by NK cells. The inhibitory receptors provide a mechanism to explain this hypothesis because inhibitory receptor engagement by target cell MHC class I tends to dominate NK cell functions. On the other hand, it is possible to overcome MHC class I inhibition by upregulating target cell expression of ligands for activation receptors. For example, stress-induced expression of ligands for NKG2D can activate NK cell function even when the targets express MHC class I molecules that are recognized by the relevant NK cells (Bauer et al. 1999; Diefenbach et al. 2000). Thus current studies suggest that NK cell function can be triggered by either downregulation of MHC class I ligands for inhibitory receptors or upregulation of stress-induced ligands for activation receptors.

In this review, we focus our discussion on two families of lectin-like molecules, Nkrp1 and Clr, that provide novel modes of regulating NK cell functions that are related but distinct from other known mechanisms.

2
Nkrp1 and Clr Families

The NK1.1 (Nkrp1c) molecule is the best known serological marker on NK cells in C57BL/6 mice (Ryan et al. 1992). Lymphocytes that express the NK1.1 antigen and do not express the TCR receptor are generally considered to be bona fide NK cells (Lanier et al. 1986). Interestingly, some mouse strains such as BALB/c, SJL, AKR, CBA, C3H and A do not express the NK1.1 antigen. [Identification of NK cells in these strains relies on use of an integrin molecule (DX5, $\alpha_2\beta_1$) expressed selectively on NK cells (Arase et al. 2001).] In C57BL/6 mice, five Nkrp1 transcripts have been identified (Table 1) (Giorda and Trucco 1991; Plougastel et al. 2001b; Ryan et al. 1992; Yokoyama et al. 1991). The corresponding genes are localized on distal mouse chromosome 6 in a cluster extending an estimated 650 kb (Fig. 1). The Nkrp1c molecule is a dimer present on the surface of NK cells. The Nkrp1d molecule has been shown recently to have a similar expression pattern (Iizuka et al. 2003). Because of the lack of monoclonal antibodies specific for the Nkrp1a and Nkrp1f molecules, no protein expression data are yet available for these molecules.

The structurally related Ly49, Nkg2, and Cd94 molecules are encoded by genetically linked loci within the NKC. Each family, however, spans independent chromosomal regions (Ho et al. 1998; Lohwasser et al. 1999; Plougastel and Trowsdale 1998; Yokoyama and Seaman 1993). Analysis of the Nkrp1 sequences available in the databases indicates that the members of the Nkrp1 family, unlike those of the Ly49 family, do not display high degrees of allelic polymorphism (Iizuka et al. 2003). The Nkrp1d molecule presents, for example, only one amino acid difference between the BALB/c and C57BL/6 strains, whereas there is extensive allelic polymorphism of the Ly49 molecules that affect ligand specificities and functions (Mehta et al. 2001; Wilhelm et al. 2002).

Recently, another low-polymorphism gene family has been localized in the same chromosomal region (Fig. 1). This new family encodes C-type lectin-related molecules (Clr) that display homology with the CD69 molecule. In C57BL/6 mice, seven Clr genes have been identified at the genomic level (Table 2). Three of them are expressed in interleukin-2-activated NK cells: *Clrb*, *Clrf*, and *Clrg*. RT-PCR analysis indicates that *Clrb* is broadly expressed, whereas *Clrg* and *Clrf* genes are present on restricted and nonoverlapping

Table 1 Nkrp1 nomenclature

Species	Strains	Genes	Other names	Ligands	References
Mouse	C57BL/6J	*Nkrp1a*	Klrb1a	?	Giorda 1991
			Ly55a		
		Nkrp1c	Klrb1c	?	Giorda and Trucco 1991
			Ly55c		Ryan et al. 1992
			CD161		Yokoyama et al. 1991
		Nkrp1d	Klrb1d	Clrb	Plougastel et al. 2001b
			Ly55d		Kung et al. 1999
		Nkrp1e			Plougastel et al. 2001b
		Nkrp1f	Klrb1f	Clrg	Plougastel et al. 2001b
	SJL/j	*Nkrp1b*	Klrb1b	?	Giorda and Trucco 1991
					Kung et al. 1999
					Carlyle et al. 1999
Rat	BN/ SsNHsdMCW	*Klrb1a*	NKR-P1.3.2.3		Ryan et al. 1991
			NKRP1A		Li et al. 2003
	F344	*Klrb1b*	NKRP1B		Dissen 1996
Human		*KLRB1A*	CD161		Lanier et al. 1994
			hNKRP1A		Exley et al. 1998
			NKRP1A		

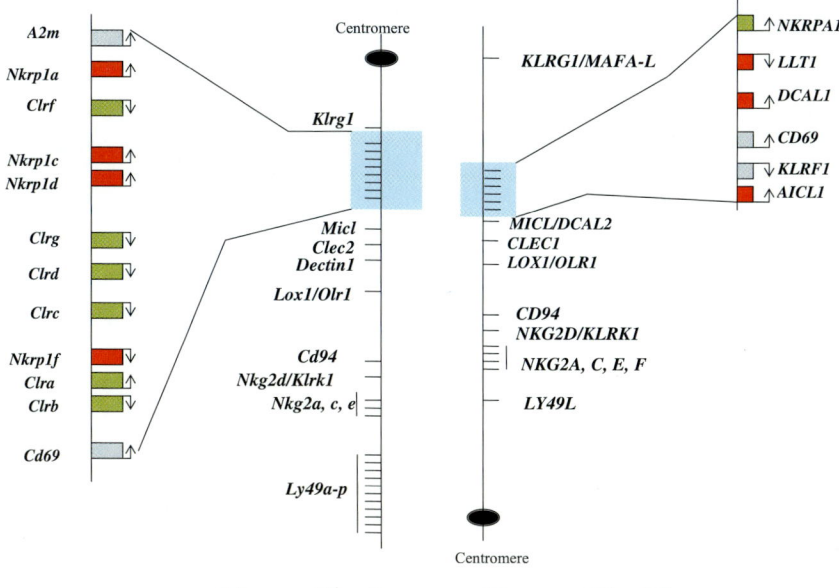

Fig. 1 Schematic representation of the NKC in mice and humans. Shown in more detail are the *Nkrp1* and *Clr* genes that are intertwined in the centromeric portion of the mouse NKC. The syntenic region of the human NKC is also shown. *Arrows* indicate transcriptional orientation

tissues (Plougastel et al. 2001a). The *Clre* sequence, a probable pseudogene, demonstrates numerous stop codons in its expected open reading frame. Transcripts for the *Clra* and *Clrc* genes have not been identified yet. The Clr genes encode proteins that do not display amino acid differences between the 129/sv, BALB/c, and C57BL/6J strains of mice. At the nucleotide level, they present as little as one difference in their coding sequence. Analysis of the rat genomic database indicates the existence of a rat *Clr* family of genes intertwined in the *Nkrp1* cluster. In human, three genes, *LLT1* (Boles et al. 1999), *AICL* (Hamann et al. 1997), and *DCAL-1* (Ryan et al. 2002), are localized next to CD69 and could be related to the Clr family of genes. Thus the Clr family appears to consist of a set of conserved, relatively nonpolymorphic molecules.

Table 2 Clr nomenclature

Species	Genes	Other names	References
Mouse	*Clra*		Plougastel et al. 2001a
	Clrb	OCIL	Plougastel et al. 2001a
			Zhou et al. 2001
			Zhou et al. 2002
			Carlyle et al. 2004
	Clrc		Plougastel et al. 2001a
	Clrd	OCILrp1	Plougastel et al. 2001a
			Zhou et al. 2002
	Clre		Plougastel et al. 2001a
	Clrf		Plougastel et al. 2001a
	Clrg	OCILrp2	Plougastel et al. 2001a
		DCL1	Zhou et al. 2002
Human	*LLT1*		Hammann et al. 1997
	AICL		Boles et al. 1999
	DCAL1		Ryan et al. 2002

2.1
Nkrp1 and Clr Molecular Interactions

The interactions between the Nkrp1 and Clr families of molecules have been determined with a system that was originally developed to detect ligand-induced T cell activation (Carlyle et al. 2004; Iizuka et al. 2003; Sanderson and Shastri 1994). Briefly, the BWZ.36 cell line that expresses an NFAT-inducible lacZ construct was transduced with retroviral constructs for chimeric molecules consisting of each Nkrp1 ectodomain and the CD3ζ cytoplasmic domain (Iizuka et al. 2003). Ligand-induced Nkrp1-expressing cell activation was then measured by a simple nonradioactive lacZ assay. Cell lines expressing putative ligands for the Nkrp1f molecule were thus identified. Moreover, such cells also bound recombinant, soluble Nkrp1f tetramers that also blocked the Nkrp1f reporter cell assay. Ligands were then cloned by transducing a ligand-negative cell line with a retrovirus cDNA library prepared from one of the cell lines that clearly expressed the ligand for the Nkrp1f molecule. The Nkrp1f tetramer was used to enrich for cDNAs for Nkrp1f ligand-expressing clones by flow cytometry. PCR extraction of cDNA sequences from tetramer-positive clones indicated that the Clrg molecule was consistently found. Deliberate transfection of the

Clrg cDNA into ligand-negative cells conferred reactivity with the Nkrp1f reporter cells and Nkrp1f tetramers, indicating that the ligand of the Nkrp1f molecule was Clrg. A specific interaction between the Nkrp1d and Clrb molecules was then identified in the latter manner. The Nkrp1b molecule has been shown to interact with the Clrb molecule (Carlyle et al. 2004). A recent paper suggests that oligosaccharides linked to Nkrp1 could play a role in Clr recognition (Gange et al. 2004), but this must be mediated in a manner distinct from authentic C-type lectins because the Nkrp1 molecules lack residues for coordinate binding of Ca^{2+}, which is required for Ca^{2+}-dependent carbohydrate interactions (Weis et al. 1992). Thus interactions between the Clr and Nkrp1 family of molecule represent the only known cases in which the NK receptors and their ligands are both lectin-like molecules.

2.2
Nkrp1 and Clr Functions

Consistent with the absence of an ITIM and the presence of a charged residue in its membrane-spanning domain, the Nkrp1c molecule behaves as an activation receptor on mouse NK cells. The mouse Nkrp1a and Nkrp1f molecules are also predicted from their protein sequences to be activation receptors, but no functional data are yet available. Nkrp1c cross-linking activates NK cells that exhibit cytotoxicity and interferon-γ (IFN-γ) production (Arase et al. 1996; Karlhofer and Yokoyama 1991; Kim and Yokoyama 1998). Interestingly, NKT cells that secrete both IFN-γ and interleukin 4 (IL-4) on T cell receptor cross-linking, produce IFN-γ but not IL-4 on Nkrp1c cross-linking, (Arase et al. 1996). The other activation receptors encoded in the NKC that have been functionally investigated (Ly49H, -D, Nkg2c, or Nkg2d molecules) all associate with the KARAP/DAP12 or DAP10 adaptor molecules. However, in the case of the mouse Nkrp1c molecules, association with the FcRγ chain has been shown with coimmunoprecipitation experiments (Arase et al. 1997). Furthermore, NK cells from FcRγ chain-deficient mice did not show cytotoxicity or IFN-γ production on Nkrp1c cross-linking, but NK1.1 expression was normal. These findings demonstrate that the FcRγ chain plays an important role in activation of NK cells via the Nkrp1c molecule but not in its expression, unlike the case for other activation receptors such as Ly49H, which requires KARAP/DAP12 for cell surface expression as well as function.

The rat and the human Nkrp1 activating molecules have also been shown to mediate transmembrane signaling (Ryan et al. 1995; Cerny et al. 1997). They all have conserved tyrosine and serine residues in their cytoplasmic domains. These residues are potential phosphorylation sites.

The mouse Nkrp1b and Nkrp1d molecules possess cytoplasmic tails with an ITIM. The Nkrp1b molecule has been shown to act as an inhibitory receptor in the SWR or SJL/J strain. Association of Nkrp1b with Src homology 2-containing protein tyrosine phosphatase-1 (SHP1) provides a molecular mechanism for this inhibition (Carlyle et al. 1999,2004; Kung et al. 1999). The Nkrp1d molecule, which is likely the allelic form of the Nkrp1b molecule in C57BL/6 mice, has also been shown to function as an inhibitory receptor on primary NK cells. Transduced expression of Clrb in susceptible cells reduces killing by C57BL/6 LAK cells. The inhibition of killing can be reversed with a blocking antibody directed against the Nkrp1d molecule (Iizuka et al. 2003). In rat, the NKRP1B molecule contains an ITIM in its cytoplasmic tail such that it functions also as an inhibitory receptor (Li et al. 2003).

The signaling molecules responsible for inducing phosphorylation of the ITAM and ITIM in Nkrp1 molecules remain unknown. The presence of conserved Cys-X-Cys-Pro sequence in the Nkrp1 molecules suggest that Src family tyrosine kinases may play a role. In rat, the Nkrp1a molecule (Ryan et al. 1991) has been shown to bind the $p56^{lck}$ Src family tyrosine kinase (Campbell and Giorda 1997; Giorda and Trucco 1991). In human, the NKRP1A molecule (CD161) does not contain the cytoplasmic tail $p56^{lck}$ binding motif, and an association with $p56^{lck}$ is therefore unlikely. In contrast to results in mouse, anti-CD161 mAb does not directly activate human T cells that express NKRP1A. Activation with limiting quantities of anti-CD3 mAb revealed costimulatory activity after CD161 ligation (Exley et al. 1998). Finally, in mouse, it is not clear whether $p56^{lck}$ is involved in inhibition by ITIM-containing Nkrp1 receptors.

Transcripts of Clr molecules are broadly expressed, but perhaps what is most interesting is the expression of Clr molecules in dendritic cell and macrophage populations. This expression is apparently regulated at the transcriptional level (Iizuka et al. 2003). Also, transcripts for the *Clrb* and *Clrg* genes (OCIL and OCILrp2, respectively) have been identified in osteoblasts. It has been suggested that these molecules could inhibit osteoclast formation in in vitro cocultures of osteoblastic stromal cells with hemopoietic cells. This inhibition would be lymphocyte independent. The authors suggest that OCIL/Clr might have a direct action to oppose RANKL in the control of osteoclastogenesis (Zhou et al. 2001, 2002), independent of IL-4 (Mirosavljevic et al. 2003). Thus the Nkrp1-Clr interactions may be especially important in the interactions of innate immune cells.

The human LLT1 and the mouse Clrb molecules are broadly expressed in peripheral blood (Carlyle et al. 1999, 2004; Mathew et al. 2004; Plougastel et al. 2001a). Biochemical analysis indicates that LLT1, like most of the lectin-like molecules encoded in the NKC, is expressed on the cell surface as a dimer (Mathew et al. 2004). LLT1 has a short cytoplasmic tail that lacks an ITIM or other tyrosine motif. However, it possesses a basic residue in its transmembrane domain that could associate with a signaling adapter chain. A monoclonal antibody specific for LLT1 does not induce activation or inhibition of lysis by NK cells but does induce IFN-γ production by a human NK cell line (YT), and by resting or activated NK cells (Mathew et al. 2004). No interaction between the human NKRP1A molecule (Lanier et al. 1994) and LLT1 has been demonstrated so far. Nkrp1-Clr interactions may, however, be indicative of the functions of related molecules that are just beginning to be understood.

Inasmuch as the expression of Nkrp1d is similar on NK cells from both wild-type and MHC class I-deficient mice, and Nkrp1d-dependent inhibition occurs in the absence of MHC class I on targets, these data indicate that NK cells utilize an MHC class I-independent mechanism to regulate their function (Iizuka et al. 2003). Interestingly, this mechanism is similar in principle to MHC class I-dependent responses conferred by Ly49 and related receptors. Indeed, the receptors involved in both MHC class I-dependent and -independent inhibitions are structurally similar, despite differences in structural features of the ligands. It is therefore tempting to speculate that MHC class I-independent regulation of NK cells by Nkrp1-Clr interactions extends the missing-self hypothesis beyond MHC class I and provides another means to regulate NK cells via inhibitory receptors (Carlyle et al. 2004; Iizuka et al. 2003). Moreover, this regulation of NK cells appears to be independent of up-regulated ligands for activation receptors, such as NKG2D (Bauer et al. 1999; Diefenbach et al. 2000). Thus the Nkrp1-Clr interactions appear to reveal novel mechanisms to regulate NK cell functions.

2.3
Genetics of *Nkrp1* and *Clr*

The genes for Nkrp1 and Clr molecules are intertwined in the centromeric portion of the NKC (Iizuka et al. 2003; Plougastel et al. 2001a,b). Interestingly, these molecules are relatively nonpolymorphic, unlike the high degree of polymorphism of the Ly49 molecules encoded in the telomeric portion of the NKC (Makrigiannis et al. 2002; Wilhelm et al. 2002; Yokoyama and Plougastel 2003). Ly49 polymorphism likely reflects the extreme polymorphism of MHC class I molecules, the ligands for Ly49 molecules that are encoded on another chromosome. Because the receptors and ligand genes independently segregate, the polymorphisms appear to have evolved to permit continued interactions, despite independent mutational events. On the other hand, Nkrp1 and Clr genes cosegregate because of close genetic linkage. Furthermore, there is evidence for suppression of recombination, for we have not observed a recombination event in the region in over 6,400 meioses (Brown et al. 2001), indicating that recombination is suppressed.

These latter genetic features resemble the self-incompatibility (SI) locus in flowering plants. The SI locus contains the genes for two interacting molecules, a receptor on the pistil and its ligand on pollen. Interaction between these molecules blocks fertilization, as a means to prevent inbreeding (Ferris et al. 2002; Nasrallah 2002). Because of tight genetic linkage and recombination suppression, recombination in this genomic region is rare, suggesting that the Nkrp1-Clr region of the NKC also shares a genetic strategy with plants to preserve receptor-ligand interactions.

3
Conclusions

The features of Nkrp1-Clr interactions are somewhat unique. In particular, these molecules represent interactions between lectin-like molecules that are independent of MHC class I and appear to regulate NK cell functions independent of induced expression of ligands for activation receptors. Moreover, the Nkrp1 and Clr genes are colocalized to a genomic region that is genetically preserved, resembling a genetic strategy conserved in plants. Finally, these molecules may be important in the interactions between NK cells and dendritic cells and macrophages. Taken together, these data strongly suggest that, like other NKC-encoded receptors, the Nkrp1 and Clr molecules play important roles in innate immunity.

Acknowledgements The authors thank Koho Iizuka for his contributions while a member of the Yokoyama laboratory, and Olga Naidenko and Daved Fremont for ongoing collaborations. Work in the Yokoyama laboratory is supported by the Howard Hughes Medical Institute, the Barnes-Jewish Hospital Foundation, and grants from the National Institutes of Health.

References

Arase H, Arase N, Saito T (1996) Interferon γ production by natural killer (NK) cells and NK1.1+ T cells upon NKR-P1 cross-linking. J Exp Med 183:2391–6

Arase H, Saito T, Phillips JH, Lanier LL (2001) Cutting edge: the mouse NK cell-associated antigen recognized by DX5 monoclonal antibody is CD49b (α2 integrin, very late antigen-2). J Immunol 167:1141–4

Arase N, Arase H, Park SY, Ohno H, Ra C, Saito T (1997) Association with FcRγ is essential for activation signal through NKR-P1 (CD161) in natural killer (NK) cells and NK1.1+ T cells. J Exp Med 186:1957–63

Bauer S, Groh V, Wu J, Steinle A, Phillips JH, Lanier LL, Spies T (1999) Activation of NK cells and T cells by NKG2D, a receptor for stress-inducible MICA. Science 285:727–9

Boles KS, Barten R, Kumaresan PR, Trowsdale J, Mathew PA (1999) Cloning of a new lectin-like receptor expressed on human NK cells. Immunogenetics 50:1–7

Brown MG, Scalzo AA, Stone LR, Clark PY, Du Y, Palanca B, Yokoyama WM (2001) Natural killer gene complex (Nkc) allelic variability in inbred mice: evidence for Nkc haplotypes. Immunogenetics 53:584–91

Campbell KS, Giorda R (1997) The cytoplasmic domain of rat NKR-P1 receptor interacts with the N-terminal domain of p56(lck) via cysteine residues. Eur J Immunol 27:72–7

Carlyle JR, Jamieson AM, Gasser S, Clingan CS, Arase H, Raulet DH (2004) Missing self-recognition of Ocil/Clr-b by inhibitory NKR-P1 natural killer cell receptors. Proc Natl Acad Sci USA 101:3527–32

Carlyle JR, Martin A, Mehra A, Attisano L, Tsui FW, Zuniga-Pflucker JC (1999) Mouse NKR-P1B, a novel NK1.1 antigen with inhibitory function. J Immunol 162:5917–23

Cerny J, Fiserova A, Horvath O, Bezouska K, Pospisil M, Horejsi V (1997) Association of human NK cell surface receptors NKR-P1 and CD94 with Src-family protein kinases. Immunogenetics 46:231–6

Diefenbach A, Jamieson AM, Liu SD, Shastri N, Raulet DH (2000) Ligands for the murine NKG2D receptor: expression by tumor cells and activation of NK cells and macrophages. Nat Immunol 1:119–26

Exley M, Porcelli S, Furman M, Garcia J, Balk S (1998) CD161 (NKR-P1A) costimulation of CD1d-dependent activation of human T cells expressing invariant V α24J αQ T cell receptor αchains. J Exp Med 188:867–76

Ferris PJ, Armbrust EV, Goodenough UW (2002) Genetic structure of the mating-type locus of *Chlamydomonas reinhardtii*. Genetics 160:181–200

Gange CT, Quinn JM, Zhou H, Kartsogiannis V, Gillespie MT, Ng KW (2004) Characterization of sugar binding by osteoclast inhibitory lectin. J Biol Chem 279:29043–9

Giorda R, Trucco M (1991) Mouse NKR-P1. A family of genes selectively coexpressed in adherent lymphokine-activated killer cells. J Immunol 147:1701–8

Hamann J, Montgomery KT, Lau S, Kucherlapati R, van Lier RA (1997) AICL: a new activation-induced antigen encoded by the human NK gene complex. Immunogenetics 45:295–300

Ho EL, Heusel JW, Brown MG, Matsumoto K, Scalzo AA, Yokoyama WM (1998) Murine Nkg2d and Cd94 are clustered within the natural killer complex and are expressed independently in natural killer cells. Proc Natl Acad Sci USA 95:6320–5

Iizuka K, Naidenko OV, Plougastel BF, Fremont DH, Yokoyama WM (2003) Genetically linked C-type lectin-related ligands for the NKRP1 family of natural killer cell receptors. Nat Immunol 4:801–7

Karlhofer FM, Ribaudo RK, Yokoyama WM (1992) MHC class I alloantigen specificity of Ly-49+ IL-2-activated natural killer cells. Nature 358:66–70

Karlhofer FM, Yokoyama WM (1991) Stimulation of murine natural killer (NK) cells by a monoclonal antibody specific for the NK1.1 antigen. IL-2-activated NK cells possess additional specific stimulation pathways. J Immunol 146:3662–73

Kim S, Yokoyama WM (1998) NK cell granule exocytosis and cytokine production inhibited by Ly-49A engagement. Cell Immunol 183:106–12

Kung SK, Su RC, Shannon J, Miller RG (1999) The NKR-P1B gene product is an inhibitory receptor on SJL/J NK cells. J Immunol 162:5876–87

Lanier LL, Chang C, Phillips JH (1994) Human NKR-P1A. A disulfide-linked homodimer of the C-type lectin superfamily expressed by a subset of NK and T lymphocytes. J Immunol 153:2417–28

Lanier LL, Phillips JH, Hackett J, Jr., Tutt M, Kumar V (1986) Natural killer cells: definition of a cell type rather than a function. J Immunol 137:2735–9

Li J, Rabinovich BA, Hurren R, Shannon J, Miller RG (2003) Expression cloning and function of the rat NK activating and inhibitory receptors NKR-P1A and -P1B. Int Immunol 15:411–6

Lohwasser S, Hande P, Mager DL, Takei F (1999) Cloning of murine NKG2A, B and C: second family of C-type lectin receptors on murine NK cells. Eur J Immunol 29:755–61

Makrigiannis AP, Pau AT, Schwartzberg PL, McVicar DW, Beck TW, Anderson SK (2002) A BAC contig map of the Ly49 gene cluster in 129 mice reveals extensive differences in gene content relative to C57BL/6 mice. Genomics 79:437–44

Mason LH, Anderson SK, Yokoyama WM, Smith HR, Winkler-Pickett R, Ortaldo JR (1996) The Ly-49D receptor activates murine natural killer cells. J Exp Med 184:2119–28

Mathew PA, Chuang SS, Vaidya SV, Kumaresan PR, Boles KS, Pham HT (2004) The LLT1 receptor induces IFN-γ production by human natural killer cells. Mol Immunol 40:1157–63

Mehta IK, Wang J, Roland J, Margulies DH, Yokoyama WM (2001) Ly49A allelic variation and MHC class I specificity. Immunogenetics 53:572–83

Mirosavljevic D, Quinn JM, Elliott J, Horwood NJ, Martin TJ, Gillespie MT (2003) T-cells mediate an inhibitory effect of interleukin-4 on osteoclastogenesis. J Bone Miner Res 18:984–93

Nasrallah JB (2002) Recognition and rejection of self in plant reproduction. Science 296:305–8

Plougastel B, Dubbelde C, Yokoyama WM (2001a) Cloning of Clr, a new family of lectin-like genes localized between mouse Nkrp1a and Cd69. Immunogenetics 53:209–14

Plougastel B, Matsumoto K, Dubbelde C, Yokoyama WM (2001b) Analysis of a 1-Mb BAC contig overlapping the mouse Nkrp1 cluster of genes: cloning of three new Nkrp1 members, Nkrp1d, Nkrp1e, and Nkrp1f. Immunogenetics 53:592–8

Plougastel B, Trowsdale J (1998) Sequence analysis of a 62-kb region overlapping the human KLRC cluster of genes. Genomics 49:193–9

Ryan EJ, Marshall AJ, Magaletti D, Floyd H, Draves KE, Olson NE, Clark EA (2002) Dendritic cell-associated lectin-1: a novel dendritic cell-associated, C-type lectin-like molecule enhances T cell secretion of IL-4. J Immunol 169:5638–48

Ryan JC, Niemi EC, Goldfien RD, Hiserodt JC, Seaman WE (1991) NKR-P1, an activating molecule on rat natural killer cells, stimulates phosphoinositide turnover and a rise in intracellular calcium. J Immunol 147:3244–50

Ryan JC, Niemi EC, Nakamura MC, Seaman WE (1995) NKR-P1A is a target-specific receptor that activates natural killer cell cytotoxicity

Ryan JC, Turck J, Niemi EC, Yokoyama WM, Seaman WE (1992) Molecular cloning of the NK1.1 antigen, a member of the NKR-P1 family of natural killer cell activation molecules. J Immunol 149:1631–5

Sanderson S, Shastri N (1994) LacZ inducible, antigen/MHC-specific T cell hybrids. Int Immunol 6:369–76

Smith HR, Chuang HH, Wang LL, Salcedo M, Heusel JW, Yokoyama WM (2000) Nonstochastic coexpression of activation receptors on murine natural killer cells. J Exp Med 191:1341–54

Vivier E, Daeron M (1997) Immunoreceptor tyrosine-based inhibition motifs. Immunol Today 18:286–91

Weis WI, Drickamer K, Hendrickson WA (1992) Structure of a C-type mannose-binding protein complexed with an oligosaccharide. Nature 360:127–34

Wilhelm BT, Gagnier L, Mager DL (2002) Sequence analysis of the ly49 cluster in C57BL/6 mice: a rapidly evolving multigene family in the immune system. Genomics 80:646–61

Yokoyama WM, Plougastel BF (2003) Immune functions encoded by the natural killer gene complex. Nat Rev Immunol 3:304–16

Yokoyama WM, Ryan JC, Hunter JJ, Smith HR, Stark M, Seaman WE (1991) cDNA cloning of mouse NKR-P1 and genetic linkage with LY-49. Identification of a natural killer cell gene complex on mouse chromosome 6. J Immunol 147:3229–36

Yokoyama WM, Seaman WE (1993) The Ly-49 and NKR-P1 gene families encoding lectin-like receptors on natural killer cells: the NK gene complex. Annu Rev Immunol 11:613–35

Zhou H, Kartsogiannis V, Hu YS, Elliott J, Quinn JM, McKinstry WJ, Gillespie MT, Ng KW (2001) A novel osteoblast-derived C-type lectin that inhibits osteoclast formation. J Biol Chem 276:14916–23

Zhou H, Kartsogiannis V, Quinn JM, Ly C, Gange C, Elliott J, Ng KW, Gillespie MT (2002) Osteoclast inhibitory lectin, a family of new osteoclast inhibitors. J Biol Chem 277:48808–15

The CD2 Family of Natural Killer Cell Receptors

M. E. McNerney · V. Kumar (✉)

Department of Pathology, Committee on Immunology, University of Chicago, 5841 S. Maryland Ave., S-315 MC3083, Chicago, IL 60637, USA
vkumar@bsd.uchicago.edu

1	CD2 Family Members	92
2	CD2 Receptor Family Signaling and X-Linked Lymphoproliferative Disease	97
3	The Regulation of NK Cell Function by CD2 Family Members	99
3.1	2B4 (CD244)	99
3.2	CD2	102
3.3	CD229	104
3.4	CS1	104
3.5	NTB-A	105
3.6	CD84-H1	107
3.7	CD48	107
3.8	CD58	108
3.9	CD2 Receptors with Unknown Functions on NK Cells	108
4	CD2 Family Receptors and Infection	109
5	Conclusions	109
	References	110

Abstract The CD2 family of receptors is evolutionarily conserved and widely expressed on cells within the hematopoietic compartment. In recent years several new members have been identified with important roles in the immune system. CD2 family members regulate natural killer (NK) cell lytic activity and inflammatory cytokine production when engaged by ligands on tumor cells. Furthermore, a subfamily of CD2 receptors, the CD150-like molecules, has been implicated in the pathogenesis of X-linked lymphoproliferative disease (XLP). Many of these receptors have now been shown to bind homophilically or heterophilically to other molecules within the family. With these discoveries a novel mechanism for lymphocyte regulation has emerged: CD2 family members on NK cells engage ligands on neighboring NK cells, leading to NK cell stimulation. Moreover, heterotypic stimulatory interactions between NK cells and other leukocytes also occur. In this manner, CD2 family members may provide interlymphocyte communication that maintains organization within the hematopoietic compartment and amplifies immune responses. This review discusses these multiple roles for CD2 family members, focusing specifically on the regulation of NK cells.

Abbreviations

BLAME	B lymphocyte activator macrophage expressed
EBV	Epstein-Barr virus
CD85-H1	CD84-homolog 1
CRACC	CD2-like receptor activating cytotoxic cells
CS1	CD2 subset 1
DC	Dendritic cell
EAT-2	Ewing sarcoma-activated transcript-2
GPI	Glycosylphosphatidylinositol
IFNγ	Interferon-γ
Ig	Immunoglobulin
ITAM	Immunoreceptor tyrosine-based activation motif
ITIM	Immunoreceptor tyrosine-based inhibitory motif
ITSM	Immunoreceptor tyrosine-based switch motif
NK cell	Natural killer cell
NTB-A	NK-T-B-antigen
SAP	Signaling lymphocyte activation molecule-associated molecule
SH2 domain	Src homology 2 domain
SHP-1	Src homology 2 domain-containing protein tyrosine phosphatase-1
SLAM	Signaling lymphocyte activation molecule
TNFα	Tumor necrosis factor-α
XLP	X-linked lymphoproliferative disease

1
CD2 Family Members

The CD2 family of receptors belongs to the immunoglobulin (Ig) superfamily. There are currently eleven members in this group: 2B4 (CD244), BLAME (B lymphocyte activator macrophage expressed), CD2 (lymphocyte function-associated antigen-2, LFA-2), CD48, CD58 (LFA-3), CD84, CD84-H1 (CD84-homolog 1, CD2 family member-10, CD2F-10, SF2001), CD150 (signaling lymphocyte activation molecule, SLAM, IPO-3), CD229 (Ly9), CS1 (CD2 subset 1, CD2-like receptor activating cytotoxic cells, CRACC, novel Ly9), and NTB-A (NK-T-B-antigen, SF2000, Ly108) (Table 1) (Durda et al. 1979; Bierer et al. 1989; Sidorenko and Clark 1993; de la Fuente et al. 1997; Peck and Ruley 2000; Boles and Mathew 2001; Boles et al. 2001; Bottino et al. 2001; Bouchon et al. 2001; Fennelly et al. 2001; Kingsbury et al. 2001; Zhang et al. 2001). In general, members of this family are type I transmembrane proteins, with a single extracellular N-terminal variable (V)-set Ig domain and a single constant (C)-2-set Ig domain with conserved patterns of disulfide bonds (Killeen et al. 1988). The exceptions are CD48 and an isoform of CD58, which are GPI linked, and CD229, which has an additional pair of V and C2 Ig domains

(Dustin et al. 1987; Staunton et al. 1989; Sandrin et al. 1992). Human CD2 and CD58 are located at chromosome 1p13, and the other nine genes are located closely together on chromosome 1q21–q24 (Boles et al. 2001). Murine CD2 family members are closely linked on chromosome 1 as well, with the exception of the CD2 gene on chromosome 3. The close homology and genetic linkage of the genes suggests that CD2 family members are derived from gene duplications of a founding gene (Wong et al. 1990). The parental receptor likely engaged in homophilic interactions, as all of the CD2 family members with known ligands bind in homophilic interactions, or heterophilic interactions with other receptors within the family. Six receptors, 2B4, CD150, CD84, CD229, NTB-A, and CS1, constitute the CD150 subfamily of the CD2 family of receptors. These six receptors all have two or more conserved tyrosine-based cytoplasmic motifs consisting of TxYxxV/I (in single-letter amino acid code, where x is any amino acid), also known as immunoreceptor tyrosine-based switch motifs (ITSMs) (Shlapatska et al. 2001) .

With the exception of CD48 and CD58, which can be expressed on some nonhematopoietic tissues (Smith and Thomas 1990; Boles et al. 2001), receptor expression is restricted to immune cells (Fig. 1). Interestingly, each receptor has a distinct profile of leukocyte distribution. To date, BLAME has the most restricted pattern of expression, limited to dendritic cells (DCs) and monocytes (Kingsbury et al. 2001); in contrast, CD48 is expressed on all nucleated hematopoietic cells (Boles et al. 2001). Eight of the eleven CD2 family receptors are expressed by NK cells. Unlike most other NK receptors, such as Ly49 or KIRs (killer cell immunoglobulin-like receptors) which are expressed on subsets of NK cells (Lanier 2005), the CD2 family of receptors have pan-NK cell expression. The exception to this is CD150, which is only found on a subset of NK cells after murine cytomegalovirus infection (Sayos et al. 2000).

The expression of many of these receptors is altered by cell activation, transformation, and infection (Thorley-Lawson et al. 1982; Fletcher et al. 1998; Sayos et al. 2000; Romero et al. 2004; Pende et al. 2005). Furthermore, isoforms for seven of the CD2 receptors have been identified that vary in the number of cytoplasmic tyrosines present, the type of transmembrane linkage, or whether the protein is expressed in soluble form (Dustin et al. 1987; Smith et al. 1997; Schatzle et al. 1999; Peck and Ruley 2000; de la Fuente et al. 2001; Wang et al. 2001; Lee et al. 2004a; Wandstrat et al. 2004). Thus there are numerous contexts for CD2 family receptor ligation, such as the cell type expressing the receptor, the receptor isoform expressed, and the state of activation of the receptor-bearing cell.

Table 1 CD2 family members and their functions on NK cells

	Other names	CD150 subfamily	Isoforms	Ligand	SAP/EAT-2 binding	Function on NK cells	References
BLAME				Unknown		Not known to be expressed on NK cells	Kingsbury et al. 2001
CD2	LFA-2, OX-34			hCD58, mCD48*		Activation and adhesion	Siliciano et al. 1985; Timonen et al. 1990; Davis et al. 1998
CD48			Soluble and GPI-linked forms	2B4, CD2		Activation, NK cell homotypic stimulation	Smith et al. 1997; Kubin et al. 1999; Assarsson et al. 2004
CD58	LFA-3		GPI-linked and transmembrane forms	hCD2		Unknown	Dustin et al. 1987
CD84-H1	CD2F-10, SF2001			Unknown		Unknown expression on NK cells	Fennelly et al. 2001; Zhang et al. 2001; Fraser et al. 2002
h2B4*	CD244	Yes		CD48	SAP and EAT-2?	SAP-dependent activation, inhibition in the absence of SAP	Valiante and Trinchieri 1993; Brown et al. 1998; Latchman et al. 1998; Benoit et al. 2000; Nakajima et al. 2000; Parolini et al. 2000; Tangye et al. 2000b; Sivori et al. 2002

Table 1 (continued)

	Other names	CD150 subfamily	Isoforms	Ligand	SAP/EAT-2 binding	Function on NK cells	References
m2B4-long		Yes	Four ITSMs	CD48	SAP and EAT-2	Inhibition in the presence or absence of SAP, NK homotypic stimulation	Garni-Wagner et al. 1993; Schatzle et al. 1999; Morra et al. 2001; Assarsson et al. 2004; Lee et al. 2004b; Mooney et al. 2004; Vaidya et al. 2005
m2B4-short		Yes	One ITSM	CD48		Activation or null	Schatzle et al. 1999; Stepp et al. 1999; Lee et al. 2004b
CD84		Yes		Self	SAP and EAT-2	Low or absent expression on NK cells, function on NK cells unknown, SAP independent signaling	de la Fuente et al. 1997; Martin et al. 2001; Tangye et al. 2002; Tangye et al. 2003; Romero et al. 2004
CD150	SLAM, IPO-3	Yes	Uncharacterized mRNA isoforms	Self	SAP and EAT-2	Induced on a subset of NK cells by MCMV, function on NK cells unknown	Sidorenko and Clark 1993; Mavaddat et al. 2000; Sayos et al. 2000; Morra et al. 2001; Wang et al. 2001

Table 1 (continued)

	Other names	CD150 subfamily	Isoforms	Ligand	SAP/EAT-2 binding	Function on NK cells	References
CD229	Ly9	Yes	Uncharacterized mRNA isoforms	Self	SAP and EAT-2	Unknown	Durda et al. 1979; de la Fuente et al. 2001; Morra et al. 2001; Sayos et al. 2001; Romero et al. 2004; Wandstrat et al. 2004; Romero et al. 2005
hCS1-long	CRACC, novel Ly9, 19A	Yes	Two ITSMs	Self	SAP	NK activation, NK homotypic stimulation, SAP independent signaling	Boles and Mathew 2001; Bouchon et al. 2001; Kumaresan et al. 2002; Tovar et al. 2002; Lee et al. 2004a
hCS1-short		Yes	No ITSMs	Self		Null	Lee et al. 2004a
NTB-A	Ly108, SF2000	Yes	mLy108-1 has two ITSM and Ly108-2 has three ITSM	Self	SAP and EAT-2	SAP-dependent activation, inhibition in the absence of SAP, NK homotypic stimulation	Peck and Ruley 2000; Bottino et al. 2001; Fraser et al. 2002; Falco et al. 2004; Flaig et al. 2004; Valdez et al. 2004

* h, human; m, mouse. Abbreviations: BLAME, B lymphocyte activator macrophage expressed; CD2F-10, CD2 family member 10; CD84-H1, CD84-homolog 1; CS1, CD2 subset 1; CRACC, CD2-like receptor activating cytotoxic cells; EAT-2, EWS-activated transcript-2; ITSM, immunoreceptor tyrosine-based switch motif; LFA-2; lymphocyte function-associated antigen 2; MCMV, murine cytomegalovirus; NTB-A, NK-T-B-antigen; SAP, signaling lymphocyte activation molecule-associated molecule; SLAM, signaling lymphocyte activation molecule

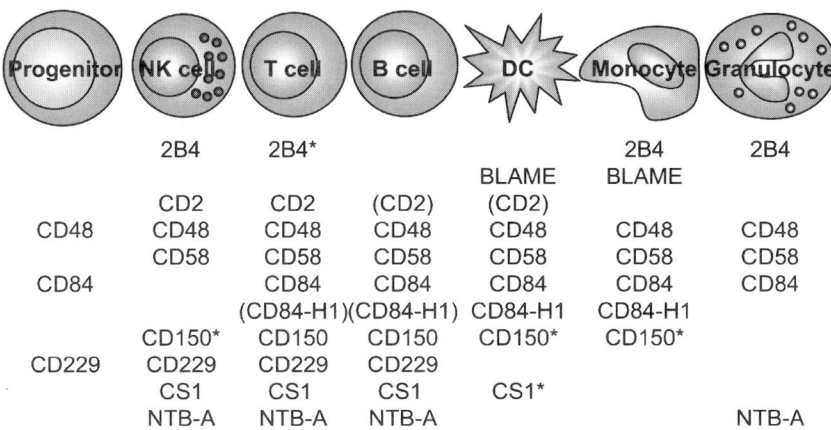

Fig. 1 CD2 family member expression on immune cells. CD2 family members have distinct distributions on hematopoietic cells. Some receptors, such as CD48 and CD58 (in humans) are widely expressed, whereas others, such as BLAME, have limited expression patterns. *CD150 on NK cells, 2B4 on CD8$^+$ T cells, CS1 and CD150 on DCs, and CD150 on monocytes are detected after cell activation. Receptors expressed on only subpopulations of cells are expressed in *parentheses*. *BLAME*, B lymphocyte activator macrophage expressed; *CD84-H1*, CD84-homolog 1; *CS1*, CD2 subset 1; *DC*, dendritic cell; *NTB-A*, NK-T-B-antigen; *SLAM*, signaling lymphocyte activation molecule

2
CD2 Receptor Family Signaling and X-Linked Lymphoproliferative Disease

Receptors in the CD2 family have diverse signaling pathways that are not completely understood. The CD150 subfamily members have cytoplasmic ITSMs, which suggests that they have a common signaling pathway. By contrast, non-CD150 subfamily members, CD2, CD48, CD58, CD84-H1, and BLAME, lack tyrosine-based cytoplasmic signaling motifs. CD48 and an isoform of CD58 have GPI linkages that may signal by association with lipid raft domains and lipid raft-associated kinases (Stefanova et al. 1991; Garnett et al. 1993; Solomon et al. 1996; Dykstra et al. 2003). CD84-H1, BLAME, and a transmembrane-containing form of CD58 have short cytoplasmic tails, which may indicate that these molecules act primarily as ligands for as yet undetermined receptors (Dustin et al. 1987; Fennelly et al. 2001; Kingsbury et al. 2001).

The ITSM-containing receptors 2B4, CD150, CD84, CD229, NTB-A, and CS1 have several common signaling characteristics. Cytoplasmic ITSM tyrosines are phosphorylated on ligation, leading to recruitment of SLAM-associated protein (SAP, SH2D1A) and (Ewing sarcoma-activated transcript-

2 (EAT-2), with the exception of CD150 and CS1, for which SAP binding is phosphorylation independent (Sayos et al. 1998, 2001; Tangye et al. 1999, 2002; Parolini et al. 2000; Bottino et al. 2001; Morra et al. 2001; Fraser et al. 2002; Lee et al. 2004a). CS1 binding to SAP remains controversial, and CS1 binding of EAT-2 is not detected (Bouchon et al. 2001; Tovar et al. 2002; Lee et al. 2004a). ITSMs bind a number of signaling molecules that historically are known to associate with immunoreceptor tyrosine-based inhibitory motifs (ITIMs) and immunoreceptor tyrosine-based activating motifs (ITAMs), including activating kinases and inhibitory phosphatases. Among the tyrosine-based motifs, ITSMs are unique for their recognition by SAP and EAT-2, and it is this association that has drawn the most attention to the CD150 subfamily. This is because of the finding that mutations in SAP are associated with X-linked lymphoproliferative disease (XLP) (Coffey et al. 1998; Nichols et al. 1998; Sayos et al. 1998) and because SAP/EAT-2 adaptors dictate unique function-switching capabilities by ITSM-bearing receptors.

XLP patients have complicated clinical features, often triggered by Epstein-Barr virus (EBV) infection (Purtilo et al. 1975). The disease most frequently manifests as fulminant infectious mononucleosis, and less commonly as B cell lymphoma and dysgammaglobulinemia (Purtilo et al. 1975). The SAP gene is mutated in these patients, affecting the functions of T cells, NK cells, and some B cells, which express SAP (Coffey et al. 1998; Nichols et al. 1998; Sayos et al. 1998; Nichols et al. 2005). SAP mutations prevent the development of NK T cells in humans and mice (Chung et al. 2005; Nichols et al. 2005; Pasquier et al. 2005). Abnormal NK cell function in XLP patients is not global but limited to the activity of SAP-binding NK receptors. SAP is thought to act as an adaptor, mediating activating signals by recruiting and activating Fyn kinase (Chan et al. 2003; Latour et al. 2003). Fyn kinase induces further phosphorylation of the ITSM-bearing receptors, leading to recruitment of other activating molecules to the receptors.

The absence of functional SAP leads to alternate signaling pathways depending on the receptor. For SLAM and 2B4, it has been argued that, in the absence of SAP, there is no receptor signaling (Benoit et al. 2000; Tangye et al. 2000b; Latour et al. 2001). In other cases, the absence of SAP leads to inhibitory outcomes, for example, NTB-A and other studies on 2B4 (Nakajima et al. 2000; Parolini et al. 2000; Bottino et al. 2001). However, SAP-independent activating signals also exist—CS1 and CD84 are activating even in NK cells and T cells of XLP patients, respectively (Bouchon et al. 2001; Tangye et al. 2003).

EAT-2 has an SH2 domain, and it is structurally similar to SAP (Morra et al. 2001). At least at the transcriptional level, it is expressed in B cells, macrophages, DCs, activated T cells, and NK cells as well as some non-hematopoietic cells (Thompson et al. 1996; Morra et al. 2001; Tangye et al.

2003; Lee et al. 2004b). EAT-2 protein is reported in murine primary NK cells (Chen et al. 2004). Unlike SAP, which binds to the SH3 domain of Fyn, EAT-2 likely does not bind Fyn (Latour et al. 2003); thus EAT-2 may function by blocking other molecules from binding to the receptor or by recruiting unknown signaling molecules. SAP and EAT-2 bind to the same receptors and are both present in NK cells, but it remains unknown what the relative importance of each of these molecules is. Although much progress has been made, SAP-dependent and -independent ITSM signaling pathways are still being defined.

3
The Regulation of NK Cell Function by CD2 Family Members
3.1
2B4 (CD244)

Of the receptors discussed in this review, 2B4 (CD244) is the best characterized with respect to NK cell function. It is expressed on NK cells, $CD8^+$ activated T cells, γδ T cells, monocytes, basophils, eosinophils, and mast cells (Boles et al. 2001; Kubota 2002; Munitz et al. 2005). In mice, 2B4 has two isoforms generated by alternative splicing. 2B4-long has four ITSMs, and 2B4-short has one ITSM; human 2B4 is only found as the long form (Boles et al. 1999; Stepp et al. 1999). CD48, the ligand for 2B4, is expressed on all nucleated hematopoietic cells and on human endothelium (Brown et al. 1998; Latchman et al. 1998). CD48 is GPI linked, and is also the ligand for CD2. However, 2B4 binds CD48 with higher affinity than does CD2 (Brown et al. 1998).

Early studies on 2B4 function evaluated the effects of anti-2B4 antibodies on the cytolytic activity of mouse NK cells (Garni-Wagner et al. 1993). In these experiments, addition of anti-2B4 antibodies enhanced the lysis of a variety of target cells. Along with the finding that plate-bound anti-2B4 triggered the release of granules and IFNγ, these studies suggested that 2B4 activates NK cells. Further studies on human NK cells corroborated these findings and in addition revealed that 2B4 does not act as a primary cytotoxicity receptor, but as a coreceptor that depends on collaboration with other triggering receptors for human NK activation (Valiante and Trinchieri 1993; Sivori et al. 2000). Human 2B4 relies on SAP for activating signals—in the absence of functional SAP, as occurs in XLP NK cells, 2B4 either fails to signal (Benoit et al. 2000; Tangye et al. 2000b) or mediates inhibitory signaling (Nakajima et al. 2000; Parolini et al. 2000).

The inhibitory role for mouse 2B4 first came to light through the use of RNK-16 rat leukemia cells transfected with the two murine 2B4 isoforms. It was found that 2B4-short activates NK cells whereas 2B4-long inhibits NK cells (Schatzle et al. 1999). This finding was perplexing, particularly because human NK cells are activated by 2B4 but only express the homologous long isoform. After this report appeared, human 2B4 was demonstrated to be inhibitory in XLP patients (Nakajima et al. 2000; Parolini et al. 2000) and in immature human NK cells that have not yet acquired SAP (Sivori et al. 2002). However, the inhibitory role of 2B4 in XLP patients could not be confirmed by other studies (Tangye et al. 2000b). The clearest evidence for the dominant inhibitory function of 2B4 was revealed by experiments in 2B4-deficient mice (Lee et al. 2004b; Mooney et al. 2004; Vaidya et al. 2005). These studies have shown that 2B4-deficient NK cells exhibit higher killing of $CD48^+$ tumor cells both in vitro and in vivo. NK cell IFNγ production is inhibited by coculture with CD48-expressing target cells. Furthermore, 2B4-deficient NK cells have higher killing of nontransformed $CD48^+$ allogeneic and syngeneic cells (Lee et al. 2004b; McNerney et al. 2005). In confirmation of previous studies (Schatzle et al. 1999), transducing 2B4-deficient primary NK cells with the 2B4-long isoform restored inhibition in response to CD48. By contrast, the 2B4-short isoform did not restore inhibition or cause activation (Lee et al. 2004b). It has recently been found that primary murine NK cells preferentially express 2B4-long transcripts as compared to 2B4-short transcripts, confirming the dominant role of 2B4-long in murine NK cells (Mooney et al. 2004).

Studies with 2B4 in mice have indicated that NK cells can be inhibited both by MHC-binding as well as MHC-independent receptors. 2B4-mediated inhibition of NK cells is nonredundant with Ly49-MHC class I-directed inhibition. Furthermore, in class I-deficient mice as well as Ly49 nonexpressing mouse NK cells, self-tolerance is maintained largely by 2B4-CD48 interactions (McNerney et al. 2005). Thus emerging evidence (reviewed in Kumar and McNerney 2005) suggests two layers of NK cell self-tolerance, executed by MHC-dependent as well as MHC-independent receptors.

It is unclear why 2B4 is activating is some circumstances and inhibitory in others. One possible explanation is that the nature of the experiments themselves is different. Cross-linking with antibody may give ambiguous results as anti-2B4 may act as an agonist or antagonist. In the initial experiments with murine NK cells, not only whole anti-2B4 antibody but also anti-2B4 Fab fragments were found to augment murine NK cell cytotoxicity against $CD48^+$ target cells (Garni-Wagner et al. 1993). This indicates that 2B4 cross-linking was not necessary for enhanced NK cell killing; instead, anti-2B4 may have been acting as an antagonist, blocking 2B4 ligation and thereby permitting activation. We believe that the use of 2B4-deficient mice and CD48-expressing or -nonexpressing targets circumvents these types of variables. Most of the studies on human 2B4 have relied on antibody cross-linking. In fact, there are few examples of 2B4-dependent activation of primary human NK cells by CD48-expressing targets (Tangye et al. 2000a,b). Another difference in the human and mouse studies is that human experiments use peripheral NK cells in vitro, whereas in mice splenic NK cells are utilized. Additionally, studies in mice have the advantage of studying NK cell function in vivo.

An alternative, and not mutually exclusive, explanation for how 2B4 is activating in some cases and inhibitory in others may be the differential influence of SAP. Unlike in humans, 2B4 inhibitory signaling in mice occurs independently of SAP expression (Lee et al. 2004b; Mooney et al. 2004). It is conceivable that human 2B4 and SAP interaction evolved in response to pathogen pressure, converting 2B4 into an activating receptor in humans. A pathogen, such as EBV, that infects the majority of humans and upregulates CD48 (Thorley-Lawson et al. 1982) could elicit such adaptation by 2B4.

Whereas 2B4 engagement by CD48 on a target cell inhibits murine NK cells, 2B4-CD48 engagement among murine NK cells themselves promotes NK cell functions. The first evidence of this was from the report in which anti-CD48 treatment of splenic cell cultures with IL-2 inhibited the generation of NK cell activity (Chavin et al. 1994). A subsequent study demonstrated that NK cell proliferation is compromised by anti-2B4 or anti-CD48 treatment (Assarsson et al. 2004). To study the role of 2B4-CD48 interactions among NK cells, we have used CD48-negative targets, thus circumventing the dominant inhibitory signals that arise when 2B4-positive NK cells engage CD48-positive tumor cells. In these experiments, 2B4-deficient NK cells, or wild-type NK cells treated with anti-2B4 or anti-CD48, reveal significant proliferative, cytotoxic, and IFNγ production defects in vitro and in vivo (Lee et al. 2005).

A role for 2B4-CD48 in murine T cell-T cell stimulation has also been elucidated. 2B4-expressing CD8$^+$ T cells have higher lysis of tumor cells (Lee et al. 2003) and proliferation (Kambayashi et al. 2001) because of interaction with CD48 on neighboring T cells. Furthermore, NK cells can stimulate T cells via 2B4-CD48 interaction (Assarsson et al. 2004). Ljunggren and colleagues have proposed that 2B4 is not the signaling receptor for activation in these homotypic interactions; instead, it acts as a ligand for CD48 (Kambayashi et al. 2001; Assarsson et al. 2004). This is probable, as CD48 is known to stimulate T cells and to associate with signaling molecules (Stefanova et al. 1991; Garnett et al. 1993; Moran and Miceli 1998).

2B4 signaling is initiated, on ligation, by phosphorylation of 2B4 cytoplasmic tyrosines. This initial phosphorylation can be mediated by Fyn and Lck Src family kinases (Nakajima et al. 2000; Sayos et al. 2000). SH2 domain-containing proteins SAP, EAT-2, SHP-1 (SH2 domain-containing protein tyrosine phosphatase-1), and SHP-2 have all been shown to subsequently associate with 2B4, and it is at this stage where the activating and inhibitory pathways diverge (Schatzle et al. 1999; Tangye et al. 1999; Parolini et al. 2000; Morra et al. 2001). Downstream activating signals rely in part on 2B4 association with LAT (linker for activation of T cells), as well as SAP recruitment of Fyn (Bottino et al. 2000; Latour et al. 2001; Klem et al. 2002). Fyn further phosphorylates 2B4 tyrosines (Chen et al. 2004), which recruit additional positive signaling molecules leading to Vav, phospholipase Cγ (PLCγ), PI3K, and MAP kinase activation (Watzl et al. 2000; Chuang et al. 2001; Aoukaty and Tan 2002). In the inhibitory pathway, in addition to SHP-1 and SHP-2, 2B4 has recently been shown to bind c-Src tyrosine kinase (Csk) and to mitigate c-cbl and SH2 domain-containing inositol-5-phosphatase (SHIP) phosphorylation (Chen et al. 2004; Eissmann et al. 2005). The functional requirement for each of these molecules in 2B4 inhibition remains undetermined. Despite significant progress, a number of studies have shown conflicting results concerning the inhibitory and activating pathways of murine and human 2B4, and many questions remain. However, the following seem to be established: in mice: (a) When NK cells engage CD48-expressing target cells, 2B4 inhibits NK cell function; (b) when NK cells engage other NK cells during IL-2 or polyI:C-induced activation, 2B4-CD48 interactions promote NK cytotoxicity; (c) 2B4-CD48 interactions among CD8$^+$ T cells increase cytolytic activity in an MHC-TCR-dependent fashion; and (d) CD48 expressed on T cells and NK cells can enhance proliferation when ligated by 2B4 on other NK or T cells.

3.2
CD2

CD2 (LFA-2) is the founding member of the CD2 family. It is primarily expressed on NK cells and T cells, and in humans it is also found on a subset of monocyte-derived dendritic cells, thymic B cells, and some B cell neoplasms (Bierer et al. 1989; Punnonen and de Vries 1993; Crawford et al. 1999; Kingma et al. 2002). In mice, CD2 is found on the majority of B cells (Yagita et al. 1989). CD2 binds CD58 in humans; mice do not have a CD58 homolog (Davis et al. 1998). In mice CD2 binds CD48; in humans the affinity of CD2 for human CD48 is considered unphysiologically low (Davis et al. 1998). The CD2 cytoplasmic domain does not have tyrosine-based motifs but is large and rich in prolines and basic residues (Bierer et al. 1989), which are important for signaling. CD2 ligation recruits the Src family kinases Src, Fyn, and Lck, as well as PI3K (Bell et al. 1992; Collins et al. 1994; Shimizu et al. 1995). The binding of CD2 with Lck has been mapped to the proline-rich regions in CD2, which are recognized by the SH3 domain of Lck, and leads to Lck activation (Collins et al. 1994; Bell et al. 1996). CD2 signaling also depends on CD3ζ and LAT signaling (Vivier et al. 1991; Moingeon et al. 1992; Martelli et al. 2000).

More distal signaling events involve PLCγ, inositol trisphosphate production, and Tec family kinase IL-2-inducible T-cell kinase (ITK) activity (Seaman et al. 1987; Collins et al. 1994; King et al. 1996). In T cells, CD2 binds the adaptor molecule CD2-associated protein (CD2AP) and other CD2AP family members (Dustin et al. 1998; Nishizawa et al. 1998). CD2AP family members have GYF and SH3 domains, which bind proline-rich regions of CD2 and contribute to CD2-dependent T cell receptor clustering and polarization (Dustin et al. 1998; Nishizawa et al. 1998; Dikic 2002; Tibaldi and Reinherz 2003). It will be interesting to determine how CD2 signaling in NK cells may be guided by these adaptor molecules.

Early studies demonstrated that CD2 cross-linking on human NK cells activated NK lytic activity against tumor cells and nontransformed allogeneic cells (Siliciano et al. 1985; Schmidt et al. 1987). In some studies, anti-CD2 plus a secondary cross-linking antibody or FcR^+ targets were necessary for anti-CD2-mediated activation (Bolhuis et al. 1986; van de Griend et al. 1987), whereas other studies found that anti-CD2 $(Fab')_2$ alone caused activation (Schmidt et al. 1988). In other reports, anti-CD2 blocked NK activation against certain tumors (Bolhuis et al. 1986; Seaman et al. 1987; van de Griend et al. 1987). Murine NK cells are less reliant on CD2 for killing of targets, as CD2 blocking leads to a small decrease in target killing (Nakamura et al. 1990). The most definitive demonstration for the function of CD2 on human NK cells was the use of targets that express, or do not express, the ligand, CD58 (Lanier et al. 1997). Transfection of CD58 into targets activates human NK cells, and this lysis is blocked with anti-CD2 plus anti-CD58 $F(ab')_2$ fragments (Lanier et al. 1997).

Contrary to expectations, NK and T cell function is essentially normal in CD2-deficient mice (Killeen et al. 1992; Lanier 1998). More sensitive assays have revealed defects in CD2-deficient T cells (Teh et al. 1997), suggesting that there may also be a subtle NK defect in CD2-deficient mice that has yet to be uncovered. Alternatively, in the absence of CD2, there may be compensation specifically by other CD2-like receptors, such as 2B4. In contrast to CD2-deficient mice, T and NK cells from CD48-deficient mice are more overtly impaired (Gonzalez-Cabrero et al. 1999; Lee et al. 2005), supporting the hypothesis that CD48-binding receptors may have partial redundancy, but the ligand, CD48, does not.

CD2 influences not only lytic events, but other processes as well. For instance, CD2 promotes T cell conjugation with antigen-presenting cells (Springer et al. 1987), and T cell cytokine mRNA stability is increased by CD2-CD48 interaction (Musgrave et al. 2003, 2004). Likewise, CD2 is important in NK-target adhesion (Timonen et al. 1990; Voltarelli et al. 1993; Barber and Long 2003), and because NK cells are activated by antigen-presenting cells (Degli-Esposti and Smyth 2005), CD2 engagement may also enhance these interactions. The importance of DC-NK interaction is becoming better understood; however, the molecules involved in DC-NK cell interactions are still being characterized (Degli-Esposti and Smyth 2005). It seems likely that CD2 family members will prove to be important in NK-DC cross talk.

3.3
CD229

CD229 (Ly9) is found on B- and T lymphocytes, and at low levels on 40% of human NK cells (Durda et al. 1979; Hogarth et al. 1980; Mathieson et al. 1980; de la Fuente et al. 2001; Romero et al. 2004). This molecule has two ITSMs and an additional ITSM-like sequence (AxYxxV) and is unique in the CD2 family, as it has four Ig domains instead of two (Sandrin et al. 1992; Tovar et al. 2000; de la Fuente et al. 2001). CD229 has two alleles in mice; Ly-9.1 is found in most strains, and Ly9.2 is only in C57BL/6 strains (Hogarth et al. 1980; Kozak et al. 1984; Tovar et al. 2000). Human and mouse CD229 mRNA both have uncharacterized splice variants (de la Fuente et al. 2001; Wandstrat et al. 2004).

On phosphorylation of one or both ITSMs, CD229 binds SHIP, SAP, and EAT-2 (Morra et al. 2001; Sayos et al. 2001; Li et al. 2003). SAP and EAT-2 recruitment prevent SHP-2 binding to CD229, and SAP further acts by recruiting Fyn, thus enhancing CD229 phosphorylation (Morra et al. 2001; Simarro et al. 2004). It has recently been determined that CD229 engages in homophilic interactions (Romero et al. 2005). CD229 attenuates T cell receptor signaling (Martin et al. 2005), but its function on NK cells is undetermined.

3.4
CS1

NK cells, T cells, B cells, and mature dendritic cells express CS1 (CD2 subset 1, CD2-like receptor activating cytotoxic cells, CRACC, novel Ly9) (Boles and Mathew 2001; Bouchon et al. 2001). Human CS1 has two splice isoforms: CS1-long has two ITSMs and an ITSM-like sequence (FVYxxV), and CS1-short lacks ITSMs (Boles and Mathew 2001; Lee et al. 2004a). Human NK cells express both transcripts, and expression levels do not change on stimulation (Lee et al. 2004a). Murine CS1 also has two isoforms: CS1-long has one consensus ITSM sequence and an ITSM-like sequence (ADYxxI) and murine CS1-short has only the ITSM motif (Tovar et al. 2002).

CS1 has been shown to engage in stimulatory homophilic interactions as a self-ligand (Bouchon et al. 2001; Kumaresan et al. 2002). Activation is due to the long isoform of CS1, as the short isoform does not effect NK cytotoxicity or calcium mobilization (Lee et al. 2004a). Because it contains ITSMs, CS1 is likely to interact with SAP. However, human NK cell cytotoxicity is activated by CS1 even in XLP NK cells; thus CS1 signaling is SAP independent (Bouchon et al. 2001). Whether CS1 binds SAP is controversial; Colonna and colleagues found that human CS1 does not associate with SAP or EAT-2 (Bouchon et al. 2001). However Mathew and colleagues noted that human CS1-long binds SAP, but this association occurs only in the absence of pervanadate, suggesting that CS1-SAP interaction occurs in the absence of phosphorylation (Lee et al. 2004a). On the other hand, Engel and colleagues demonstrated that although murine CS1 does not bind SAP, human CS1 does binds SAP but only in the presence of Fyn, suggesting that SAP association is dependent on CS1 phosphorylation (Tovar et al. 2002). CS1 does not interact with LAT, so how CS1 mediates SAP-independent activating signals remains to be determined (Bouchon et al. 2001). CS1 also does not associate with SHP-1, SHP-2, or SHIP (Bouchon et al. 2001; Lee et al. 2004a).

Interestingly, RNK-16 cells transfected with human CS1-long have increased basal cytotoxicity in the absence of CS1 cross-linking with antibody, whereas RNK-16 cells transfected with CS1-short do not (Lee et al. 2004a). As CS1 is a self-ligand, this phenomenon may be the product of NK-NK cell homophilic interaction. Possibly stimulation also occurs in heterotypic interactions, such as those between DCs and NK cells. It will important to determine what isoforms of CS1 other cell types express, and whether interlymphocyte CS1 engagement leads to bidirectional activation.

3.5
NTB-A

NTB-A (NK-T-B-antigen, SF2000, Ly108) is an activating receptor expressed on mouse and human T and B lymphocytes, human NK cells, and human eosinophils (Peck and Ruley 2000; Bottino et al. 2001; Munitz et al. 2005). It was first identified as Ly108 in mice, and in this study, Ly108 transcripts were not detected in murine NK cells (Peck and Ruley 2000). Murine Ly108 has two splice forms: Ly108-1 has two ITSMs and Ly108-2 has an additional ITSM-like sequence (TxYxxP) (Peck and Ruley 2000; Wandstrat et al. 2004). C57BL/6 mice preferentially express Ly108-2 transcripts (Wandstrat et al. 2004). In humans, NTB-A has two ITSMs and one ITIM (Bottino et al. 2001; Fraser et al. 2002).

The ligand for NTB-A has recently been determined to be NTB-A itself (Falco et al. 2004; Flaig et al. 2004; Valdez et al. 2004). NTB-A-expressing target cells are more susceptible to NK cell killing, and soluble NTB-A or anti-NTB-A blocks this susceptibility (Falco et al. 2004; Flaig et al. 2004). Antibody cross-linking of NTB-A activates NK cell lytic activity in redirected lysis assays (Bottino et al. 2001). However, NTB-A cross-linking is not sufficient for NK cell activation, indicating that NTB-A may act as a coreceptor, rather than a principal activating receptor. Indeed, NK cell lysis of EBV-infected B cells was mediated cooperatively by NTB-A, 2B4, and NKp46 (Bottino et al. 2001). Interestingly, NTB-A expression is often downregulated on leukemic cells as compared to nontransformed counterparts, suggesting immune selection for NTB-A-low tumor variants (Pende et al. 2005).

NTB-A also regulates NK cell proliferation (Flaig et al. 2004). Soluble, antagonistic NTB-A isoleucine fusion protein inhibited NK cell proliferation in the presence and absence of IL-2, suggesting a role for NTB-A in NK-NK cell homophilic interactions (Flaig et al. 2004). However, NTB-A-expressing fibroblasts inhibited NK cell proliferation, suggesting that NTB-A ligation on NK cells by NTB-A on targets may have a different outcome than when NTB-A is ligated among NK cells themselves. Thus, as with 2B4-CD48 interactions, NTB-A signaling may be context dependent (Flaig et al. 2004).

NTB-A basally binds SHP-1 and binds SAP, EAT-2, and SAP on phosphorylation (Bottino et al. 2001; Fraser et al. 2002). SAP is required for activation, as NTB-A is inhibitory in NK cells from XLP patients; NK cells from XLP patients exhibited low levels of killing against EBV-infected B cells, but killing is restored by blocking NTB-A engagement with antibody (Bottino et al. 2001). Unlike NK cells from healthy donors, NK cells from XLP patients do not produce IFNγ or TNFα on NTB-A engagement (Falco et al. 2004). NTB-A is also inhibitory on developing immature human NK cells, which lack SAP protein (Sivori et al. 2002). Thus, like 2B4, early expression of NTB-A may prevent NK cell autoreactivity until MHC-binding NK cell inhibitory receptors are acquired.

On T cells, NTB-A has been thought to be a Th1 promoting receptor. In vitro, NTB-A cross-linking costimulates T cell Th1 IFNγ production, but not IL-4 production (Valdez et al. 2004). In vivo, NTB-A-Fc fusion protein inhibits B cell isotype switching to IgG2a and IgG3, and delays the onset of experimental autoimmune encephalomyelitis, a Th1-mediated disease (Valdez et al. 2004). Recent analysis of NTB-A/Ly108 deficient mice, however, indicates that Ly108 is required for Th2 cytokine production and immune responses, and not Th1 cytokine production (Howie et al. 2005).

In another autoimmune model, systemic lupus erythematosus, a locus associated with the disease in mice has been identified as the CD150 cluster of genes (Wandstrat et al. 2004). Polymorphisms of several CD150 family members and expression level differences have been identified, which may potentially contribute to the lupus phenotype. The strongest single-gene candidate for susceptibility was identified as *Ly108/NTB-A*. Lupus-prone mice preferentially express the Ly108-1 isoform, leading to a fivefold difference in Ly108-1 to Ly108-2 transcript ratio as compared to wild-type mice. It will be interesting to determine how Ly108 splice variations specifically differ in their signaling pathways. Before the onset of lupus, $CD4^+$ T cells in lupus-prone mice demonstrate higher Ca^{2+} flux in response to stimulation as compared to wild-type mice, but the specific role for Ly108 or other CD150 family members on lymphocytes in lupus-prone mice has not been analyzed (Wandstrat et al. 2004).

3.6
CD84-H1

CD84-H1 (CD84-homolog 1) is also known as CD2F-10 (CD2 family member 10) and SF2001 (Fennelly et al. 2001; Zhang et al. 2001; Fraser et al. 2002). The human and mouse cytoplasmic tails are short and basic, and they lack known signaling motifs (Fennelly et al. 2001). Human CD84-H1 mRNA has been found in monocytes, T cells, B cells, and DCs by one group (Zhang et al. 2001), whereas another group identified human CD84-H1 mRNA in macrophages but not other lymphocytes, including NK cells (Fennelly et al. 2001). Antibodies to CD84-H1 will aid in identifying CD84-H1 protein expression and function, as well as the putative ligand.

3.7
CD48

CD48 is a GPI-linked member of the CD2 family (Staunton et al. 1989). In mice, it is the low-affinity ligand for CD2 and the high-affinity ligand for 2B4; it is expressed on all nucleated hematopoietic cells in mice and humans and on human endothelium (Boles et al. 2001). Recent data suggest that 2B4-expressing cells, including NK cells or 2B4-transfected tumors, provide activating signals by ligating CD48 on T cells and other NK cells (Assarsson et al. 2004). CD48 signals by associating with Fyn and Lck kinases and GTP-binding proteins (Stefanova et al. 1991; Garnett et al. 1993; Solomon et al. 1996). Indeed, CD2 on antigen-presenting cells engages CD48 on T cells, promoting T cell activation (Moran and Miceli 1998); thus it seems likely that CD48 may similarly enhance NK cell function when ligated. Furthermore, 2B4-fusion protein stimulates B cell proliferation and DC cytokine production (Kubin et al. 1999); thus emerging data indicate that 2B4-CD48 interaction provides bidirectional stimulatory signals among cytotoxic cells themselves and between cytotoxic and antigen-presenting cells.

3.8
CD58

CD58 (LFA-3) binds CD2 in humans and is found on all nucleated hematopoietic cells, red blood cells, and some nonhematopoietic tissues including endothelial cells and fibroblasts (Smith and Thomas 1990). Mice do not appear to have a CD58 homolog. CD58 has a GPI-linked form as well as an isoform with a transmembrane domain (Dustin et al. 1987). To our knowledge, CD58 is not known to directly signal on NK cells, but with a GPI linkage and raft association (Dykstra et al. 2003) the possibility exists. Interestingly, CD58 on T cells ligates CD2 on DCs, leading to DC maturation, which in turn increases T cell activation (Crawford et al. 2003). A parallel interaction between NK cells and DCs is also possible.

3.9
CD2 Receptors with Unknown Functions on NK Cells

B lymphocyte activator macrophage expressed (BLAME) has a short cytoplasmic tail with no known signaling motifs (Kingsbury et al. 2001). It is conserved in humans and mice and expressed on DCs and monocytes. BLAME expression on NK cells is unknown, and the ligand remains undetermined.

CD84 engages in homophilic interactions (Martin et al. 2001) and is expressed on B cells, T cells, DCs, monocytes, platelets, and granulocytes (Krause et al. 2000; Zaiss et al. 2003; Romero et al. 2004). CD84 expression is either very low or absent on resting human NK cells (Tangye et al. 2002; Romero et al. 2004). It has two ITSMs (de la Fuente et al. 1997) and binds SAP and EAT-2 (Tangye et al. 2002) but can signal independently of SAP (Tangye et al. 2003).

Signaling lymphocyte activation molecule (SLAM, CD150, IPO-3) is expressed on activated T cells, activated macrophages, B cells, and DCs (Sidorenko and Clark 1993; Cocks et al. 1995; Kruse et al. 2001; Romero et al. 2004). SLAM engages in homophilic interactions (Mavaddat et al. 2000). As evidenced by the study of SLAM-deficient mice, SLAM appears to promote Th2, and not Th1, immune responses (Wang et al. 2004). SLAM is not expressed on resting human NK cells (Romero et al. 2004) or resting murine NK cells (Sayos et al. 2000) but is induced on 15% of murine NK cells in response to murine cytomegalovirus infection in vivo (Sayos et al. 2000). How SLAM may regulate NK cells is unknown.

4
CD2 Family Receptors and Infection

Why are there so many CD2-like receptors? One possible explanation is that innate immune receptors must maintain diversity in response to changing pathogen pressures without somatic gene rearrangement. The CD2 family of receptors is involved in the immune response to a number of infections, giving credence to this hypothesis. The most direct example is the CD150 receptor, which is utilized by the measles virus for cellular entry (Tatsuo et al. 2000). Thus the multiple receptors in the CD2 family, and their variations, may be a product of pathogen pressure.

The *molluscum contagiosum* virus genome encodes a CD150 homolog (Senkevich et al. 1997). One possible function of this protein may be to compete with host CD150 for ligand binding and thereby block antiviral responses (Sidorenko and Clark 2003). Similarly, a CD2 homolog is encoded by African Swine Fever virus, and deletion of this gene decreases the severity of the infection (Borca et al. 1998). The mechanism of action of the protein is unknown, but data from in vitro experiments suggest that it is immunosuppressive.

Patients with XLP are susceptible to fulminant EBV infections (Purtilo et al. 1975). Similarly, mice deficient in SAP are more susceptible to lymphocyte choriomeningitis virus and murine gammaherpesvirus-68 infections (Czar et al. 2001; Wu et al. 2001; Yin et al. 2003). In these cases, all of the receptors that signal through SAP are candidates for contributing to immunodeficiency and susceptibility to infection. 2B4 and NTB-A in particular may play an important role in humans, as these receptors are critical in NK cell killing of EBV-infected B cells (Bottino et al. 2001).

Cytomegalovirus has evolved numerous mechanisms to evade NK cells (Lodoen and Lanier 2005). It has been reported that downregulation of CD58 on fibroblasts results from CMV infection and that this decreases NK cell lysis of the infected targets (Fletcher et al. 1998). As EBV modulates CD48 expression (Thorley-Lawson et al. 1982), it is possible that influencing CD2 family immune receptors is common among herpes viruses. Because there is a strong association between CD2-like receptors and infection, responding to pathogens may be a principal role for these receptors.

5
Conclusions

NK cell inhibition, activation, costimulation, and adhesion are all regulated by CD2 family members. Significant advances have been made in identifying new receptors and their ligands, and how these receptor-ligand pairs regulate antitumor and antiviral responses of NK cells. At least one human disease, XLP, is causally related to defective signaling via members of the CD2 family of molecules. In addition, polymorphisms in CD2 family members may also contribute to autoimmunity in lupus-prone mice. A feature that seems characteristic of this family of molecules is stimulatory homotypic interactions between NK cells: 2B4, CD48, CS1, and NTB-A are all involved in such interactions. Furthermore, analysis of ITSM and SAP signaling has yielded the description of a novel signaling pathway that impacts not only NK cells but also numerous other cell types that express ITSM-bearing receptors. Gene-deficient mouse models have been particularly informative for the CD2 family and have sometimes given surprising results, possibly due to the complexity and multitude of functions these receptors have (Killeen et al. 1992; Gonzalez-Cabrero et al. 1999; Lee et al. 2004b; Wang et al. 2004; Howie et al. 2005). Generation of mice deficient for newly identified receptors and testing their responses to infection in vivo will yield further valuable insights.

References

Aoukaty A, Tan R (2002) Association of the X-linked lymphoproliferative disease gene product SAP/SH2D1A with 2B4, a natural killer cell-activating molecule, is dependent on phosphoinositide 3-kinase. J Biol Chem 277:13331–13337

Assarsson E, Kambayashi T, Schatzle JD, Cramer SO, von Bonin A, Jensen PE, Ljunggren HG, Chambers BJ (2004) NK cells stimulate proliferation of T and NK cells through 2B4/CD48 interactions. J Immunol 173:174–180

Barber DF, Long EO (2003) Coexpression of CD58 or CD48 with intercellular adhesion molecule 1 on target cells enhances adhesion of resting NK cells. J Immunol 170:294–299

Bell GM, Bolen JB, Imboden JB (1992) Association of Src-like protein tyrosine kinases with the CD2 cell surface molecule in rat T lymphocytes and natural killer cells. Mol Cell Biol 12:5548–5554

Bell GM, Fargnoli J, Bolen JB, Kish L, Imboden JB (1996) The SH3 domain of p56lck binds to proline-rich sequences in the cytoplasmic domain of CD2. J Exp Med 183:169–178

Benoit L, Wang X, Pabst HF, Dutz J, Tan R (2000) Defective NK cell activation in X-linked lymphoproliferative disease. J Immunol 165:3549–3553

Bierer BE, Sleckman BP, Ratnofsky SE, Burakoff SJ (1989) The biologic roles of CD2, CD4, and CD8 in T-cell activation. Annu Rev Immunol 7:579–599

Boles KS, Mathew PA (2001) Molecular cloning of CS1, a novel human natural killer cell receptor belonging to the CD2 subset of the immunoglobulin superfamily. Immunogenetics 52:302–307

Boles KS, Nakajima H, Colonna M, Chuang SS, Stepp SE, Bennett M, Kumar V, Mathew PA (1999) Molecular characterization of a novel human natural killer cell receptor homologous to mouse 2B4. Tissue Antigens 54:27–34

Boles KS, Stepp SE, Bennett M, Kumar V, Mathew PA (2001) 2B4 (CD244) and CS1: novel members of the CD2 subset of the immunoglobulin superfamily molecules expressed on natural killer cells and other leukocytes. Immunol Rev 181:234–249

Bolhuis RL, Roozemond RC, van de Griend RJ (1986) Induction and blocking of cytolysis in CD2+, CD3- NK and CD2+, CD3+ cytotoxic T lymphocytes via CD2 50 KD sheep erythrocyte receptor. J Immunol 136:3939–3944

Borca MV, Carrillo C, Zsak L, Laegreid WW, Kutish GF, Neilan JG, Burrage TG, Rock DL (1998) Deletion of a CD2-like gene, 8-DR, from African swine fever virus affects viral infection in domestic swine. J Virol 72:2881–2889

Bottino C, Augugliaro R, Castriconi R, Nanni M, Biassoni R, Moretta L, Moretta A (2000) Analysis of the molecular mechanism involved in 2B4-mediated NK cell activation: evidence that human 2B4 is physically and functionally associated with the linker for activation of T cells. Eur J Immunol 30:3718–3722

Bottino C, Falco M, Parolini S, Marcenaro E, Augugliaro R, Sivori S, Landi E, Biassoni R, Notarangelo LD, Moretta L, Moretta A (2001) NTB-A, a novel SH2D1A-associated surface molecule contributing to the inability of natural killer cells to kill Epstein-Barr virus-infected B cells in X-linked lymphoproliferative disease. J Exp Med 194:235–246

Bouchon A, Cella M, Grierson HL, Cohen JI, Colonna M (2001) Activation of NK cell-mediated cytotoxicity by a SAP-independent receptor of the CD2 family. J Immunol 167:5517–5521

Brown MH, Boles K, van der Merwe PA, Kumar V, Mathew PA, Barclay AN (1998) 2B4, the natural killer and T cell immunoglobulin superfamily surface protein, is a ligand for CD48. J Exp Med 188:2083–2090

Chan B, Lanyi A, Song HK, Griesbach J, Simarro-Grande M, Poy F, Howie D, Sumegi J, Terhorst C, Eck MJ (2003) SAP couples Fyn to SLAM immune receptors. Nat Cell Biol 5:155–160

Chavin KD, Qin L, Lin J, Woodward J, Baliga P, Kato K, Yagita H, Bromberg JS (1994) Anti-CD48 (murine CD2 ligand) mAbs suppress cell mediated immunity in vivo. Int Immunol 6:701–709

Chen R, Relouzat F, Roncagalli R, Aoukaty A, Tan R, Latour S, Veillette A (2004) Molecular dissection of 2B4 signaling: implications for signal transduction by SLAM-related receptors. Mol Cell Biol 24:5144–5156

Chuang SS, Kumaresan PR, Mathew PA (2001) 2B4 (CD244)-mediated activation of cytotoxicity and IFN-γ release in human NK cells involves distinct pathways. J Immunol 167:6210–6216

Chung B, Aoukaty A, Dutz J, Terhorst C, Tan R (2005) Signaling lymphocytic activation molecule-associated protein controls NKT cell functions. J Immunol 174:3153–3157

Cocks BG, Chang CC, Carballido JM, Yssel H, de Vries JE, Aversa G (1995) A novel receptor involved in T-cell activation. Nature 376:260–263

Coffey AJ, Brooksbank RA, Brandau O, Oohashi T, Howell GR, Bye JM, Cahn AP, Durham J, Heath P, Wray P, Pavitt R, Wilkinson J, Leversha M, Huckle E, Shaw-Smith CJ, Dunham A, Rhodes S, Schuster V, Porta G, Yin L, Serafini P, Sylla B, Zollo M, Franco B, Bentley DR, et al. (1998) Host response to EBV infection in X-linked lymphoproliferative disease results from mutations in an SH2-domain encoding gene. Nat Genet 20:129–135

Collins TL, Kassner PD, Bierer BE, Burakoff SJ (1994) Adhesion receptors in lymphocyte activation. Curr Opin Immunol 6:385–393

Crawford K, Gabuzda D, Pantazopoulos V, Xu J, Clement C, Reinherz E, Alper CA (1999) Circulating CD2+ monocytes are dendritic cells. J Immunol 163:5920–5928

Crawford K, Stark A, Kitchens B, Sternheim K, Pantazopoulos V, Triantafellow E, Wang Z, Vasir B, Larsen CE, Gabuzda D, Reinherz E, Alper CA (2003) CD2 engagement induces dendritic cell activation: implications for immune surveillance and T-cell activation. Blood 102:1745–1752

Czar MJ, Kersh EN, Mijares LA, Lanier G, Lewis J, Yap G, Chen A, Sher A, Duckett CS, Ahmed R, Schwartzberg PL (2001) Altered lymphocyte responses and cytokine production in mice deficient in the X-linked lymphoproliferative disease gene SH2D1A/DSHP/SAP. Proc Natl Acad Sci USA 98:7449–7454

Davis SJ, Ikemizu S, Wild MK, van der Merwe PA (1998) CD2 and the nature of protein interactions mediating cell-cell recognition. Immunol Rev 163:217–236

de la Fuente MA, Pizcueta P, Nadal M, Bosch J, Engel P (1997) CD84 leukocyte antigen is a new member of the Ig superfamily. Blood 90:2398–2405

de la Fuente MA, Tovar V, Villamor N, Zapater N, Pizcueta P, Campo E, Bosch J, Engel P (2001) Molecular characterization and expression of a novel human leukocyte cell-surface marker homologous to mouse Ly-9. Blood 97:3513–3520

Degli-Esposti MA, Smyth MJ (2005) Close encounters of different kinds: dendritic cells and NK cells take centre stage. Nat Rev Immunol 5:112–124

Dikic I (2002) CIN85/CMS family of adaptor molecules. FEBS Lett 529:110–115

Durda PJ, Boos SC, Gottlieb PD (1979) T100: a new murine cell surface glycoprotein detected by anti-Lyt-2.1 serum. J Immunol 122:1407–1412

Dustin ML, Olszowy MW, Holdorf AD, Li J, Bromley S, Desai N, Widder P, Rosenberger F, van der Merwe PA, Allen PM, Shaw AS (1998) A novel adaptor protein orchestrates receptor patterning and cytoskeletal polarity in T-cell contacts. Cell 94:667–677

Dustin ML, Selvaraj P, Mattaliano RJ, Springer TA (1987) Anchoring mechanisms for LFA-3 cell adhesion glycoprotein at membrane surface. Nature 329:846–848

Dykstra M, Cherukuri A, Sohn HW, Tzeng SJ, Pierce SK (2003) Location is everything: lipid rafts and immune cell signaling. Annu Rev Immunol 21:457–481

Eissmann P, Beauchamp L, Wooters J, Tilton JC, Long EO, Watzl C (2005) Molecular basis for positive and negative signaling by the natural killer cell receptor 2B4 (CD244). Blood 105:4722–4729

Falco M, Marcenaro E, Romeo E, Bellora F, Marras D, Vely F, Ferracci G, Moretta L, Moretta A, Bottino C (2004) Homophilic interaction of NTBA, a member of the CD2 molecular family: induction of cytotoxicity and cytokine release in human NK cells. Eur J Immunol 34:1663–1672

Fennelly JA, Tiwari B, Davis SJ, Evans EJ (2001) CD2F-10: a new member of the CD2 subset of the immunoglobulin superfamily. Immunogenetics 53:599–602

Flaig RM, Stark S, Watzl C (2004) Cutting edge: NTB-A activates NK cells via homophilic interaction. J Immunol 172:6524–6527

Fletcher JM, Prentice HG, Grundy JE (1998) Natural killer cell lysis of cytomegalovirus (CMV)-infected cells correlates with virally induced changes in cell surface Lymphocyte Function-Associated Antigen-3 (LFA-3) expression and not with the CMV-induced down-regulation of cell surface class I HLA. J Immunol 161:2365–2374

Fraser CC, Howie D, Morra M, Qiu Y, Murphy C, Shen Q, Gutierrez-Ramos JC, Coyle A, Kingsbury GA, Terhorst C (2002) Identification and characterization of SF2000 and SF2001, two new members of the immune receptor SLAM/CD2 family. Immunogenetics 53:843–850

Garnett D, Barclay AN, Carmo AM, Beyers AD (1993) The association of the protein tyrosine kinases p56lck and p60fyn with the glycosyl phosphatidylinositol-anchored proteins Thy-1 and CD48 in rat thymocytes is dependent on the state of cellular activation. Eur J Immunol 23:2540–2544

Garni-Wagner BA, Purohit A, Mathew PA, Bennett M, Kumar V (1993) A novel function-associated molecule related to non-MHC-restricted cytotoxicity mediated by activated natural killer cells and T cells. J Immunol 151:60–70

Gonzalez-Cabrero J, Wise CJ, Latchman Y, Freeman GJ, Sharpe AH, Reiser H (1999) CD48-deficient mice have a pronounced defect in $CD4^+$ T cell activation. Proc Natl Acad Sci USA 96:1019–1023

Hogarth PM, Craig J, McKenzie IF (1980) A monoclonal antibody detecting the Ly-9.2 (Lgp 100) cell-membrane alloantigen. Immunogenetics 11:65–74

Howie D, Laroux FS, Morra M, Satoskar AR, Rosas LE, Faubion WA, Julien A, Rietdijk S, Coyle AJ, Fraser C, Terhorst C (2005) Cutting Edge: The SLAM family receptor Ly108 controls T cell and neutrophil functions. J Immunol 174:5931–5935

Kambayashi T, Assarsson E, Chambers BJ, Ljunggren HG (2001) Cutting edge: Regulation of $CD8^+$ T cell proliferation by 2B4/CD48 interactions. J Immunol 167:6706–6710

Killeen N, Moessner R, Arvieux J, Willis A, Williams AF (1988) The MRC OX-45 antigen of rat leukocytes and endothelium is in a subset of the immunoglobulin superfamily with CD2, LFA-3 and carcinoembryonic antigens. EMBO J 7:3087–3091

Killeen N, Stuart SG, Littman DR (1992) Development and function of T cells in mice with a disrupted CD2 gene. EMBO J 11:4329–4336

King PD, Sadra A, Han A, Liu XR, Sunder-Plassmann R, Reinherz EL, Dupont B (1996) CD2 signaling in T cells involves tyrosine phosphorylation and activation of the Tec family kinase, EMT/ITK/TSK. Int Immunol 8:1707–1714

Kingma DW, Imus P, Xie XY, Jasper G, Sorbara L, Stewart C, Stetler-Stevenson M (2002) CD2 is expressed by a subpopulation of normal B cells and is frequently present in mature B-cell neoplasms. Cytometry 50:243–248

Kingsbury GA, Feeney LA, Nong Y, Calandra SA, Murphy CJ, Corcoran JM, Wang Y, Prabhu Das MR, Busfield SJ, Fraser CC, Villeval JL (2001) Cloning, expression, and function of BLAME, a novel member of the CD2 family. J Immunol 166:5675–5680

Klem J, Verrett PC, Kumar V, Schatzle JD (2002) 2B4 is constitutively associated with linker for the activation of T cells in glycolipid-enriched microdomains: properties required for 2B4 lytic function. J Immunol 169:55–62

Kozak CA, Davidson WF, Morse HC, 3rd (1984) Genetic and functional relationships of the retroviral and lymphocyte alloantigen loci on mouse chromosome 1. Immunogenetics 19:163–168

Krause SW, Rehli M, Heinz S, Ebner R, Andreesen R (2000) Characterization of MAX.3 antigen, a glycoprotein expressed on mature macrophages, dendritic cells and blood platelets: identity with CD84. Biochem J 346:729–736

Kruse M, Meinl E, Henning G, Kuhnt C, Berchtold S, Berger T, Schuler G, Steinkasserer A (2001) Signaling lymphocytic activation molecule is expressed on mature CD83+ dendritic cells and is up-regulated by IL-1β. J Immunol 167:1989–1995

Kubin MZ, Parshley DL, Din W, Waugh JY, Davis-Smith T, Smith CA, Macduff BM, Armitage RJ, Chin W, Cassiano L, Borges L, Petersen M, Trinchieri G, Goodwin RG (1999) Molecular cloning and biological characterization of NK cell activation-inducing ligand, a counterstructure for CD48. Eur J Immunol 29:3466–3477

Kubota K (2002) A structurally variant form of the 2B4 antigen is expressed on the cell surface of mouse mast cells. Microbiol Immunol 46:589–592

Kumar V, McNerney ME (2005) A new self: MHC-class-I-independent natural-killer-cell self-tolerance. Nat Rev Immunol 5:363–374

Kumaresan PR, Lai WC, Chuang SS, Bennett M, Mathew PA (2002) CS1, a novel member of the CD2 family, is homophilic and regulates NK cell function. Mol Immunol 39:1–8

Lanier LL (1998) NK cell receptors. Annu Rev Immunol 16:359–393

Lanier LL (2005) NK cell recognition. Annu Rev Immunol 23:225–274.

Lanier LL, Corliss B, Phillips JH (1997) Arousal and inhibition of human NK cells. Immunol Rev 155:145–154

Latchman Y, McKay PF, Reiser H (1998) Identification of the 2B4 molecule as a counter-receptor for CD48. J Immunol 161:5809–5812

Latour S, Gish G, Helgason CD, Humphries RK, Pawson T, Veillette A (2001) Regulation of SLAM-mediated signal transduction by SAP, the X-linked lymphoproliferative gene product. Nat Immunol 2:681–690

Latour S, Roncagalli R, Chen R, Bakinowski M, Shi X, Schwartzberg PL, Davidson D, Veillette A (2003) Binding of SAP SH2 domain to FynT SH3 domain reveals a novel mechanism of receptor signalling in immune regulation. Nat Cell Biol 5:149–154

Lee JK, Boles KS, Mathew PA (2004a) Molecular and functional characterization of a CS1 (CRACC) splice variant expressed in human NK cells that does not contain immunoreceptor tyrosine-based switch motifs. Eur J Immunol 34:2791–2799

Lee KM, Bhawan S, Majima T, Wei H, Nishimura MI, Yagita H, Kumar V (2003) Cutting edge: the NK cell receptor 2B4 augments antigen-specific T cell cytotoxicity through CD48 ligation on neighboring T cells. J Immunol 170:4881–4885

Lee KM, Forman JP, McNerney ME, Stepp SE, Kuppireddi S, Guzior D, Latchman YE, Sayegh MH, Yagita H, Oh SB, Wulfing C, Schatzle J, Mathew PA, Sharpe AH, Kumar V (2005) Requirement of homotypic NK cell interactions through 2B4(CD244)/CD48 in the generation of NK effector functions. Blood:DOI 10.1182/blood-2005-1101-0185

Lee KM, McNerney ME, Stepp SE, Mathew PA, Schatzle JD, Bennett M, Kumar V (2004b) 2B4 acts as a non-major histocompatibility complex binding inhibitory receptor on mouse natural killer cells. J Exp Med 199:1245–1254

Li C, Iosef C, Jia CY, Han VK, Li SS (2003) Dual functional roles for the X-linked lymphoproliferative syndrome gene product SAP/SH2D1A in signaling through the signaling lymphocyte activation molecule (SLAM) family of immune receptors. J Biol Chem 278:3852–3859

Lodoen MB, Lanier LL (2005) Viral modulation of NK cell immunity. Nat Rev Microbiol 3:59–69

Martelli MP, Lin H, Zhang W, Samelson LE, Bierer BE (2000) Signaling via LAT (linker for T-cell activation) and Syk/ZAP70 is required for ERK activation and NFAT transcriptional activation following CD2 stimulation. Blood 96:2181–2190

Martin M, Del Valle JM, Saborit I, Engel P (2005) Identification of Grb2 as a novel binding partner of the signaling lymphocytic activation molecule-associated protein binding receptor CD229. J Immunol 174:5977–5986

Martin M, Romero X, de la Fuente MA, Tovar V, Zapater N, Esplugues E, Pizcueta P, Bosch J, Engel P (2001) CD84 functions as a homophilic adhesion molecule and enhances IFN-γ secretion: adhesion is mediated by Ig-like domain 1. J Immunol 167:3668–3676

Mathieson BJ, Sharrow SO, Bottomly K, Fowlkes BJ (1980) Ly 9, an alloantigenic marker of lymphocyte differentiation. J Immunol 125:2127–2136

Mavaddat N, Mason DW, Atkinson PD, Evans EJ, Gilbert RJ, Stuart DI, Fennelly JA, Barclay AN, Davis SJ, Brown MH (2000) Signaling lymphocytic activation molecule (CDw150) is homophilic but self-associates with very low affinity. J Biol Chem 275:28100–28109

McNerney ME, Guzior D, Kumar V (2005) 2B4 (CD244)-CD48 interactions provide a novel MHC class I-independent system for NK cell self-tolerance in mice. Blood:DOI 10.1182/blood-2005-1101-0357

Moingeon P, Lucich JL, McConkey DJ, Letourneur F, Malissen B, Kochan J, Chang HC, Rodewald HR, Reinherz EL (1992) CD3ζ dependence of the CD2 pathway of activation in T lymphocytes and natural killer cells. Proc Natl Acad Sci USA 89:1492–1496

Mooney JM, Klem J, Wulfing C, Mijares LA, Schwartzberg PL, Bennett M, Schatzle JD (2004) The murine NK receptor 2B4 (CD244) exhibits inhibitory function independent of signaling lymphocytic activation molecule-associated protein expression. J Immunol 173:3953–3961

Moran M, Miceli MC (1998) Engagement of GPI-linked CD48 contributes to TCR signals and cytoskeletal reorganization: a role for lipid rafts in T cell activation. Immunity 9:787–796

Morra M, Lu J, Poy F, Martin M, Sayos J, Calpe S, Gullo C, Howie D, Rietdijk S, Thompson A, Coyle AJ, Denny C, Yaffe MB, Engel P, Eck MJ, Terhorst C (2001) Structural basis for the interaction of the free SH2 domain EAT-2 with SLAM receptors in hematopoietic cells. EMBO J 20:5840–5852

Munitz A, Bachelet I, Fraenkel S, Katz G, Mandelboim O, Simon HU, Moretta L, Colonna M, Levi-Schaffer F (2005) 2B4 (CD244) is expressed and functional on human eosinophils. J Immunol 174:110–118

Musgrave BL, Watson CL, Haeryfar SM, Barnes CA, Hoskin DW (2004) CD2-CD48 interactions promote interleukin-2 and interferon-γ synthesis by stabilizing cytokine mRNA. Cell Immunol 229:1–12

Musgrave BL, Watson CL, Hoskin DW (2003) CD2-CD48 interactions promote cytotoxic T lymphocyte induction and function: anti-CD2 and anti-CD48 antibodies impair cytokine synthesis, proliferation, target recognition/adhesion, and cytotoxicity. J Interferon Cytokine Res 23:67–81

Nakajima H, Cella M, Bouchon A, Grierson HL, Lewis J, Duckett CS, Cohen JI, Colonna M (2000) Patients with X-linked lymphoproliferative disease have a defect in 2B4 receptor-mediated NK cell cytotoxicity. Eur J Immunol 30:3309–3318

Nakamura T, Takahashi K, Fukazawa T, Koyanagi M, Yokoyama A, Kato H, Yagita H, Okumura K (1990) Relative contribution of CD2 and LFA-1 to murine T and natural killer cell functions. J Immunol 145:3628–3634

Nichols KE, Harkin DP, Levitz S, Krainer M, Kolquist KA, Genovese C, Bernard A, Ferguson M, Zuo L, Snyder E, Buckler AJ, Wise C, Ashley J, Lovett M, Valentine MB, Look AT, Gerald W, Housman DE, Haber DA (1998) Inactivating mutations in an SH2 domain-encoding gene in X-linked lymphoproliferative syndrome. Proc Natl Acad Sci USA 95:13765–13770

Nichols KE, Hom J, Gong SY, Ganguly A, Ma CS, Cannons JL, Tangye SG, Schwartzberg PL, Koretzky GA, Stein PL (2005) Regulation of NKT cell development by SAP, the protein defective in XLP. Nat Med 11:340–345

Nishizawa K, Freund C, Li J, Wagner G, Reinherz EL (1998) Identification of a proline-binding motif regulating CD2-triggered T lymphocyte activation. Proc Natl Acad Sci USA 95:14897–14902

Parolini S, Bottino C, Falco M, Augugliaro R, Giliani S, Franceschini R, Ochs HD, Wolf H, Bonnefoy JY, Biassoni R, Moretta L, Notarangelo LD, Moretta A (2000) X-linked lymphoproliferative disease. 2B4 molecules displaying inhibitory rather than activating function are responsible for the inability of natural killer cells to kill Epstein-Barr virus-infected cells. J Exp Med 192:337–346

Pasquier B, Yin L, Fondaneche MC, Relouzat F, Bloch-Queyrat C, Lambert N, Fischer A, de Saint-Basile G, Latour S (2005) Defective NKT cell development in mice and humans lacking the adapter SAP, the X-linked lymphoproliferative syndrome gene product. J Exp Med 201:695–701

Peck SR, Ruley HE (2000) Ly108: a new member of the mouse CD2 family of cell surface proteins. Immunogenetics 52:63–72

Pende D, Spaggiari GM, Marcenaro S, Martini S, Rivera P, Capobianco A, Falco M, Lanino E, Pierri I, Zambello R, Bacigalupo A, Mingari MC, Moretta A, Moretta L (2005) Analysis of the receptor-ligand interactions in the natural killer-mediated lysis of freshly isolated myeloid or lymphoblastic leukemias: evidence for the involvement of the Poliovirus receptor (CD155) and Nectin-2 (CD112). Blood 105:2066–2073

Punnonen J, de Vries JE (1993) Characterization of a novel CD2+ human thymic B cell subset. J Immunol 151:100–110

Purtilo DT, Cassel CK, Yang JP, Harper R (1975) X-linked recessive progressive combined variable immunodeficiency (Duncan's disease). Lancet 1:935–940

Romero X, Benitez D, March S, Vilella R, Miralpeix M, Engel P (2004) Differential expression of SAP and EAT-2-binding leukocyte cell-surface molecules CD84, CD150 (SLAM), CD229 (Ly9) and CD244 (2B4). Tissue Antigens 64:132–144

Romero X, Zapater N, Calvo M, Kalko SG, de la Fuente MA, Tovar V, Ockeloen C, Pizcueta P, Engel P (2005) CD229 (Ly9) lymphocyte cell surface receptor interacts homophilically through its N-terminal domain and relocalizes to the immunological synapse. J Immunol 174:7033–7042

Sandrin MS, Gumley TP, Henning MM, Vaughan HA, Gonez LJ, Trapani JA, McKenzie IF (1992) Isolation and characterization of cDNA clones for mouse Ly-9. J Immunol 149:1636–1641

Sayos J, Martin M, Chen A, Simarro M, Howie D, Morra M, Engel P, Terhorst C (2001) Cell surface receptors Ly-9 and CD84 recruit the X-linked lymphoproliferative disease gene product SAP. Blood 97:3867–3874

Sayos J, Nguyen KB, Wu C, Stepp SE, Howie D, Schatzle JD, Kumar V, Biron CA, Terhorst C (2000) Potential pathways for regulation of NK and T cell responses: differential X-linked lymphoproliferative syndrome gene product SAP interactions with SLAM and 2B4. Int Immunol 12:1749–1757

Sayos J, Wu C, Morra M, Wang N, Zhang X, Allen D, van Schaik S, Notarangelo L, Geha R, Roncarolo MG, Oettgen H, De Vries JE, Aversa G, Terhorst C (1998) The X-linked lymphoproliferative-disease gene product SAP regulates signals induced through the co-receptor SLAM. Nature 395:462–469

Schatzle JD, Sheu S, Stepp SE, Mathew PA, Bennett M, Kumar V (1999) Characterization of inhibitory and stimulatory forms of the murine natural killer cell receptor 2B4. Proc Natl Acad Sci USA 96:3870–3875

Schmidt RE, Caulfield JP, Michon J, Hein A, Kamada MM, MacDermott RP, Stevens RL, Ritz J (1988) T11/CD2 activation of cloned human natural killer cells results in increased conjugate formation and exocytosis of cytolytic granules. J Immunol 140:991–1002

Schmidt RE, Michon JM, Woronicz J, Schlossman SF, Reinherz EL, Ritz J (1987) Enhancement of natural killer function through activation of the T11 E rosette receptor. J Clin Invest 79:305–308

Seaman WE, Eriksson E, Dobrow R, Imboden JB (1987) Inositol trisphosphate is generated by a rat natural killer cell tumor in response to target cells or to crosslinked monoclonal antibody OX-34: possible signaling role for the OX-34 determinant during activation by target cells. Proc Natl Acad Sci USA 84:4239–4243

Senkevich TG, Koonin EV, Bugert JJ, Darai G, Moss B (1997) The genome of molluscum contagiosum virus: analysis and comparison with other poxviruses. Virology 233:19–42

Shimizu Y, Mobley JL, Finkelstein LD, Chan AS (1995) A role for phosphatidylinositol 3-kinase in the regulation of $\beta 1$ integrin activity by the CD2 antigen. J Cell Biol 131:1867–1880

Shlapatska LM, Mikhalap SV, Berdova AG, Zelensky OM, Yun TJ, Nichols KE, Clark EA, Sidorenko SP (2001) CD150 association with either the SH2-containing inositol phosphatase or the SH2-containing protein tyrosine phosphatase is regulated by the adaptor protein SH2D1A. J Immunol 166:5480–5487

Sidorenko SP, Clark EA (1993) Characterization of a cell surface glycoprotein IPO-3, expressed on activated human B and T lymphocytes. J Immunol 151:4614–4624

Sidorenko SP, Clark EA (2003) The dual-function CD150 receptor subfamily: the viral attraction. Nat Immunol 4:19–24

Siciliano RF, Pratt JC, Schmidt RE, Ritz J, Reinherz EL (1985) Activation of cytolytic T lymphocyte and natural killer cell function through the T11 sheep erythrocyte binding protein. Nature 317:428–430

Simarro M, Lanyi A, Howie D, Poy F, Bruggeman J, Choi M, Sumegi J, Eck MJ, Terhorst C (2004) SAP increases FynT kinase activity and is required for phosphorylation of SLAM and Ly9. Int Immunol 16:727–736

Sivori S, Falco M, Marcenaro E, Parolini S, Biassoni R, Bottino C, Moretta L, Moretta A (2002) Early expression of triggering receptors and regulatory role of 2B4 in human natural killer cell precursors undergoing in vitro differentiation. Proc Natl Acad Sci USA 99:4526–4531

Sivori S, Parolini S, Falco M, Marcenaro E, Biassoni R, Bottino C, Moretta L, Moretta A (2000) 2B4 functions as a co-receptor in human NK cell activation. Eur J Immunol 30:787–793

Smith GM, Biggs J, Norris B, Anderson-Stewart P, Ward R (1997) Detection of a soluble form of the leukocyte surface antigen CD48 in plasma and its elevation in patients with lymphoid leukemias and arthritis. J Clin Immunol 17:502–509

Smith ME, Thomas JA (1990) Cellular expression of lymphocyte function associated antigens and the intercellular adhesion molecule-1 in normal tissue. J Clin Pathol 43:893–900

Solomon KR, Rudd CE, Finberg RW (1996) The association between glycosylphosphatidylinositol-anchored proteins and heterotrimeric G protein αsubunits in lymphocytes. Proc Natl Acad Sci USA 93:6053–6058

Springer TA, Dustin ML, Kishimoto TK, Marlin SD (1987) The lymphocyte function-associated LFA-1, CD2, and LFA-3 molecules: cell adhesion receptors of the immune system. Annu Rev Immunol 5:223–252

Staunton DE, Fisher RC, LeBeau MM, Lawrence JB, Barton DE, Francke U, Dustin M, Thorley-Lawson DA (1989) Blast-1 possesses a glycosyl-phosphatidylinositol (GPI) membrane anchor, is related to LFA-3 and OX-45, and maps to chromosome 1q21–23. J Exp Med 169:1087–1099

Stefanova I, Horejsi V, Ansotegui IJ, Knapp W, Stockinger H (1991) GPI-anchored cell-surface molecules complexed to protein tyrosine kinases. Science 254:1016–1019

Stepp SE, Schatzle JD, Bennett M, Kumar V, Mathew PA (1999) Gene structure of the murine NK cell receptor 2B4: presence of two alternatively spliced isoforms with distinct cytoplasmic domains. Eur J Immunol 29:2392–2399

Tangye SG, Cherwinski H, Lanier LL, Phillips JH (2000a) 2B4-mediated activation of human natural killer cells. Mol Immunol 37:493–501

Tangye SG, Lazetic S, Woollatt E, Sutherland GR, Lanier LL, Phillips JH (1999) Cutting edge: human 2B4, an activating NK cell receptor, recruits the protein tyrosine phosphatase SHP-2 and the adaptor signaling protein SAP. J Immunol 162:6981–6985

Tangye SG, Nichols KE, Hare NJ, van de Weerdt BCM (2003) Functional requirements for interactions between CD84 and Src Homology 2 domain-containing proteins and their contribution to human T cell activation. J Immunol 171:2485–2495

Tangye SG, Phillips JH, Lanier LL, Nichols KE (2000b) Functional requirement for SAP in 2B4-mediated activation of human natural killer cells as revealed by the X-linked lymphoproliferative syndrome. J Immunol 165:2932–2936

Tangye SG, van de Weerdt BC, Avery DT, Hodgkin PD (2002) CD84 is up-regulated on a major population of human memory B cells and recruits the SH2 domain containing proteins SAP and EAT-2. Eur J Immunol 32:1640–1649

Tatsuo H, Ono N, Tanaka K, Yanagi Y (2000) SLAM (CDw150) is a cellular receptor for measles virus. Nature 406:893–897

Teh S-J, Killeen N, Tarakhovsky A, Littman DR, Teh H-S (1997) CD2 regulates the positive selection and function of antigen-specific CD4-CD8+ T cells. Blood 89:1308–1318

Thompson AD, Braun BS, Arvand A, Stewart SD, May WA, Chen E, Korenberg J, Denny C (1996) EAT-2 is a novel SH2 domain containing protein that is up regulated by Ewing's sarcoma EWS/FLI1 fusion gene. Oncogene 13:2649–2658

Thorley-Lawson DA, Schooley RT, Bhan AK, Nadler LM (1982) Epstein-Barr virus superinduces a new human B cell differentiation antigen (B-LAST 1) expressed on transformed lymphoblasts. Cell 30:415–425

Tibaldi EV, Reinherz EL (2003) CD2BP3, CIN85 and the structurally related adaptor protein CMS bind to the same CD2 cytoplasmic segment, but elicit divergent functional activities. Int Immunol 15:313–329

Timonen T, Gahmberg CG, Patarroyo M (1990) Participation of CD11a-c/CD18, CD2 and RGD-binding receptors in endogenous and interleukin-2-stimulated NK activity of CD3-negative large granular lymphocytes. Int J Cancer 46:1035–1040

Tovar V, de la Fuente MA, Pizcueta P, Bosch J, Engel P (2000) Gene structure of the mouse leukocyte cell surface molecule Ly9. Immunogenetics 51:788–793

Tovar V, del Valle J, Zapater N, Martin M, Romero X, Pizcueta P, Bosch J, Terhorst C, Engel P (2002) Mouse novel Ly9: a new member of the expanding CD150 (SLAM) family of leukocyte cell-surface receptors. Immunogenetics 54:394–402

Vaidya SV, Stepp SE, McNerney ME, Lee JK, Bennett M, Lee KM, Stewart CL, Kumar V, Mathew PA (2005) Targeted disruption of the 2B4 gene in mice reveals an in vivo role of 2B4 (CD244) in the rejection of B16 melanoma cells. J Immunol 174:800–807

Valdez PA, Wang H, Seshasayee D, van Lookeren Campagne M, Gurney A, Lee WP, Grewal IS (2004) NTB-A, a new activating receptor in T cells that regulates autoimmune disease. J Biol Chem 279:18662–18669

Valiante NM, Trinchieri G (1993) Identification of a novel signal transduction surface molecule on human cytotoxic lymphocytes. J Exp Med 178:1397–1406

van de Griend RJ, Bolhuis RL, Stoter G, Roozemond RC (1987) Regulation of cytolytic activity in CD3- and CD3+ killer cell clones by monoclonal antibodies (anti-CD16, anti-CD2, anti-CD3) depends on subclass specificity of target cell IgG-FcR. J Immunol 138:3137–3144

Vivier E, Morin PM, O'Brien C, Schlossman SF, Anderson P (1991) CD2 is functionally linked to the zeta-natural killer receptor complex. Eur J Immunol 21:1077–1080

Voltarelli JC, Gjerset G, Anasetti C (1993) Adhesion of CD16+ K cells to antibody-coated targets is mediated by CD2 and CD18 receptors. Immunology 79:509–511

Wandstrat AE, Nguyen C, Limaye N, Chan AY, Subramanian S, Tian XH, Yim YS, Pertsemlidis A, Garner HR, Jr., Morel L, Wakeland EK (2004) Association of extensive polymorphisms in the SLAM/CD2 gene cluster with murine lupus. Immunity 21:769–780

Wang N, Morra M, Wu C, Gullo C, Howie D, Coyle T, Engel P, Terhorst C (2001) CD150 is a member of a family of genes that encode glycoproteins on the surface of hematopoietic cells. Immunogenetics 53:382–394

Wang N, Satoskar A, Faubion W, Howie D, Okamoto S, Feske S, Gullo C, Clarke K, Sosa MR, Sharpe AH, Terhorst C (2004) The cell surface receptor SLAM controls T cell and macrophage functions. J Exp Med 199:1255–1264

Watzl C, Stebbins CC, Long EO (2000) NK cell inhibitory receptors prevent tyrosine phosphorylation of the activation receptor 2B4 (CD244). J Immunol 165:3545–3548

Wong YW, Williams AF, Kingsmore SF, Seldin MF (1990) Structure, expression, and genetic linkage of the mouse BCM1 (OX45 or Blast-1) antigen. Evidence for genetic duplication giving rise to the BCM1 region on mouse chromosome 1 and the CD2/LFA3 region on mouse chromosome 3. J Exp Med 171:2115–2130

Wu C, Nguyen KB, Pien GC, Wang N, Gullo C, Howie D, Sosa MR, Edwards MJ, Borrow P, Satoskar AR, Sharpe AH, Biron CA, Terhorst C (2001) SAP controls T cell responses to virus and terminal differentiation of TH2 cells. Nat Immunol 2:410–414

Yagita H, Nakamura T, Karasuyama H, Okumura K (1989) Monoclonal antibodies specific for murine CD2 reveal its presence on B as well as T cells. Proc Natl Acad Sci USA 86:645–649

Yin L, Al-Alem U, Liang J, Tong WM, Li C, Badiali M, Medard JJ, Sumegi J, Wang ZQ, Romeo G (2003) Mice deficient in the X-linked lymphoproliferative disease gene sap exhibit increased susceptibility to murine gammaherpesvirus-68 and hypo-gammaglobulinemia. J Med Virol 71:446–455

Zaiss M, Hirtreiter C, Rehli M, Rehm A, Kunz-Schughart LA, Andreesen R, Hennemann B (2003) CD84 expression on human hematopoietic progenitor cells. Exp Hematol 31:798–805

Zhang W, Wan T, Li N, Yuan Z, He L, Zhu X, Yu M, Cao X (2001) Genetic approach to insight into the immunobiology of human dendritic cells and identification of CD84-H1, a novel CD84 homologue. Clin Cancer Res 7:822s-829s

Immunobiology of Human NKG2D and Its Ligands

S. González · V. Groh · T. Spies (✉)

Fred Hutchinson Cancer Research Center, 1100 Fairview Ave. N.,
Seattle, WA 98109, USA
tspies@fhcrc.org

1	Introduction	122
2	Structure and Regulation of MIC	123
3	Tumor-Associated and Pathogen-Induced Expression of MIC	125
4	The ULBP Family of NKG2D Ligands	126
5	NKG2D and Its Physical Interactions with MIC and ULBP	127
6	Activating and Costimulatory Functions of NKG2D	129
7	Viral and Tumor Immune Evasion	130
8	Role of MIC-NKG2D in Autoimmune Diseases	131
9	Recognition of MIC by Intraepithelial γδ T Cells	132
10	Polymorphism of MIC and Disease Associations	133
References		134

Abstract The NKG2D-DAP10 receptor complex activates natural killer (NK) cells and costimulates effector T cell subsets upon engagement of ligands that can be conditionally expressed under physiologically harmful conditions such as microbial infections and malignancies. These characteristics have given rise to the widely embraced concept of immunorecognition of "induced or damaged self," complementing the "missing self" paradigm that is represented by MHC class I allotypes and their interactions with inhibitory receptors on NK cells. However, this notion may only be partially sustainable, as various patterns of constitutive tissue distributions have become apparent among members of one NKG2D ligand family. This review summarizes the biological properties of NKG2D and its ligands and discusses the interactions and regulation of these molecules with emphasis of their significance in microbial infections, tumor immunology, and autoimmune disease.

1
Introduction

When NK cells engage target cells, the aggregate signals from inhibitory and activating receptors are integrated into balances that control their effector functions. Among these natural killer receptors (NKR) are inhibitory or activating isoforms of the killer cell Ig-like receptors (KIR) and the inhibitory leukocyte Ig-like receptor (LIR)-1, which bind to HLA-A, -B, or -C alleles, and the C-type lectin-like inhibitory CD94-NKG2A and activating CD94-NKG2C heterodimers, which interact with HLA-E (Lee et al. 1998; Long 1999). Inhibitory receptors have higher ligand affinities than their activating isoforms and thus convey dominant-negative signals (Lanier 2001). They have cytoplasmic immunoreceptor tyrosine-based inhibition motifs (ITIM), which function by recruitment of SHP-1 tyrosine phosphatases (Ravetch and Lanier 2000). Activating KIR isoforms, which lack ITIM, and the CD94-NKG2C receptor associate with an adaptor protein, DAP12, which has a cytoplasmic immunoreceptor tyrosine-based activation motif (ITAM) and signals similar to the CD3ζ and FcεRIγ chains, by recruitment of Syk or ZAP-70 tyrosine kinases (Lanier 2001). Additional activating receptors include members of the LIR family and the Nkp30, Nkp44, and Nkp46 proteins, which are also referred to as natural cytotoxicity receptors (Borges et al. 1997; Pessino et al. 1998; Cantoni et al. 1999; Pende et al. 1999). However, the significance and ligand interactions of these molecules are less well defined. In their interactions with inhibitory NKR, MHC class I molecules function as passports certifying the integrity of cells. Because their expression is often impaired by viral infections and tumorigenesis, insufficient engagement of inhibitory NKR results in target cell susceptibility to lysis by NK cells. Because NK cells express variable arrays of inhibitory NKR with different ligand specificities, they are enabled to detect loss of individual MHC class I alleles. Additional expression of KIR or CD94-NKG2A on T cells after persistent antigen-driven stimulation results in increased T cell antigen receptor (TCR)-dependent activation thresholds and T cell anergy, thus effecting downmodulation of effector responses in chronic infections and malignancies, which may safeguard against autoimmune reactions (Noppen et al. 1998; Moser et al. 2002).

Whereas most NKR bind MHC class I molecules that are ubiquitously expressed, the activating NKG2D receptor interacts with distant relatives of MHC class I, some of which are inducibly expressed (Lanier 2001; Raulet 2003). Among these, the prototype ligands are the closely related MICA and MICB, which are regulated by cellular stress. The tissue distribution of these proteins is restricted to intestinal epithelium, but they can be induced by some microbial infections and are frequently associated with epithelial tumors of

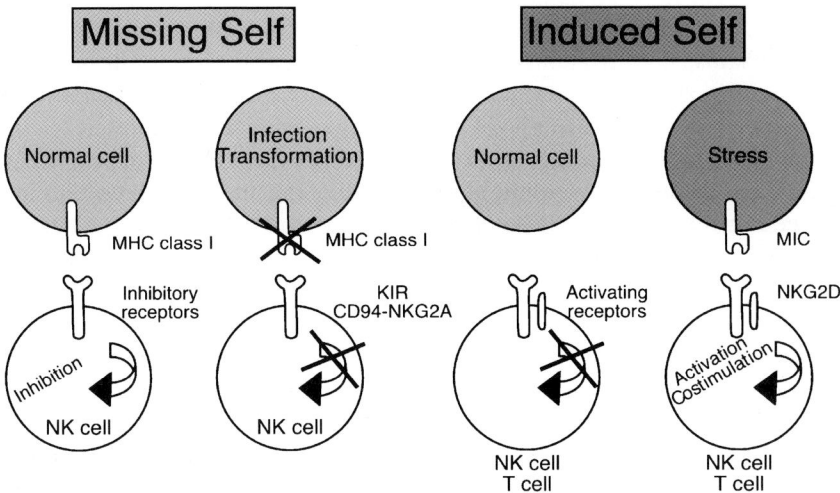

Fig. 1 Regulation of NK cell responses by inhibitory NKR interacting with MHC class I molecules and by NKG2D on engagement by its inducible MIC ligands

diverse tissue origins. NKG2D is encoded by a gene linked to the NKG2 receptor family, although it bears no sequence resemblance. Engagement of NKG2D by MIC potently activates NK cell functions and costimulates effector T cell responses. Thus MIC deliver an "induced or damaged self" signal that is coupled to cellular changes caused by microbes or malignant cell growth, thereby alerting the immune system to harmful conditions (Fig. 1) (Raulet 2003). This system bears superficial similarity to the recognition of pathogen-associated molecular patterns (PAMP) by the family of Toll-like receptors (TLR). Additional NKG2D ligands are represented by a family of at least five ULBP proteins. However, the tissue distribution, regulation, and significance of these molecules are not well defined.

2
Structure and Regulation of MIC

MICA and MICB are encoded by genes near *HLA-B*, and homologous dysfunctional pseudogene sequences are located in the vicinities of *HLA-A*, *-E*, and *-G* (Bahram et al. 1994; Bahram and Spies, 1996). The 43-kD MICA and MICB core polypeptides share 84% amino acid sequence homology and are distinctively related to mammalian MHC class I chains as compared to the class I-like CD1 and Fc-receptor molecules encoded elsewhere in the genome.

The MIC protein sequences are about equidistant from all mammalian MHC class I chains, sharing about 30% identical amino acid residues throughout the aligned extracellular α1, α2, and α3 domains. Further characteristic of these molecules are seven or eight N-linked glycosylation sites, unique transmembrane and cytoplasmic tail sequences, three extra cysteine residues in the α1 and α3 domains, and the absence of all of the amino acid residues involved in binding of CD8. Sequences orthologous to MIC are conserved in the genomes of all mammalian species examined, with the exception of rodents (Bahram et al. 1994). MIC genes are functionally expressed in diverse nonhuman primates and presumably most other mammals (Steinle et al. 1998). MIC proteins are not associated with $β_2$-microglobulin ($β_2$m), and their transport is independent of the peptide processing machinery that is required for the assembly of peptide antigen-presenting MHC class I molecules (Groh et al. 1996). Moreover, gel-filtration chromatography of acid-treated MICA isolated from cells after labeling with tritiated amino acids provided no evidence for bound peptides (Groh et al. 1998). These characteristics are reflected in the crystal structure of MICA, which shows a dramatically altered class I fold with only a shallow remnant of a peptide-binding groove and restructured α1α2 platform and α3 domain interfaces that preclude binding of $β_2$m (Li et al. 1999).

Unlike that of the ubiquitous MHC class I molecules, the tissue distribution of MIC is normally restricted to variable areas of the intestinal epithelium, with limited evidence for surface expression (Groh et al. 1996). In cultured polarized epithelial cells, the proteins are sorted to basolateral epithelial membranes by an active process that is determined by two adjacent hydrophobic amino acids, leucine and valine, at the membrane-proximal ends of their cytoplasmic tails (Suemizu et al. 2002). The immunobiology and regulatory mechanisms underlying the expression of MIC in intestinal epithelium are poorly understood. Among tissue culture cell lines, expression of MIC is mostly limited to fibroblast and epithelial cells and is not inducible by interferons. Importantly, however, *MIC* can be heat shock-induced similar to *heat shock protein 70 (hsp70)* genes, presumably because of the presence of a highly conserved heat shock response element (HSE) in the 5′-flanking regions of the corresponding genes (Groh et al. 1996, 1998). Data from electrophoretic mobility shift assays (EMSA) and in vivo genomic footprinting (IVGF) have confirmed that these motifs specifically bind heat shock factor-1 (HSF-1), which is the dominant transcription factor controlling the expression of *hsp70* genes (D. Suciu and T. Spies, unpublished data; Morimoto et al. 1992). In accord with the mode of hsp70 regulation, MIC are expressed in significant amounts on rapidly proliferating epithelial cell lines but are scarce on quiescent cells grown to high confluence. Under this condition, exposure to heat shock results in a maximal 10-fold amplification of MIC mRNAs and surface proteins (Groh et al. 1998). Hence, *MIC* can be regarded as cell stress response genes.

3
Tumor-Associated and Pathogen-Induced Expression of MIC

MIC are frequently expressed in many, but not all, lung, breast, kidney, ovarian, prostate, gastric, and colon carcinomas and melanomas (Groh et al. 1999; Vetter et al. 2002). There are high degrees of variability in the proportions of tumor cells that are positive for MIC. The physiological reasons are unknown, but they could be related to local stress-inducing conditions such as tumor cell proliferation, hypoxia, and hyperglycemia. Oxidative stress has been shown to increase *MIC* gene expression in a colon carcinoma cell line (Yamamoto et al. 2001). Modest MIC expression has also been reported in some hematopoietic malignancies (AML, ALL, and CML), perhaps most significantly in multiple myeloma (Salih et al. 2003).

MIC are strongly induced in fibroblast and endothelial cells by cytomegalovirus (CMV) and by *Mycobacterium tuberculosis* infection in dendritic and epithelial cells (Das et al. 2001; Groh et al. 2001). MICB is induced by Sendai and influenza A virus infection in macrophages (Siren et al. 2004). Skin lesions of lepromatous lepra patients are marked by large amounts of MIC (V. Groh and T. Spies, unpublished data). Intestinal epithelial expression of MIC may be inducible by bacteria, because adhesion of diarrheagenic *Escherichia coli* strains to the intestinal epithelial Caco-2 cell line induces a rapid increase of MICA (Tieng et al. 2002). This effect has been related to an interaction of the bacterial AfaE-III adhesin with the cellular CD55 receptor, a glycosylphosphatidylinositol (GPI)-anchored protein that is expressed on most human cells and inhibits complement C3b deposition. However, how this interaction might result in MIC induction has remained unclear. So far, these are the only examples establishing a connection between infectious agents and MIC expression, suggesting that the scope of a more universal function of MIC in infectious diseases remains to be fully explored. This is of particular significance because immune response systems have primarily evolved by pathogen-driven selection. In the mouse, members of the retinoic acid early inducible-1 (RAE-1) family of NKG2D ligands are induced in macrophages on stimulation of TLR by microbial products (Hamerman et al. 2004). However, similar observations have not been reported for the human MIC or ULBP ligands so far.

4
The ULBP Family of NKG2D Ligands

Binding studies utilizing recombinant IgG Fc region fusion proteins led to the discovery that the CMV UL16 transmembrane glycoprotein, which was of unknown function, specifically interacts with cell surface proteins that were termed ULBP1 and ULBP2 (Cosman et al. 2001). Three additional ULBP sequences were identified by sequence homology (Fig. 2) (Chalupny et al. 2003; Bacon et al. 2004). ULBP3 and -4 and MICA do not interact with UL16, but MICB does. ULBP share no direct sequence relationship with MIC and are encoded outside the MHC on chromosome 6q25. As with MIC, ULBP are distant members of the MHC class I family. All ULBP lack the membrane proximal α3 domain. ULBP1–3, and ULBP4 and -5 have GPI membrane anchors and transmembrane regions, respectively. None of these molecules is associated with $β_2$m or peptide ligands. The α1α2 domains of ULBP share about 50%–60% identical amino acids and are equidistant from those of MHC class I and MIC, with about 25% sequence homology. ULBP1–3 are moderately induced by CMV infection (Welte et al. 2003). Although ULBP mRNAs are quite ubiquitously expressed, little is known regarding the tissue distribution and regulation of the encoded proteins. Preliminary data indicate diverse constitutive expression patterns in epithelia, endothelia, and antigen-presenting cells (V. Groh and T. Spies, unpublished data). This may oppose the "induced or damaged self" hypothesis and warrants further investigation (Fig. 1). In outer cell membranes, the GPI-anchored ULBP are clustered in lipid raft microdomains, which may serve to create enhanced avidity because at least mouse GPI-anchored NKG2D ligands have lower receptor affinities than those with transmembrane domains (Eleme et al. 2004). Indeed, these ULBP and MICA, which is S-acylated, accumulate at NK cell immune synapses. With polarized epithelial cells, lipid rafts form preferentially at apical membrane surfaces. Disruption of epithelial tight junctions, for example, by processes of infection or tumorigenesis, could allow GPI-anchored ULBP to diffuse toward basolateral surfaces where they would become exposed to NKG2D-bearing lymphocytes. Currently, there are no experimentally validated models explaining the significance of the conservation of the two families of highly diversified NKG2D ligands. However, it seems probable that these have been selected to serve as indicators of diverse pathological conditions in different tissue environments by adoption of distinct strategies, namely, cell stress response-coupled transcriptional induction of MIC and, perhaps, induction of immunological visibility of GPI-anchored ULBP by alterations of cellular and tissue integrities.

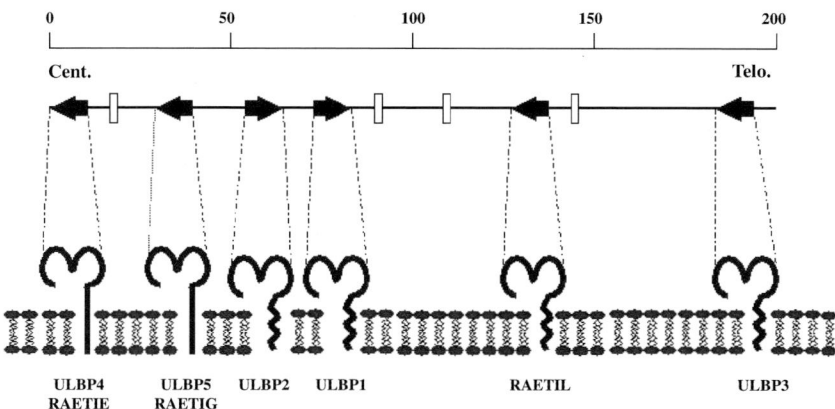

Fig. 2 Schematic depiction of the genetic organization of the *ULBP* gene family of NKG2D ligands. *Arrows* indicate transcriptional orientation of genes on 6q24.2–q25.3. RAET1L encodes a potentially functional gene but has not been further characterized

5
NKG2D and Its Physical Interactions with MIC and ULBP

Formerly an orphan receptor with unknown function (Houchins et al. 1991), NKG2D was first identified as a receptor for MICA and MICB and subsequently for the ULBP ligands (Bauer et al. 1999; Cosman et al. 2001; Chalupny et al. 2003; Bacon et al. 2004). Recombinant NKG2D binds firmly to transfectants expressing its ligands, as do recombinant ligands to lymphocyte subsets expressing NKG2D (Steinle et al. 2001). Analysis by size-exclusion chromatography showed that NKG2D homodimers form stable complexes with monomeric MICA in solution, thus demonstrating that no other components are required to facilitate this interaction. Glycosylation of NKG2D or MICA is not essential but enhances complex formation (Steinle et al. 2001). NKG2D is a type II membrane glycoprotein of 42 kD with a core polypeptide of 28 kD that is expressed on most NK cells, γδ T cells, CD8 αβ T cells, and a subset of NK T cells and thus is the most broadly distributed NKR known (Bauer et al. 1999). It shares no direct relationship with other NKG2 proteins and is not associated with CD94. Instead, NKG2D pairs via interactions between oppositely charged transmembrane amino acids with the DAP10 adaptor protein, which signals similar to CD28 by activation of the p85 subunit of phosphatidylinositol 3-kinase (PI3-K) on tyrosine phosphorylation of a YXXM motif in its cytoplasmic domain (Fig. 3) (Wu et al. 1999). In mouse NK cells, an alternatively spliced, shortened form of NKG2D can associate with DAP12 (Diefenbach et al. 2002); however, there is no corresponding vari-

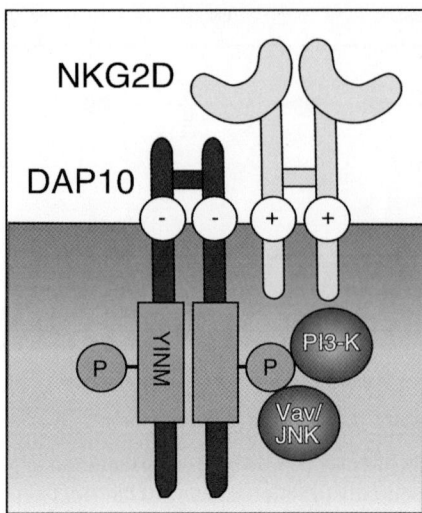

Fig. 3 Composition of the NKG2D-DAP10 receptor complex and signaling via PI3-K-dependent and -independent pathways

ant of NKG2D and alternative association with DAP12 in humans (Rosen et al. 2004).

In a complex crystal structure, the saddle-shaped NKG2D homodimer sits astride the α1α2 platform domain of MICA, with each NKG2D monomer contacting either the α1 or the α2 subdomain (Li et al. 2001). The footprint of NKG2D on MICA largely overlaps that of αβ TCR on MHC class I-peptide ligands, despite the lack of structural similarity between the Ig-like domains of TCR and the C-type lectin-like domains of NKG2D. The rigidity of the interaction of NKG2D with MICA and diverse other ligands involves an investment of the majority of the interaction energy in two binding site core tyrosines (at positions 152 and 199) that are able to make distinct, dominant interactions at each interface in the absence of conformational plasticity. This is distinct from "induced-fit" or "preexisting equilibrium" mechanisms that can be involved in αβ TCR- and antibody-mediated recognition (McFarland and Strong 2003). With the additional information obtained from a NKG2D-ULBP3 complex structure (Radaev et al. 2001), the perplexing ability of NKG2D to interact with highly diverse ligands has been suggested to involve common interfaces and distinct but overlapping sets of hydrogen bonds, hydrophobic interactions, and salt bridges, thus permitting conservation of general shape complementarities and binding energies (Radaev et al. 2002).

6
Activating and Costimulatory Functions of NKG2D

Engagement of NKG2D by any of its ligands on transfectants or by MIC on diverse epithelial tumor cells activates NK cells in the presence of inhibitory NKR and their respective MHC class I ligands (Bauer et al. 1999). Moreover, ectopic expression by transfection of murine RAE-1 ligands causes NKG2D-dependent rejection of tumor cells by NK cells and primed cytotoxic T cells in syngeneic mice, thus reinforcing the potential significance of human MIC-NKG2D in innate and adaptive immune responses against tumors (Cerwenka et al. 2001; Diefenbach et al. 2001). Whereas NKG2D has the capacity to trigger NK cells, it costimulates CD8 $\alpha\beta$ T cells and $\gamma\delta$ T cells (Das et al. 2001; Groh et al. 2001; Roberts et al. 2001). Cytotoxicity assays with CMV or melanoma antigen-specific CD8 $\alpha\beta$ T cells have shown that engagement of NKG2D by MIC strongly augments T cell responses under conditions of suboptimal MHC-peptide antigen stimulation of TCR (Groh et al. 2001, 2002; Vetter et al. 2002). Induced expression of MIC can thus overcome interference of viral gene products with antigen processing and presentation and the downmodulation of MHC class I that is frequently associated with tumors. However, even at optimal stimulation of TCR, NKG2D potently costimulates the production of cytokines, including interferon-γ (IFN-γ), tumor necrosis factor-α (TNF-α), and interleukin-2 (IL-2) and IL-4, and T cell proliferation (Groh et al. 2001). Similarly, NKG2D costimulates Vγ_2/Vδ_2 T cells, which recognize bacterial and mycobacterial soluble organic phosphate and alkamine antigens in a non-MHC-restricted manner. Infection by *Mycobacterium tuberculosis* induces expression of MIC on dendritic and epithelial cells, resulting in NKG2D-mediated costimulation of Vγ_2/Vδ_2 T cell cytotoxicity, proliferation, and release of IFN-γ and IL-2 (Das et al. 2001). The induction of MIC and function of NKG2D thus offer an explanation for why these T cells expand dramatically only during microbial infections although they are capable of recognizing antigen-related moieties that are abundant in uninfected individuals.

NKG2D can also trigger T cells in a TCR-independent manner. Normal freshly isolated intestinal intraepithelial lymphocytes (IEL) exhibit markedly diminished expression of NKG2D, which may be downmodulated to prevent chronic T cell stimulation and autoreactive bystander T cell activation. High levels of NKG2D can be induced by IL-15 (Roberts et al. 2001), which is produced by intestinal epithelial cells on external stimuli and infection. In patients with active celiac disease, however, NKG2D is strongly expressed because of high local levels of IL-15 and MIC is upregulated in intestinal epithelial cells (Hue et al. 2004; Meresse et al. 2004). Under these conditions, freshly isolated intraepithelial CD8 $\alpha\beta$ T cells lyse intestinal epithelial cell lines independent of TCR engagement. NKG2D-DAP10 signaling involves both PI3-K-dependent and -independent (Vav/JNK) pathways (Fig. 3). This activation mode was also observed with normal peripheral blood effector stage CD8 T cells cultured as lymphokine-activated killer (LAK) cells in the presence of high doses of IL-15 (Meresse et al. 2004).

7
Viral and Tumor Immune Evasion

The existence of numerous specific interactions between viral proteins and molecules of the immune system reflects the intense evolutionary pressure imposed on host-pathogen relationships. Usually, these constitute a balance between viral escape from immune control and the host defense limiting virus spread and resultant disease. Human CMV persists lifelong in a latent state with asymptomatic episodes of virus shedding. Only in immunocompromised individuals does virus reactivation result in severe disease manifestations. To maintain long-term persistence in infected hosts, CMV interferes with several stages of antigen processing and presentation by MHC class I molecules, thus compromising the ability of CD8 $\alpha\beta$ T cells to eliminate infected cells. The CMV US6 membrane protein impairs the function of TAP, which delivers peptides into the endoplasmic reticulum (ER) for binding to MHC class I molecules. The US3 protein retains class I molecules in the ER, and US2 and US11 redirect nascent class I chains back into the cytosol, where they are degraded (Ploegh 1998). Perhaps not surprisingly, CMV also has the capacity to obstruct the function of NKG2D ligands: UL16 retains ULBP1, ULBP2, and MICB intracellularly via localization to or retrieval from the *trans*-Golgi network, thus abrogating surface expression (Dunn et al. 2003; Welte et al. 2003; Wu et al. 2003). This retention is mediated by a tyrosine-based motif in the cytoplasmic tail sequence of UL16. Deletion of this motif restores surface expression of the NKG2D ligands, whereas UL16 is redirected to endosomal compartments (Wu et al. 2003). However, this mechanism of CMV immune evasion is bypassed by ULBP3 and MICA, which are not bound by UL16.

In patients with epithelial tumors that are positive for MIC, large proportions of tumor-infiltrating lymphocytes (TIL) have low levels of NKG2D as a result of ligand-induced endocytosis and at least partial lysosomal degradation (Groh et al. 2002). In addition, NKG2D is systemically diminished on matched peripheral blood T cells and NK cells. This deficiency is associated with circulating tumor-derived soluble MICA and presumably MICB, which cause the downregulation of NKG2D. As a result, the responsiveness of tumor antigen-specific effector T cells and NK cells is severely impaired (Groh et al. 2002; Doubrovina et al. 2003). Thus tumor shedding of MIC, which is probably due to the activity of metalloproteinases (Salih et al. 2002), may promote tumor immune evasion. Moreover, NKG2D is also downmodulated, albeit less substantially, by transforming growth factor β1 (TGF-β1) (Castriconi et al. 2003; Lee et al. 2004).

8
Role of MIC-NKG2D in Autoimmune Diseases

Because ligand binding unconditionally triggers NKG2D without counterbalance by a known antagonist, its dysregulation together with anomalous expression of MIC in local tissue sites may promote autoreactive T cell stimulation. Indeed, recent evidence indicates that MIC-NKG2D may play important roles in the pathogenesis of several autoimmune diseases. In rheumatoid arthritis (RA), the severity of autoimmune and inflammatory joint disease correlates with large numbers of $CD4^+CD28^-$ T cells, which are scarce in healthy individuals. Large proportions of these T cells aberrantly express NKG2D, which is absent from almost all normal CD4 T cells. NKG2D is induced by TNF-α and IL-15, which are present in RA synovia and RA patient sera. RA synoviocytes aberrantly express MIC, presumably because of pannus invasion, and thus stimulate autologous $CD4^+CD28^-$ T cell cytokine production and proliferation (Groh et al. 2003). As with cancer patients, RA serum contains substantial amounts of soluble MIC, which fails to downmodulate NKG2D because of the opposing activity of TNF-α and IL-15. Thus, by causing autoreactive T cell stimulation, MIC-NKG2D may promote the self-perpetuating pathology in RA (Groh et al. 2003). $CD4^+CD28^-$ T cells are also expanded in other autoimmune diseases and chronic inflammatory conditions, including multiple sclerosis, Wegener granulomatosis, ankylosing spondylitis, atherosclerotic coronary artery disease, and inflammatory bowel disease, suggesting the possibility of an involvement of MIC-NKG2D. In active celiac disease, upregulation of MIC on enterocytes by gliadin or its p31–49 peptide triggers NKG2D-dependent activation of IEL, resulting in cytotoxicity against epithelial targets and enhanced TCR-dependent CD8 T cell responses (Hue et al. 2004; Meresse et al. 2004). IL-15-mediated induction of NKG2D and resultant TCR-independent T cell activation may also contribute to villous atrophy (Meresse et al. 2004).

9
Recognition of MIC by Intraepithelial γδ T Cells

Although $V\gamma_2/V\delta_2$ T cells predominate in the circulation, a small subset of γδ T cells defined by the expression of $V_\delta 1$ is enriched in intestinal epithelium and other epithelial sites. Some of these T cells recognize CD1c, a member of the CD1 family of lipid antigen-presenting molecules. In addition, numerous $V_\delta 1$ γδ T cell lines and clones with substantial sequence diversity in the rearranged γ (V-N-J) and δ (V-NDN-J) chains, including variability in nontemplated (N) sequences and numbers of D segments, respond against diverse target cells expressing MICA or MICB (Groh et al. 1998, 1999). These responses are dependent on triggering of TCR and NKG2D, posing the conundrum of whether the γδ TCR recognize MIC or an unidentified surface moiety. This was resolved by demonstration of MICA tetramer binding to various $V_\delta 1$ γδ TCR expressed on transfectants of a T cell line selected for lack of NKG2D (Wu et al. 2002). Tetramer binding was restricted to TCR derived from responder T cell clones classified as reactive against a broad range of MIC-expressing epithelial tumor and transfectant target cells and was abrogated when TCR were composed of mismatched γ and δ chains. These observations, and the inability of $V_\delta 1$ γδ T cells to respond against target cells expressing ULBP ligands of NKG2D, support the model that MIC delivers both the TCR-dependent signal 1 and the NKG2D-dependent costimulatory signal 2 for activation of a subset of $V_\delta 1$ γδ T cells (Wu et al. 2002). This dual function has precedent in the manifold interactions of MHC class I molecules with αβ TCR, the CD8 coreceptor, KIR, and LIR. The γδ TCR-mediated recognition of MIC validates an earlier hypothesis derived from studies of mouse dendritic epidermal T cells, that intraepithelial γδ T cells may recognize stress-inducible self antigens (Havran et al. 1991). At least in humans, this is corroborated by the colocalization of intraepithelial $V_\delta 1$ γδ T cells and MIC in tissue environments that include the intestinal mucosa, sites of viral infection, and epithelial tumors. A potentially important role of $V_\delta 1$ γδ T cells in antitumor immune responses is supported by experiments showing that mice lacking γδ T cells are highly susceptible to carcinogen-induced skin malignancies. Exposure to carcinogens induces skin expression of RAE-1 ligands, which stimulate NKG2D-dependent γδ T cell cytotoxicity (Girardi et al. 2001). The requirement of NKG2D for activation of the human $V_\delta 1$ γδ T cells may be due to suboptimal TCR stimulation by MIC. This may not be the case with $V_\delta 1$ γδ T cells specific for CD1c, which respond against target cells lacking demonstrated expression of NKG2D ligands (Spada et al. 2000).

10
Polymorphism of MIC and Disease Associations

MICA and to a lesser extent MICB are polymorphic, comprising more than 50 and about 15 amino acid substitutions in their extracellular α1α2α3 domains, respectively (Stephens 2001). Unlike MHC class I alleles, all these substitutions are only biallelic and appear randomly distributed. Little is known regarding the functional significance of this allelic variation; however, many substitutions are not conservative, suggesting evolutionary selection instead of random fixation. Mapping onto the MICA crystal structure suggests that some variant amino acid positions may affect interactions with NKG2D whereas most are distant from the NKG2D binding platform or buried inside the folded polypeptide. Analysis of the binding strength of soluble recombinant NKG2D to transfectants expressing five of the most frequent MICA alleles has revealed substantial variations in binding affinities in the range of 10- to 50-fold. These differences are associated with a single amino acid substitution at position 129, methionine or valine, which determines strong (MICA*01 and *07) and weak binding (MICA*04, *08 and *016) alleles, respectively (Steinle et al. 2001). This polymorphism may affect thresholds of NK and T cell activation. In the crystal structure of MICA*01, position 129 is located in the β4 strand of the β-pleated sheet in the α2 domain. Because the side chain of methionine is partially buried and forms hydrophobic interactions with glutamine 136, alanine 139, and methionine 140 in the first α2 helical stretch, its substitution by valine likely affects NKG2D binding indirectly by a conformational change.

Extensive sequence diversity occurs within the MICA transmembrane region, mainly in the number of polyalanine repeats associated with different alleles (Stephens 2001). The MICA*08 allele, which has the highest frequency in Caucasians and Oriental populations, has a premature stop codon resulting in loss of part of the transmembrane region and the cytoplasmic tail. This protein is membrane anchored but fails to be properly sorted in polarized epithelial cells (Suemizu et al. 2002). Another defective allele is MICA*010, which has a single proline for arginine substitution at position 6 in the first β-strand of the α1 domain. This change blocks a β-sheet hydrogen bond with the histidine carbonyl at position 27 on the β2-strand and is incompatible with β-sheet secondary structure, thus interfering with a stable protein fold (Li et al. 2000). Of particular interest is a MIC-null haplotype associated with HLA-B*4801 that is relatively common among the Japanese and very frequent (56.5%) within an Amerindian community in Paraguay (Ota et al. 2000; Russomando et al. 2002). In this haplotype, the entire *MICA* gene is within a 100-(kb deletion and *MICB* has a stop codon in exon 3 encoding the α2 domain. Because individuals homozygous for this haplotype have no discernible immunological deficiency, and significant common disease histories are not apparent, these observations have led to the conclusion that MIC function may not be essential or part of a redundant system. However, a more compelling explanation may eventually emerge, perhaps that loss of MIC expression may confer a selective advantage under certain environmental conditions.

Numerous studies have investigated relationships between MICA alleles and susceptibility to diseases that are associated with the closely linked *HLA-B* and *-C* genes, including ankylosing spondylitis, psoriasis vulgaris, psoriatic arthritis, and Behçet disease (Stephens 2001). However, positive associations are likely secondary because of strong linkage disequilibrium between *MICA* and the two MHC class I genes nearby and have not been confirmed by analyses of different HLA haplotypes in diverse ethnic groups. MICA has also been associated with MHC class II-linked diseases such as insulin-dependent diabetes mellitus (IDDM), Addision disease, sclerosing cholangitis, and celiac disease. However, as yet there is no evidence of a primary genetic association of *MICA* or *MICB* with any disease, and the functional significance of most of the allelic variation of these genes has remained unclear.

As with MHC class I molecules, a direct consequence of MICA polymorphism is the occurrence of autoantibodies in patients with irreversible rejection of allogeneic kidney and pancreas transplants. These show epithelial expression of MIC, which is not seen with normal organs or nonrejected transplants (Hankey et al. 2002; Sumitran-Holgersson et al. 2002). Thus MIC may contribute to allograft rejection, suggesting that matching of donor and recipients may improve clinical outcomes.

Acknowledgements S.G. was supported by the Spanish Fondo de Investigaciones Sanitarias (PI030067). Work from the authors' laboratory was supported by National Institutes of Health Grants AI-30581 and AI-52319.

References

Bacon L, Eagle RA, Meyer M, Easom N, Young NT, Trowsdale J (2004) Two human ULBP/RAET1 molecules with transmembrane regions are ligands for NKG2D. J Immunol 173:1078–1084

Bahram S, Bresnahan M, Geraghty DE, Spies T (1994) A second lineage of mammalian major histocompatibility complex class I genes. Proc Natl Acad Sci USA 91:6259–6263

Bahram S, Spies T (1996) Nucleotide sequence of a human MHC class I MICB cDNA. Immunogenetics 43:230–233

Bauer S, Groh V, Wu J, Steinle A, Phillips JH, Lanier LL, Spies T (1999) Activation of NK cells and T cells by NKG2D, a receptor for stress-inducible MICA. Science 285:727–729

Borges L, Hsu M-L, Fanger N, Kubin M, Cosman D (1997) A family of human lymphoid and myeloid Ig-like receptors, some of which bind to MHC class I molecules. J Immunol 159:5192–5196

Cantoni C, Bottino C, Vitale M, Pessino A, Augugliaro R, Malaspina A, Parolini S, Moretta L, Moretta A, Biassoni R (1999) NKp44, a triggering receptor involved in tumor cell lysis by activated human natural killer cells, is a novel member of the immunoglobulin superfamily. J Exp Med 189:787–796

Castriconi R, Cantoni C, Della Chiesa M, Vitale M, Marcenaro E, Conte R, Biassoni R, Bottino C, Moretta L, Moretta A (2003) Transforming growth factor β1 inhibits expression of NKp30 and NKG2D receptors: consequences for the NK-mediated killing of dendritic cells. Proc Natl Acad Sci USA 100:4120–4125

Cerwenka A, Baron JL, Lanier LL (2001) Ectopic expression of retinoic acid early inducible-1 gene (RAE-1) permits natural killer cell-mediated rejection of a MHC class I-bearing tumor in vivo. Proc Natl Acad Sci USA 98:11521–11526

Chalupny NJ, Sutherland CL, Lawrence WA, Rein-Weston A, Cosman D (2003) ULBP4 is a novel ligand for human NKG2D. Biochem Biophys Res Commun 305:129–135

Cosman D, Müllberg J, Sutherland CL, Chin W, Armitage R, Fanslow W, Kubin M, Chalupny NJ (2001) ULBPs, novel MHC class I-related molecules, bind to CMV glycoprotein UL16 and stimulate NK cell cytotoxicity through the NKG2D receptor. Immunity 14:123–133

Das H, Groh V, Kuijl C, Sugita M, Morita CT, Spies T, Bukowski JF (2001) MICA engagement by human Vγ2Vδ2 T cells enhances their antigen-dependent effector function. Immunity 15:83–93

Diefenbach A, Jensen ER, Jamieson AM, Raulet DH (2001) Rae1 and H60 ligands of the NKG2D receptor stimulate tumour immunity. Nature 413:165–171

Diefenbach A, Tomasello E, Lucas M, Jamieson AM, Hsia JK, Vivier E, Raulet DH (2002) Selective associations with signaling proteins determine stimulatory versus costimulatory activity of NKG2D. Nat Immunol 3:1142–1149

Doubrovina ES, Doubrovin MM, Vider E, Sisson RB, O'Reilly RJ, Dupont B, Vyas YM (2003) Evasion from NK cell immunity by MHC class I-chain related molecules expressing colon carcinoma. J Immunol 171:6891–6899

Dunn C, Chalupny NJ, Sutherland CL, Dosch S, Sivakumar PV, Johnson DC, Cosman D (2003) Human cytomegalovirus glycoprotein UL16 causes intracellular sequestration of NKG2D ligands, protecting against natural killer cytotoxicity. J Exp Med 197:1427–1439

Eleme K, Taner SB, Onfelt B, Collinson LM, McCann FE, Chalupny NJ, Cosman D, Hopkins C, Magee AI, Davis DM (2004) Cell surface organization of stress-inducible proteins ULBP and MICA that stimulate human NK cells and T cells via NKG2D. J Exp Med 199:1005–1010

Girardi M, Oppenheim DE, Steele CR, Lewis JM, Glusac E, Filler R, Hobby P, Sutton B, Tigelaar RE, Hayday AC (2001) Regulation of cutaneous malignancy by γδ T cells. Science 294:605–609

Groh V, Bahram S, Bauer S, Herman A, Beauchamp M, Spies T (1996) Cell stress-regulated human major histocompatibility complex class I gene expressed in gastrointestinal epithelium. Proc Natl Acad Sci USA 93:12445–12450

Groh V, Steinle A, Bauer S, Spies T (1998) Recognition of stress-induced MHC molecules by intestinal epithelial γδ T cells. Science 279:1737–1740

Groh V, Rhinehart R, Secrist H, Bauer S, Grabstein KH, Spies T (1999) Broad tumor-associated expression and recognition by tumor-derived γδ T cells of MICA and MICB. Proc Natl Acad Sci USA 96:6879–6884

Groh V, Rhinehart R, Randolph-Habecker J, Topp MS, Riddell SR, Spies T (2001) Costimulation of CD8 αβ T cells by NKG2D via engagement by MIC induced on virus-infected cells. Nat Immunol 2:255–260

Groh V, Wu J, Yee C, Spies T (2002) Tumour-derived soluble MIC ligands impair expression of NKG2D and T-cell activation. Nature 419:734–738

Groh V, Brühl A, Nelson JL, El-Gabalawi H, Spies T (2003) Stimulation of T cell autoreactivity by anomalous expression of NKG2D and its MIC ligands in rheumatoid arthritis. Proc Natl Acad Sci USA 100, 9452–9457

Hamerman JA, Ogasawara K, Lanier LL (2004) Toll-like receptor signaling in macrophages induces ligands for the NKG2D receptor. J Immunol 172:2001–2005

Hankey KG, Drachenberg CB, Papadimitriou JC, Klassen DK, Philosophe B, Bartlett ST, Groh V, Spies T, Mann DL (2002) MIC expression in renal and pancreatic allografts. Transplantation 73:304–306

Havran WL, Chien YH, Allison JP (1991) Recognition of self antigens by skin-derived T cells with invariant γδ antigen receptors. Science 252:1430–1432

Houchins JP, Yabe T, McSherry C, Bach FH (1991) DNA sequence analysis of NKG2, a family of related cDNA clones encoding type II integral membrane proteins on human natural killer cells. J Exp Med 173:1017–1020

Hue S, Mention JJ, Monteiro RC, Zhang S, Cellier C, Schmitz J, Verkarre V, Fodil N, Bahram S, Cerf-Bensussan N, Caillat-Zucman S (2004) A direct role for NKG2D/MICA interaction in villous atrophy during celiac disease. Immunity 21:367–377

Lanier LL (2001) On guard—activating NK cell receptors. Nat Immunol 2:23–27

Lee JC, Lee KM, Kim DW, Heo DS (2004) Elevated TGF-β1 secretion and down-modulation of NKG2D underlies impaired NK cytotoxicity in cancer patients. J Immunol 172:7335–7340

Lee N, Llano M, Carretero M, Ishitani A, Navarro F, Lopez-Botet M, Geraghty DE (1998) HLA-E is a major ligand for the natural killer inhibitory receptor CD94/NKG2A. Proc Natl Acad Sci USA 95:5199–5204

Li P, Willie ST, Bauer S, Morris DL, Spies T, Strong RK (1999) Crystal structure of the MHC class I homolog MIC-A, a γδ T cell ligand. Immunity 10:577–584

Li P, Morris DL, Willcox BE, Steinle A, Spies T, Strong RK (2001) Complex structure of the activating immunoreceptor NKG2D and its MHC class I-like ligand MICA. Nat Immunol 2:443–451

Li Z, Groh V, Strong RK, Spies T (2000) A single amino acid substitution causes loss of expression of a MICA allele. Immunogenetics 51:246–248

Long EO (1999) Regulation of immune responses through inhibitory receptors. Annu Rev Immunol 17:875–904

McFarland BJ, Strong RK (2003) Thermodynamic analysis of degererate recognition by the NKG2D immunoreceptor: not induced fit but rigid adaptation. Immunity 19:803–812

Meresse B, Chen Z, Ciszewski C, Tretiakova M, Bhagat G, Krausz TN, Raulet DH, Lanier LL, Groh V, Spies T, Ebert EC, Green PH, Jabri B (2004) Coordinated Induction by IL-15 of a TCR-independent pathway converts CTL into lymphokine-activated killer cells in celiac disease. Immunity 21, 357–366

Morimoto RI, Sarge KD, Abravaya K (1992) Transcriptional regulation of heat shock genes. J Biol Chem 267:21987–21990

Moser JM, Gibbs J, Jensen PE, Lukacher AE (2002) CD94-NKG2A receptors regulate antiviral $CD8^+$ T cell responses. Nat Immunol 3:189–195

Noppen C, Schaefer C, Zajac P, Schutz A, Kocher T, Kloth J, Heberer M, Colonna M, De Libero G, Spagnoli GC (1998) C-type lectin-like receptors in peptide-specific HLA class I-restricted expression and modulation of effector functions in clones sharing identical TCR structure and epitope specificity. Eur J Immunol 28:1134–1142

Ota M, Bahram S, Katsuyama Y, Saito S, Nose Y, Sada M, Ando H, Inoko H (2000) On the MICA deleted-MICB null, HLA-B*4801 haplotype. Tissue Antigens 56:268–271

Pende D, Parolini S, Pessino A, Sivori S, Augugliaro R, Morelli L, Marcenaro E, Accame L, Malaspina A, Biassoni R, Bottino C, Moretta L, Moretta A (1999) Identification and molecular characterization of NKp30, a novel triggering receptor involved in natural cytotoxicity mediated by human natural killer cells. J Exp Med 190:1505–1516

Pessino A, Sivori S, Bottino C, Malaspina A, Morelli L, Moretta L, Biassoni R, Moretta A (1998) Molecular cloning of NKp46, a novel member of the immunoglobulin superfamily involved in triggering of natural cytotoxicity. J Exp Med 188:953–960

Ploegh HL (1998) Viral strategies of immune evasion. Science 280:248–253

Radaev S, Rostro B, Brooks AG, Colonna M, Sun PD (2001) Conformational plasticity revealed by the cocrystal structure of NKG2D and its class I MHC-like ligand ULBP3. Immunity 15:1039–1049

Radaev S, Kattah M, You Z, Colonna M, Sun PD (2002) Making sense of the diverse ligand recognition by NKG2D. J Immunol 169:6279–6285

Raulet DH (2003) Roles of the NKG2D immunoreceptor and its ligands. Nat Rev Immunol 3:781–790

Ravetch JV, Lanier LL (2000) Immune inhibitory receptors. Science 290:84–89

Roberts AI, Lee L, Schwartz E, Groh V, Spies T, Ebert EC, Jabri B (2001) NKG2D receptors induced by IL-15 costimulate CD28-negative effector CTL in the tissue microenvironment. J Immunol 167:5527–5530

Rosen, DB, Araki, M, Hamerman JA, Chen T, Yamamura T, Lanier LL (2004) A structural basis for the association of DAP12 with mouse, but not human, NKG2D. J Immunol 173:2470–2478

Russomando AK, Kikuchi M, Candia N, Franco L, Almiron M, Ubalee R, Hirayama K (2002) High frequency of MIC null haplotype (HLA-B48-MICA-del-MICB*0107N) in the Angaite Amerindian community in Paraguay. Immunogenetics 54:439–441

Salih HR, Rammensee HG, Steinle A (2002) Down-regulation of MICA on human tumors by proteolytic shedding. J Immunol 169:4098–4102

Salih HR, Antropius H, Gieseke F, Lutz SZ, Kanz L, Rammensee HG, Steinle A (2003) Functional expression and release of ligands for the activating immunoreceptor NKG2D in leukemia. Blood 102:1389–1396

Siren, J, Sareneva T, Pirhonen J, Strengell M, Veckman V, Julkunen I, Matikainen S (2004) Cytokine and contact-dependent activation of natural killer cells by influenza A or Sendai virus-infected macrophages. J. Gen Virol 85:2357–2364

Spada, FM, Grant EP, Peters PJ, Sugita M, Melian A, Leslie DS, Lee HK, van Donselaar E, Hanson DA, Krensky AM, Majdic O, Porcelli SA, Morita CT, Brenner MB (2000) Self-recognition of CD1 by γδ T cells: implications for innate immunity. J Exp Med 191:937–948

Suemizu H, Radosavljevic M, Kimura M, Sadahiro S, Yoshimura S, Bahram S, Inoko H (2002) A basolateral sorting motif in the MICA cytoplasmic tail. Proc Natl Acad Sci USA 99:2971–2976

Steinle A, Groh V, Bauer S, Spies T (1998) Diversification, expression and γδ T-cell recognition of evolutionary distant members of the MIC family of major histocompatibility complex class I-related molecules. Proc Natl Acad Sci USA 95:12510–12515

Steinle A, Li P, Morris DL, Groh V, Lanier LL, Strong RK, Spies T (2001) Interactions of human NKG2D with its ligands MICA, MICB, and homologs of the mouse RAE-1 protein family. Immunogenetics 53:279–287

Stephens HAF (2001) MICA and MICB genes: can the enigma of their polymorphism be resolved? Trends Immunol 22:378–385

Sumitran-Holgersson S, Wilczek HE, Holgersson J, Soderstrom K (2002) Identification of the nonclassical HLA molecules, MICA, as targets for humoral immunity associated with irreversible rejection of kidney allografts. Transplantation 74:268–277

Tieng V, Le Bouguenec C, du Merle L, Bertheau P, Desreumaux P, Janin A, Charron D, Toubert A (2002) Binding of *Escherichia coli* adhesin AfaE to CD55 triggers cell-surface expression of the MHC class I-related MICA. Proc Natl Acad Sci USA 5:2684–2586

Vetter CS, Groh V, thor Straten P, Spies T, Bröcker E-B, Becker J. Expression of stress-induced MIC molecules on human melanoma. J Invest Dermatol 118, 600–605, 2002

Welte SA, Sinsger C, Lutz SZ, Singh-Jasuja H, Sampaio KL, Eknigk U, Rammensee HG, Steinle A (2003) Selective intracellular retention of virally induced NKG2D ligands by the human cytomegalovirus UL16 glycoprotein. Eur J Immunol 33:194–203

Wu J, Song Y, Bakker ABH, Bauer S, Spies T, Lanier LL, Phillips JH (1999) An activating immunoreceptor complex formed by NKG2D and DAP10. Science 285:730–732

Wu J, Groh V, Spies T (2002) T cell antigen receptor engagement and specificity in the recognition of stress-inducible MIC by human epithelial γδ T cells. J Immumol 169:1236–1240

Wu J, Chalupny NJ, Manley TJ, Riddell SR, Cosman D, Spies T (2003) Intracellular retention of the MHC class I-related chain B ligand of NKG2D by the human CMV UL16 glycoprotein. J Immunol 170:4196–4200

Yamamoto K, Fujiyama Y, Andoh A, Bamba T, Okabe H (2001) Oxidative stress increases MICA and MICB gene expression in the human colon carcinoma cell line (CaCo-2). Biochim Biophys Acta 1526:10–12

NKG2 Receptor-Mediated Regulation of Effector CTL Functions in the Human Tissue Microenvironment

B. Jabri (✉) · B. Meresse

Department of Pathology, University of Chicago, 5841 South Maryland Avenue–S354, Chicago, IL 60637, USA
bjabri@bsd.uchicago.edu

1	Introduction	140
2	TCR and Activating NKRs: The TCR Primacy Rule	140
3	Assembly and Signaling Properties of NKG2D and CD94/NKG2 Receptors Expressed by CTLs	142
4	Tissue Ligands of NKG2D and CD94/NKG2 Receptors	145
5	Regulation of NKG2D and CD94/NKG2 Expression and Function in CTLs	146
5.1	Role of Tissue Environment	146
5.2	Role of TCR Specificity	147
5.3	Role of TCR Engagement	148
5.4	Role of IL-15	149
6	Role of NKG2D and CD94/NKG2 Receptors in Organ-Specific Autoimmunity	151
7	Conclusion	152
	References	153

Abstract NKG2 receptors and their ligands play an essential role in the control of CTL activation in the tissue microenvironment. We discuss the regulation of NKG2 receptor expression by CTL and how uncontrolled activation of NKG2 receptors can lead to organ-specific autoimmune and inflammatory disorders.

Abbreviations
CTL   Cytolytic T lymphocyte
NKR   Natural killer receptor
TCR   T cell receptor

1
Introduction

In human, tissue effector cytolytic T lymphocytes (CTLs) are typically $CD28^-CTLA\text{-}4^-$ but express NKG2D and frequently CD94/NKG2 NK lineage receptors (Dulphy et al. 2002; Groh et al. 2003, 2002; Jabri et al. 2000, 2002; Norris et al. 2003; Perrin et al. 2002; Roberts et al. 2001; Saruhan-Direskeneli et al. 2004; Speiser et al. 1999), indicating that they may follow different activation rules than naive and memory T cells. By recognizing conserved MHC-like ligands induced on tissue cells by stress, inflammation, and transformation, these natural killer receptors (NKRs) up- or downmodulate T cell receptor (TCR) stimulation, thus linking innate with adaptive immunity (reviewed in Lanier 2004; McMahon and Raulet 2001; Vivier and Anfossi 2004). This new layer of T cell regulation at the effector stage serves to focus adaptive effector functions on infected or transformed tissues and may also prevent chronic inflammation and unwanted responses to peripheral tissue-specific antigens, particularly those that are not efficiently cross-presented for tolerance in the draining lymph nodes.

In this review, we focus on the role of NKG2D and CD94/NKG2 receptors in the regulation of human effector CTLs in the tissue microenvironment. We also examine differences in NK receptor expression and function in the NK cell vs. the CTL. Finally, we emphasize unexpected differences between the mouse and human systems.

2
TCR and Activating NKRs: The TCR Primacy Rule

Effector CTLs, although they can express a broad panoply of NKRs, usually lack NKRs that signal through a immunomodulatory tyrosine-based activating motif (ITAM) (Table 1). These ITAMs can recruit kinases from the ZAP70/Syk family and induce alone full cellular activation. Instead, the NKRs expressed by CTLs are characterized by their capacity to modulate, positively or negatively, TCR activation. This ensures that T cell activation remains under the control of the TCR (the TCR primacy rule). For example, NKp46 protein (Moretta and Moretta 2004; Pessino et al. 1998), which associates with CD3ζ and therefore could be potentially expressed on the cell surface of CTL, is not present in CTLs, including in intracellular compartments (unpublished data). Similarly, NKG2C protein is absent in normal conditions, even though transcripts are detected (Jabri et al. 2002 and unpublished data). In addition, CTLs do not express transcripts of the ITAM-bearing adaptor

Table 1 NKRs and their adaptor molecules in human CTL: the TCR primacy rule

Gene	Receptor	Adaptor	Function	Ligand	CTL expression
KLRC2	NKG2C	DAP12	Activator	HLA-E	No
KLRC3	NKG2E	?	?	HLA-E	?
KLRC3	NKG2H	DAP12?	?	HLA-E?	?
KLRC4	NKG2F	DAP12?	?	?	?
KLRK1	NKG2D	DAP10	Costimulation/cytotoxicity	MICA/B,ULBP1,2,3,4	Yes
KLRC1	NKG2A/B	None	Inhibitor	HLA-E	Yes
KIR2DS (1–5)	CD158 (g,h,i,j),nkat7	DAP12	Activator	HLA-C?	No
KIR3DS1	CD158e2	DAP12?	Activator	?	No
KIR2DL (1–5)	CD158 (a,b1,b2,d,f)	None	Inhibitor	HLA-C	Yes
KIR3DL (1–3)	CD158 (k,z,e1)	None	Inhibitor	HLA-A?	Yes
NCR3	NKp30	CD3ζ/FcεR1γ	Activator	?	No
NCR2	NKp44	DAP12	Activator	?	No
NCR1	NKp46	CD3ζ/FcεR1γ	Activator	?	No
NKR-P1A	CD161	?	Costimulation?	?	Yes
CD244	2B4	SAP	Costimulation?	CD48	Yes
CD226	DNAM-1	?	Costimulation	CD112,CD155	Yes
CD96	TACTILE	?	Costimulation	CD155	Yes
LILRB1	ILT2/LIR-1	None	Inhibitor	HLA A,B,C,E,F,G, CMV UL18	Yes

molecule DAP12 (also called KARAP; Olcese et al. 1997), which is required for the expression of NKG2C (Lanier et al. 1998) and NKp44 (Moretta and Moretta 2004; Vitale et al. 1998). Furthermore, even when DAP12 transcripts are induced in T cells in pathological conditions, their presence does not signify that DAP12 protein is expressed, suggesting that DAP12 is also regulated at the translational level. Altogether, these observations suggest that there is a transcriptional and translational regulatory network, involving probably also epigenetic modifications (Uhrberg 2005), that prevents the expression of NKRs associated with ITAM-bearing adaptor molecules in T cells.

Some important exceptions to the TCR primacy rule, however, have emerged. For example during CMV infection CTLs were reported to express surface NKG2C, and similar observations were obtained in conditions of chronic T cell activation in vitro (Ortega et al. 2004) or inflammation in vivo (Guma et al. 2004 and unpublished data). These changes, which may effectively convert the CTL into an NK cell, have major physiopathological implications that are discussed later. Although they could transiently benefit the host in case of infection, they are detrimental in the case of chronic inflammation and may lead to severe immunopathology, as suggested in celiac disease.

3
Assembly and Signaling Properties of NKG2D and CD94/NKG2 Receptors Expressed by CTLs

CD94, NKG2D, and the NKG2 family comprised of A, C, E, and F are genetically and structurally related type II transmembrane proteins with a C-type lectin domain. They are encoded within the NK complex (NKC) on human chromosome 12p12.3–p13.1 (Houchins et al. 1991; Plougastel and Trowsdale 1997; Renedo et al. 1997) and overall display very low levels of polymorphism, CD94 and NKG2A being the most conserved (Shum et al. 2002). NKG2A and NKG2E have splice variants, NKG2B and NKG2E, respectively. The signaling receptors expressed on the cell surface include CD94/NKG2A (Brooks et al. 1997; Carretero et al. 1997; Lazetic et al. 1996) and CD94/NKG2C (Lazetic et al. 1996) disulfide-linked heterodimers, and NKG2D homodimers (Bauer et al. 1999), as well as a yet-undefined CD94/NKG2x/adaptor immunoreceptor complex with coactivating properties (unpublished data) (Fig. 1). CD94 homodimers exist (Lazetic et al. 1996) but probably have no signaling properties. Although transcripts for NKG2E, NKG2H, and NKG2F have been detected in primary human CTLs (Jabri et al. 2002 and unpublished data), their expression pattern remains to be clarified by specific antibodies. In mouse, NKG2E was found to

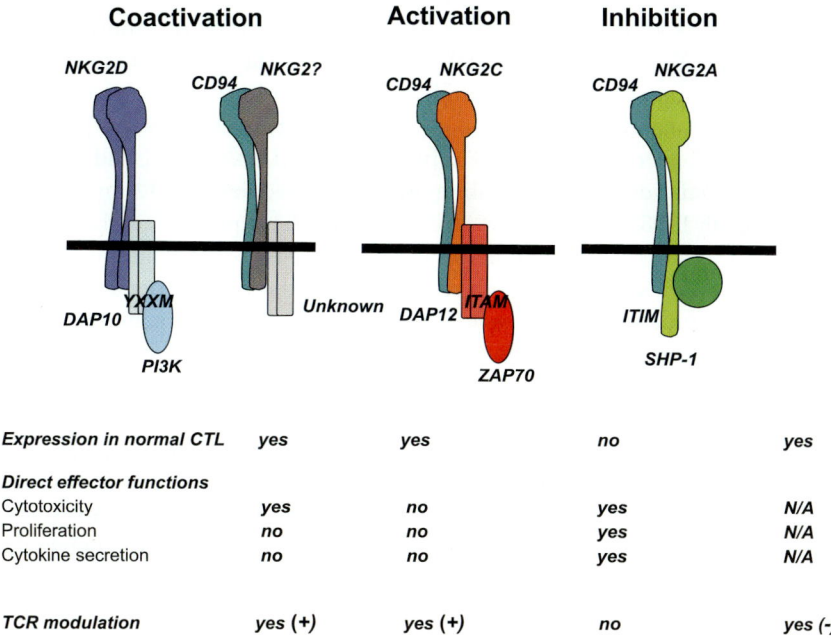

Fig. 1 Expression of CD94/NKG2x and NKG2D receptors in tissue CTL. Under normal conditions, effector CTLs in tissue express NKG2D and may express an inhibitory CD94/NKG2A receptor or a yet-undefined coactivating CD94/NKG2x receptor. However, under pathological conditions, CD94/NKG2C/DAP12 receptors can be induced on CTLs

be expressed on the cell surface in association with DAP12 (Vance et al. 1999). In humans the situation is more complex. In theory, NKG2E and NKG2H could be expressed on the surface, because NKG2E and H transcripts are present and their transmembrane region is identical to the one found in NKG2C, that is, it also contains a lysine residue. However, transfection of NKG2E with CD94 and any of the classic adaptor molecules with a negative charge in the transmembrane, namely, DAP12, CD3ζ, and FcεRIγ, did not result in NKG2E surface expression in various cell types (unpublished data). There is one report suggesting that NKG2H could be expressed on the surface with DAP12 in RBL cells (Bellon et al. 1999). NKG2F, which lacks a extracellular region, is expressed in human NK cells and can associate with DAP12 (Kim et al. 2004; Plougastel and Trowsdale 1997). However, its expression seems confined to the intracellular compartment (Kim et al. 2004) and its role in human T cells remains to be determined.

NKG2A has an immunoreceptor tyrosine-based inhibitory motif (ITIM) that recruits the phosphatase SHP-1 and SHP-2 (SH2 domain-containing protein tyrosine phosphatase) and confers inhibitory properties to the CD94/NKG2A receptor (Carretero et al. 1997; Halary et al. 1997; Houchins et al. 1997; Le Drean et al. 1998). In contrast, CD94/NKG2C and NKG2D require association to the signaling adaptor molecules DAP12 and DAP10 (Lanier et al. 1998; Wu et al. 1999) in order (a) to be expressed on the surface and (a) to signal. DAP12 contains an ITAM, whereas DAP10 contains a PI3-K binding motif, YXXM. Thus both receptors transduce activating signals, but they differ fundamentally in that CD94/NKG2C can fully activate the cell to divide and produce cytokines, whereas NKG2D costimulates in a manner similar to CD28 (Groh et al. 2001; Roberts et al. 2001). Consistent with the TCR primacy rule, CD94/NKG2C is usually not expressed by CTLs, although exceptions were reported in CMV infections (Guma et al. 2004) and on chronic CD4 T cell activation in vitro (Ortega et al. 2004).

Most NKR expression and function is usually restricted to effector CTLs. An apparent exception is NKG2D, which in humans is expressed by virtually all CD8 T cells (Bauer et al. 1999), whereas in mouse it is induced after TCR stimulation (Jamieson et al. 2002). However, NKG2D seems not to be fully functional in human primary naive CD8 T cells (Ehrlich et al. 2005). Another potentially important difference between mouse and human is the induction, on activation of mouse NK cells and T cells, of a short NKG2D splice variant capable of associating with DAP12 (Diefenbach et al. 2002). Consequently, NKG2D stimulation can sometimes result in the recruitment of ZAP70 and the acquisition of new functions, namely, the capacity to mediate cytokine secretion and proliferation. Such transcripts have not been identified in humans yet, and even if they existed, the transmembrane region of NKG2D is predicted to preclude pairing with DAP12 (Rosen et al. 2004). An apparent exception to the TCR primacy rule is the ability of NKG2D to mediate direct cytolysis (although proliferation and cytokine secretion are never observed) (Meresse et al. 2004; Verneris et al. 2003). The NKG2D cytolytic pathway involves PLC-γ, Vav, PI3-kinase, and the MAP kinases JNK and ERK (Billadeau et al. 2003; Meresse et al. 2004). This cytolytic property, however, is restricted to effector CTLs pre-exposed to IL-15 or high doses of IL-2, suggesting temporal control at a defined, transient stage of the CD8 T cell history (Meresse et al. 2004).

4
Tissue Ligands of NKG2D and CD94/NKG2 Receptors

The ligands of NKG2D and CD94/NKG2 belong to families of MHC-like molecules that share the important property of being inducible on solid tissue cells upon stress, transformation, and inflammation (reviewed in Lanier 2004; Raulet 2003). This is highly consistent with a role of these NKRs in focusing the activation of effector CTLs on the appropriate tissue target, namely, a cell that not only is expressing antigen but also exhibits signs of distress.

Thus human NKG2D ligands comprise MICA, MICB (Groh et al. 1996) and ULBP1, -2, -3, and -4 (Cosman et al. 2001; Jan Chalupny et al. 2003), which are distantly related to MHC class I, do not bind peptides, and do not require β2-microglobulin for expression. MIC molecules are highly expressed in embryonic tissue but are poorly expressed in adult tissue, with the exception of the colon, which is constitutively colonized by bacteria. MIC molecules can be induced on transformation, infection, or stress in adult tissue (Groh et al. 1996). MICA and MICB are MHC encoded (Bahram et al. 1994) and do not have a homolog in mouse, whereas ULBP genes are non-MHC encoded and are the orthologs of the mouse RAE-1 genes (Radosavljevic et al. 2002). The other mouse NKG2D ligands comprise H60 and MULT-1, which demonstrate relative low homology to RAE-1 (reviewed in Raulet 2003).

The ligand of CD94/NKG2A and CD94/NKG2C receptors is the nonclassic MHC class I molecule HLA-E (Braud et al. 1998; Llano et al. 1998) and its Qa-1 homolog in mouse (Vance et al. 1999) combined with conserved leader peptides of MHC class I molecules. In human, CD94/NKG2A and CD94/NKG2C also recognize HLA-E with the HLA-G leader peptide (Llano et al. 1998; Vales-Gomez et al. 1999). Because CD94/NKG2C is poorly expressed by CTLs, ligand induction should generally translate into an inhibitory signal when target cells express normal levels of MHC class I. In disease conditions such as CMV (Guma et al. 2004) and severe celiac disease (manuscript in preparation) CTLs can express CD94/NKG2C, but they do not express CD94/NKG2A, thus avoiding a conflict between these opposite forms of signaling. Intriguingly, human NKG2E and its splice variant H differ significantly from the other mouse and human NKG2 molecules in the putative ligand binding site, suggesting that they may display specificities in addition to their ability to bind HLA-E with the classic MHC class I leader peptides (Kaiser et al. 2005). The hsp60 leader peptide, which binds HLA-E but is not recognized by CD94/NKG2A or CD94/NKG2C (Michaelsson et al. 2002), or other viral and stress induced peptides might be interesting candidates because they would allow targeting of CTL responses against damaged or infected tissue cells. Interestingly, as reported for MIC (Wu et al. 2002), HLA-E recognition can also be TCR mediated (Garcia et al. 2002; Pietra et al. 2001), in particular, HLA-E-restricted CTLs with TCR specificity for hsp60 leader peptide (Davies et al. 2003) and CMV peptides (Romagnani et al. 2004) have been identified in mouse and human, respectively.

5
Regulation of NKG2D and CD94/NKG2 Expression and Function in CTLs

Because NKRs are expressed or become functional only at the effector CTL stage, they have the potential to considerably alter the tolerance thresholds established for naive CTL precursors in the thymus and in the periphery. Hence, local and transient induction of their ligands is essential to prevent damaging, chronic autoreactivity in the case of coactivating NKRs. Conversely, expression of inhibitory NKRs (CD94/NKG2A) could play an important role in the prevention of protracted inflammatory processes. There is surprisingly little understanding of the mechanisms that determine the type (coactivating or inhibitory) and specificity of NKRs expressed by a CTL. It is also unclear whether the pattern of NKRs expressed is stable or variable.

5.1
Role of Tissue Environment

There are only limited studies determining the expression pattern of NK receptors in resident tissue effector T cells, because most tissues in humans, with the exception of the intestine and the liver, are difficult to access. In general, CD8 T cells from tissues (e.g., intestine and liver) express more NKRs than CD8 T cells in the blood. For instance, CD94 and NKR-P1A are expressed on more than 30% and 60% of intestinal intraepithelial CTL, respectively, whereas they are expressed by less than 10% of peripheral blood CTL (Jabri et al. 2000). This may be due in part to their effector status as well as to local, tissue-specific influences that increase NKR expression. Conversely, NKRs might in some cases be expressed at lower levels in a tissue than in the peripheral blood. For example, NKG2D expression by CTL in tumor and intestine is lower than in the blood (Lee et al. 2004; Roberts et al. 2001) and might reflect the high level of TGFβ expression in these tissues (Castriconi et al. 2003; Lee et al. 2004).

Further attesting to the impact of the tissue environment on NKR expression is the evidence that NKR expression varies between different tissues. Strikingly, CD56 is expressed by more than 50% of liver CTL and less than 25% of intestinal intraepithelial CTL. Moreover, KIR receptors are significantly expressed in the liver (where more than 12% of liver T cells are CD158b[+] and more than 7% are CD158a⁺), whereas they are present on less than 3% of intraepithelial CTL (Jabri et al. 2000; Norris et al. 2003). Altogether these observations suggest that tissue-specific signals regulate NKR expression in CTL and thus contribute to adapt the effector CTL response to a given tissue environment.

5.2
Role of TCR Specificity

Because NKG2A, unlike KIRs, could be induced in vitro on TCR stimulation in combination with various cytokines (Bertone et al. 1999; Derre et al. 2002; Mingari et al. 1998), it was suggested that NKG2A might be an activation-induced event with no link to TCR specificity. However, if NKRs do modulate TCR signaling during the course of natural immune responses, it is logical to expect some signature distribution of these NKRs based on antigen specificity. Indeed, analysis of naturally expanded CTL clones in the human intestinal epithelium and in peripheral blood not only showed clonal homogeneity with respect to expression of NKG2A but also demonstrated that CTLs expressing TCRs with different but related sequences, that is, sharing the same antigenic specificity, also shared the same NKG2A pattern (Jabri et al. 2002). Conversely, NKG2A was conspicuously absent on activated peripheral T lymphocytes during acute EBV infection (Mingari et al. 1997) and on CMV- and EBV-specific CTLs during chronic infection (Ince et al. 2004) in humans, whereas it was found to be induced on mouse CTLs in all viral infections studied, for example, polyoma virus and LCMV (McMahon et al. 2002; Moser et al. 2002). However, the link between NKR and TCR specificity has not yet been studied in detail in mice. Finally, CD94/NKG2A is not coexpressed with activating CD94/NKG2 receptors in human CTLs (Arlettaz et al. 2004; Guma et al. 2004; Jabri et al. 2002), suggesting that they may not be stochastically expressed. Altogether, these observations indicate that in human CD94/NKG2A expression is tightly regulated. Studies of the KIR system have shown that members of the same in vitro derived human CTL clones could express different KIR patterns (Uhrberg et al. 2001; Vely et al. 2001), revealing a stochastic component in the expression of these receptors. However, it is difficult to draw final conclusions because of the great complexity of the KIR system (due in part to common expression of KIRs in absence of the relevant MHC ligand) and the lack of a complete panel of anti-KIR antibodies, rendering in vivo studies difficult. Further studies examining natural CTL expansions in human natural and disease conditions, as well as experimental systems in mice, are critically needed to better understand this complex but fundamental issue. A key question to be answered is whether expression of various NKRs is instructed by

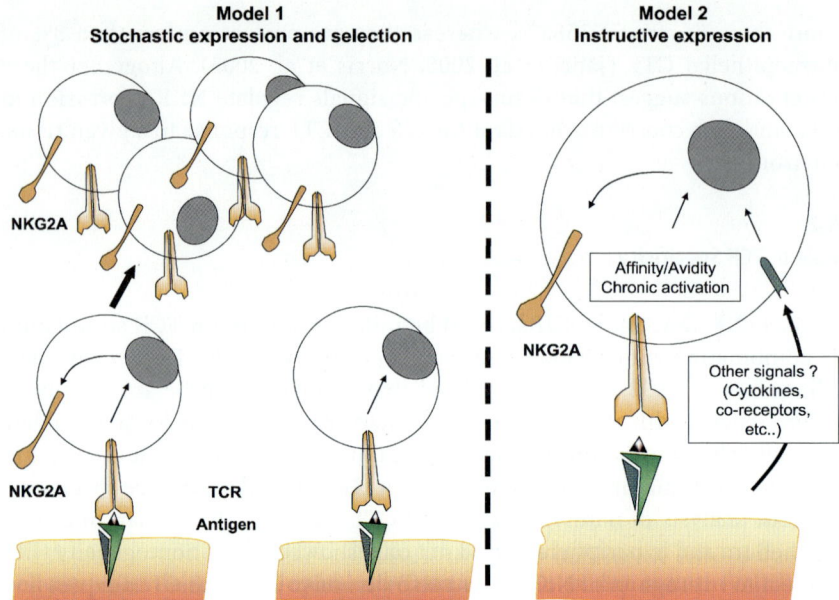

Fig. 2 NKG2A commitment in CTLs. NKG2A expression is determined by the context in which antigen-specific CD8 cells are primed or expanded during the differentiation process into effector/memory CTLs. In the stochastic model 1, NKG2A is induced randomly among naive CTLs stimulated by TCR and plays an important role in their expansion or survival. In the instructive model 2, TCR affinity for the peptide/MHC complex, antigen concentration, cytokine milieu and coreceptors expressed by antigen-presenting cells are among the potential signals that might play a role in NKG2A commitment in naive T cells

the antigenic environment (e.g., antigen concentration, chronicity, cytokines, coreceptors expressed by antigen presenting cells) or stochastic and then selected consequently to the impact of NKRs on CTL expansion or survival as suggested in mice (Gunturi et al. 2003; Ugolini et al. 2001) (Fig. 2).

5.3
Role of TCR Engagement

There is strong evidence suggesting that human effector CTLs expressing a given NKG2A or C isotype are stably committed to that isotype. The stability of NKG2A *expression* seems to vary (Arlettaz et al. 2004; Jabri et al. 2002). However, individual CTLs lacking NKG2A expression, despite a TCR specificity known to be associated with NKG2A in vivo, can be reinduced to express NKG2A within 48 h of TCR engagement in vitro, indicating stable *commitment*

(Jabri et al. 2002). Like CTLA-4, NKG2A may therefore participate in a negative feedback loop in which TCR stimulation upregulates NKG2A expression and, in turn, NKG2A downmodulates TCR activation. This property may explain why some NKG2A induction could be induced in vitro on TCR stimulation on a limited subset of peripheral blood T lymphocytes, representing less than 25% of total T cells (Bertone et al. 1999; Derre et al. 2002; Mingari et al. 1998). Importantly, IL-15, TGF-β, and IL-12 could induce CD94, but not NKG2A, in the absence of concomitant TCR stimulation (Bertone et al. 1999; Derre et al. 2002; Jabri et al. 2000; Jabri et al. 2002; Mingari et al. 1998), further suggesting control of TCR over NKG2A expression. The regulation of NKG2C, NKG2E, and H is still poorly understood. Although transcripts of these genes are found in most memory T cells (Jabri et al. 2002), NKG2C proteins do not seem to be expressed under physiological conditions by human CTLs, as determined by staining with specific antibodies (unpublished data). In vitro studies suggest that NKG2C expression may require chronic T cell activation (Ortega et al. 2004).

5.4
Role of IL-15

IL-15 is an essential cytokine controlling several steps of NKR expression and function. Rather than being released, it is expressed on the cell surface (e.g., APCs, keratinocytes, synovial cells, and intestinal epithelial cells; Jabri et al. 2000; Kurowska et al. 2002; Mention et al. 2003; Neely et al. 2001; Ruckert et al. 2000) bound to the IL-15Rα chain (Dubois et al. 2002). IL-15 protein expression is induced on stress and infection and, in addition to its role in CTL proliferation and homeostasis, has the unique property of upregulating the expression of activating NKR expression and enhancing the effector functions of CTL (Fig. 3). IL-15 increases the level of surface expression of NKG2D and CD94 in otherwise unstimulated CTLs (Jabri et al. 2000; Meresse et al. 2004; Mingari et al. 1998; Roberts et al. 2001). This effect is mediated in part by its capacity to activate CD94, NKG2D, and DAP10 transcription (Groh et al. 2003; Lieto et al. 2003; Meresse et al. 2004). The mechanisms by which IL-15 impacts on the transcription of these molecules is still poorly understood and may involve several mechanisms. For instance, GAS/EBS elements, which are potentially responsive to IL-15 stimulation, have been identified in the CD94 promoter (Lieto et al. 2003). In contrast, IL-15 cannot induce the transcription of NKG2A in the absence of TCR engagement but was found to synergize with TCR for NKG2A expression (Mingari et al. 1998). Its contribution to the expression of the other NKG2 molecules remains to be determined. IL-15 also increases NKG2D expression at the cell surface by preventing NKG2D

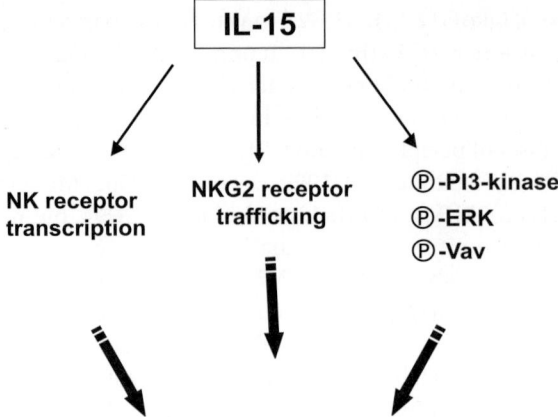

Fig. 3 IL-15 upregulates CTL effector functions by upregulating activating NKRs. IL-15 acts at multiple levels, increasing the expression of NKRs such as CD94 and NKG2D/Dap10 and preventing NKG2D downregulation on receptor engagement. IL-15 also directly activates Vav, PI3-K, and ERK involved in cytolytic signaling pathways. Ultimately, TCR- and IL-15-stimulated CTLs can kill targets expressing NKG2D ligands independently of TCR specificity (LAK conversion)

downregulation by its ligands (Groh et al. 2003). This conspicuous effect might be essential for tumor rejection because many tumors abundantly express and shed NKG2D ligands (Groh et al. 2002). Conversely, preventing NKG2D downregulation may be quite detrimental in chronic conditions and could favor protracted activation of CTLs and autoimmunity.

The physiological importance of IL-15 is exemplified by its remarkably coordinated effects in inducing or activating several components of the NKG2D cytolytic signaling pathway in CTL. Thus, in addition to its effect on NKG2D/DAP10 expression, IL-15 rapidly induces Vav and PI3-kinase dependent ERK phosphorylation in effector CTLs (Meresse et al. 2004 and unpublished data). In fact, exposure to IL-15 alone (or high doses of IL-2) is sufficient to convert CTLs into lymphokine-activated killer (LAK)-like cells that efficiently kill MIC+ targets through NKG2D (Meresse et al. 2004; Verneris et al. 2003). This property not only explains previous reports of CTL conversion into LAK cells in vitro (Brooks 1983; Gamero et al. 1995) but also underlies the aberrant cytolytic properties of intestinal CTLs chronically exposed to IL-15 in the intestinal epithelium of celiac disease patients in vivo. It is highly likely therefore that IL-15 and LAK activity might play an important role in the pathogenesis of celiac diseases and other complex immunopathological disorders.

6
Role of NKG2D and CD94/NKG2 Receptors in Organ-Specific Autoimmunity

Whereas the role of KIR expression by CTLs is suggested mostly by genetic reports and studies performed on peripheral blood lymphocytes (Martin et al. 2002; Momot et al. 2004; Namekawa et al. 2000; Snyder et al. 2003; Yen et al. 2001), there is now strong, converging evidence indicating that NKG2D and CD94/NKG2 receptors play essential roles in the control of effector CTLs in tissues, controlling important disease processes. The presence of abundant melanoma-specific CTLs in patients with progressive tumor has been correlated with expression of inhibitory NKG2A, suggesting that tumors can escape rejection by inducing and engaging inhibitory NKRs (Speiser et al. 1999). Conversely, several studies provide evidence for a role of activating CD94/NKG2 and NKG2D receptors in organ-specific autoimmunity. In rheumatoid arthritis patients, NKG2D was found to be induced on autoreactive CD4 T cells in joint fluid whereas MIC was expressed on synovial cells. High IL-15 expression by synovial cells prevented the downregulation of NKG2D on engagement with molecules, hence sustaining chronic NKG2D activation (Groh et al. 2003). In NOD mice with type I diabetes, islet cells expressed NKG2D ligands and NKG2D function was critical for their destruction by autoreactive CTLs (Ogasawara et al. 2004). In celiac disease patients, activating CD94 receptors are highly upregulated in intraepithelial CTLs (Jabri et al. 2000 and manuscript in preparation) and high expression of IL-15 and MIC by intestinal epithelial cells appeared to prime their killing by intraepithelial CTLs through a TCR-independent, NKG2D-mediated pathway (Hue et al. 2004; Meresse et al. 2004). Altogether, these studies suggest the following model (Fig. 4). Exogenous stress (gluten in celiac disease or viral infection) or endogenous stress (type I diabetes) induces expression of IL-15 and nonclassic MHC class I molecules by tissue cells, initiating a feedback loop resulting in the arming of activating NKRs on CTLs and aberrant tissue destruction. The role of activating NKRs could be to lower the TCR activation threshold for cross-reactive self-antigen or to confer LAK properties against target cells expressing stress markers.

Importantly, the arming of NKG2D is restricted to cytolytic function. NKG2D cannot induce CTLs to secrete cytokines or proliferate, even on IL-15

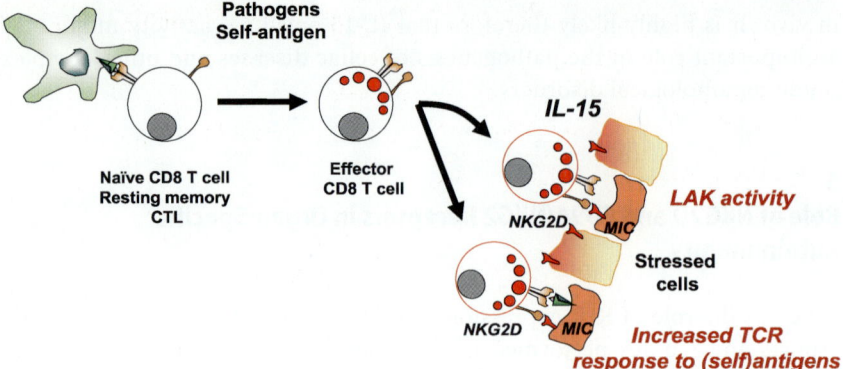

Fig. 4 Tissue control of CTL effector functions by NKG2D and IL-15. NKG2D ligands and IL-15 are expressed by tissue cells in stress and infectious conditions. IL-15 arms the NKG2D cytolytic signaling pathway in effector CTLs, focusing cytolytic activity on tissue targets undergoing stress and infection. This regulation is beneficial for host defense but may also lead to chronic autoimmune and inflammatory disorders

stimulation (Groh et al. 2001; Roberts et al. 2001). Thus NKG2D alone does not explain how CTLs can undergo expansion and secrete IFN-γ in celiac disease. The recent discovery that CTLs could also express CD94/NKG2C/DAP12 immunoreceptor complexes under pathological conditions suggests that another, more severe level of dysregulation occurs in some situations (Guma et al. 2004; Ortega et al. 2004). Ultimately, the loss of TCR control over proliferation might be involved in the malignant transformation of CTLs, as observed in celiac disease (reviewed in Green and Jabri 2003) or in IL-15-overexpressing mice (Fehniger et al. 2001).

7
Conclusion

There is growing evidence that NKRs expressed by CTLs play a fundamental role in tissue immunity, modulating their activation properties based on recognition of stress- and transformation-induced ligands. This dialog between the killers and their victims ensures optimal focusing of adaptive immunity on appropriate targets that express not only infectious antigens but also signs of distress. This new level of regulation of adaptive immunity by innate immunity has obvious benefits for host defense and for self-tolerance. However, increasing evidence points to dysregulation of these mechanisms in the pathology of tumor and autoimmune and inflammatory disorders. Detailed understanding of the regulation of IL-15 and nonclassic MHC class I molecules and their effect on CTL signaling in tissues might illuminate longstanding enigmas in tissue specific immunopathology and suggest new avenues for therapeutic intervention in these widespread diseases.

References

Arlettaz, L., Villard, J., de Rham, C., Degermann, S., Chapuis, B., Huard, B., and Roosnek, E. (2004). *Eur J Immunol* **34,** 3456–64.
Bahram, S., Bresnahan, M., Geraghty, D. E., and Spies, T. (1994). *Proc Natl Acad Sci USA* **91,** 6259–63.
Bauer, S., Groh, V., Wu, J., Steinle, A., Phillips, J. H., Lanier, L. L., and Spies, T. (1999). *Science* **285,** 727–9.
Bellon, T., Heredia, A. B., Llano, M., Minguela, A., Rodriguez, A., Lopez-Botet, M., and Aparicio, P. (1999). *J Immunol* **162,** 3996–4002.
Bertone, S., Schiavetti, F., Bellomo, R., Vitale, C., Ponte, M., Moretta, L., and Mingari, M. C. (1999). *Eur J Immunol* **29,** 23–9.
Billadeau, D. D., Upshaw, J. L., Schoon, R. A., Dick, C. J., and Leibson, P. J. (2003). *Nat Immunol* **4,** 557–64.
Braud, V. M., Allan, D. S., O'Callaghan, C. A., Soderstrom, K., D'Andrea, A., Ogg, G. S., Lazetic, S., Young, N. T., Bell, J. I., Phillips, J. H., Lanier, L. L., and McMichael, A. J. (1998). *Nature* **391,** 795–9.
Brooks, A. G., Posch, P. E., Scorzelli, C. J., Borrego, F., and Coligan, J. E. (1997). *J Exp Med* **185,** 795–800.
Brooks, C. G. (1983). *Nature* **305,** 155–8.
Carretero, M., Cantoni, C., Bellon, T., Bottino, C., Biassoni, R., Rodriguez, A., Perez-Villar, J. J., Moretta, L., Moretta, A., and Lopez-Botet, M. (1997). *Eur J Immunol* **27,** 563–7.
Castriconi, R., Cantoni, C., Della Chiesa, M., Vitale, M., Marcenaro, E., Conte, R., Biassoni, R., Bottino, C., Moretta, L., and Moretta, A. (2003). *Proc Natl Acad Sci USA* **100,** 4120–5.
Cosman, D., Mullberg, J., Sutherland, C. L., Chin, W., Armitage, R., Fanslow, W., Kubin, M., and Chalupny, N. J. (2001). *Immunity* **14,** 123–133.
Davies, A., Kalb, S., Liang, B., Aldrich, C. J., Lemonnier, F. A., Jiang, H., Cotter, R., and Soloski, M. J. (2003). *J Immunol* **170,** 5027–33.
Derre, L., Corvaisier, M., Pandolfino, M. C., Diez, E., Jotereau, F., and Gervois, N. (2002). *J Immunol* **168,** 4864–70.
Diefenbach, A., Tomasello, E., Lucas, M., Jamieson, A. M., Hsia, J. K., Vivier, E., and Raulet, D. H. (2002). *Nat Immunol* **3,** 1142–9.
Dubois, S., Mariner, J., Waldmann, T. A., and Tagaya, Y. (2002). *Immunity* **17,** 537–47.
Dulphy, N., Rabian, C., Douay, C., Flinois, O., Laoussadi, S., Kuipers, J., Tamouza, R., Charron, D., and Toubert, A. (2002). *Int Immunol* **14,** 471–9.
Ehrlich, L. I., Ogasawara, K., Hamerman, J. A., Takaki, R., Zingoni, A., Allison, J. P., and Lanier, L. L. (2005). *J Immunol* **174,** 1922–31.

Fehniger, T. A., Suzuki, K., Ponnappan, A., VanDeusen, J. B., Cooper, M. A., Florea, S. M., Freud, A. G., Robinson, M. L., Durbin, J., and Caligiuri, M. A. (2001). *J Exp Med* **193,** 219–31.

Gamero, A. M., Ussery, D., Reintgen, D. S., Puleo, C. A., and Djeu, J. Y. (1995). *Cancer Res* **55,** 4988–94.

Garcia, P., Llano, M., de Heredia, A. B., Willberg, C. B., Caparros, E., Aparicio, P., Braud, V. M., and Lopez-Botet, M. (2002). *Eur J Immunol* **32,** 936–44.

Green, P. H., and Jabri, B. (2003). *Lancet* **362,** 1419.

Groh, V., Bahram, S., Bauer, S., Herman, A., Beauchamp, M., and Spies, T. (1996). *Proc Natl Acad Sci USA* **93,** 12445–50.

Groh, V., Bruhl, A., El-Gabalawy, H., Nelson, J. L., and Spies, T. (2003). *Proc Natl Acad Sci USA* **100,** 9452–7.

Groh, V., Rhinehart, R., Randolph-Habecker, J., Topp, M. S., Ridell, S. R., and Spies, T. (2001). *Nat Immunol* **2,** 255–260.

Groh, V., Wu, J., Yee, C., and Spies, T. (2002). *Nature* **419,** 734–8.

Guma, M., Angulo, A., Vilches, C., Gomez-Lozano, N., Malats, N., and Lopez-Botet, M. (2004). *Blood* **104,** 3664–71.

Gunturi, A., Berg, R. E., and Forman, J. (2003). *J Immunol* **170,** 1737–45.

Halary, F., Peyrat, M. A., Champagne, E., Lopez-Botet, M., Moretta, A., Moretta, L., Vie, H., Fournie, J. J., and Bonneville, M. (1997). *Eur J Immunol* **27,** 2812–21.

Houchins, J. P., Lanier, L. L., Niemi, E. C., Phillips, J. H., and Ryan, J. C. (1997). *J Immunol* **158,** 3603–9.

Houchins, J. P., Yabe, T., McSherry, C., and Bach, F. H. (1991). *J Exp Med* **173,** 1017–20.

Hue, S., Mention, J. J., Monteiro, R. C., Zhang, S., Cellier, C., Schmitz, J., Verkarre, V., Fodil, N., Bahram, S., Cerf-Bensussan, N., and Caillat-Zucman, S. (2004). *Immunity* **21,** 367–77.

Ince, M. N., Harnisch, B., Xu, Z., Lee, S. K., Lange, C., Moretta, L., Lederman, M., and Lieberman, J. (2004). *Immunology* **112,** 531–42.

Jabri, B., de Serre, N. P., Cellier, C., Evans, K., Gache, C., Carvalho, C., Mougenot, J. F., Allez, M., Jian, R., Desreumaux, P., Colombel, J. F., Matuchansky, C., Cugnenc, H., Lopez-Botet, M., Vivier, E., Moretta, A., Roberts, A. I., Ebert, E. C., Guy-Grand, D., Brousse, N., Schmitz, J., and Cerf-Bensussan, N. (2000). *Gastroenterology* **118,** 867–79.

Jabri, B., Selby, J. M., Negulescu, H., Lee, L., Roberts, A. I., Beavis, A., Lopez-Botet, M., Ebert, E. C., and Winchester, R. J. (2002). *Immunity* **17,** 487–99.

Jamieson, A. M., Diefenbach, A., McMahon, C. W., Xiong, N., Carlyle, J. R., and Raulet, D. H. (2002). *Immunity* **17,** 19–29.

Jan Chalupny, N., Sutherland, C. L., Lawrence, W. A., Rein-Weston, A., and Cosman, D. (2003). *Biochem Biophys Res Commun* **305,** 129–35.

Kaiser, B. K., Barahmand-Pour, F., Paulsene, W., Medley, S., Geraghty, D. E., and Strong, R. K. (2005). *J Immunol* **174,** 2878–84.

Kim, D. K., Kabat, J., Borrego, F., Sanni, T. B., You, C. H., and Coligan, J. E. (2004). *Mol Immunol* **41,** 53–62.

Kurowska, M., Rudnicka, W., Kontny, E., Janicka, I., Chorazy, M., Kowalczewski, J., Ziolkowska, M., Ferrari-Lacraz, S., Strom, T. B., and Maslinski, W. (2002). *J Immunol* **169,** 1760–7.

Lanier, L. L. (2005). *Annu Rev Immunol* **23,** 225–74.

Lanier, L. L., Corliss, B., Wu, J., and Phillips, J. H. (1998). *Immunity* **8**, 693–701.
Lazetic, S., Chang, C., Houchins, J. P., Lanier, L. L., and Phillips, J. H. (1996). *J Immunol* **157**, 4741–5.
Le Drean, E., Vely, F., Olcese, L., Cambiaggi, A., Guia, S., Krystal, G., Gervois, N., Moretta, A., Jotereau, F., and Vivier, E. (1998). *Eur J Immunol* **28**, 264–76.
Lee, J. C., Lee, K. M., Kim, D. W., and Heo, D. S. (2004). *J Immunol* **172**, 7335–40.
Lieto, L. D., Borrego, F., You, C. H., and Coligan, J. E. (2003). *J Immunol* **171**, 5277–86.
Llano, M., Lee, N., Navarro, F., Garcia, P., Albar, J. P., Geraghty, D. E., and Lopez-Botet, M. (1998). *Eur J Immunol* **28**, 2854–63.
Martin, M. P., Nelson, G., Lee, J. H., Pellett, F., Gao, X., Wade, J., Wilson, M. J., Trowsdale, J., Gladman, D., and Carrington, M. (2002). *J Immunol* **169**, 2818–22.
McMahon, C. W., and Raulet, D. H. (2001). *Curr Opin Immunol* **13**, 465–70.
McMahon, C. W., Zajac, A. J., Jamieson, A. M., Corral, L., Hammer, G. E., Ahmed, R., and Raulet, D. H. (2002). *J Immunol* **169**, 1444–52.
Mention, J. J., Ben Ahmed, M., Begue, B., Barbe, U., Verkarre, V., Asnafi, V., Colombel, J. F., Cugnenc, P. H., Ruemmele, F. M., McIntyre, E., Brousse, N., Cellier, C., and Cerf-Bensussan, N. (2003). *Gastroenterology* **125**, 730–45.
Meresse, B., Chen, Z., Ciszewski, C., Tretiakova, M., Bhagat, G., Krausz, T. N., Raulet, D. H., Lanier, L. L., Groh, V., Spies, T., Ebert, E. C., Green, P. H., and Jabri, B. (2004). *Immunity* **21**, 357–66.
Michaelsson, J., Teixeira de Matos, C., Achour, A., Lanier, L., Karre, K., and Soderstrom, K. (2002). *J. Exp. Med.* **196**, 1–13.
Mingari, M. C., Ponte, M., Bertone, S., Schiavetti, F., Vitale, C., Bellomo, R., Moretta, A., and Moretta, L. (1998). *Proc Natl Acad Sci USA* **95**, 1172–7.
Mingari, M. C., Ponte, M., Cantoni, C., Vitale, C., Schiavetti, F., Bertone, S., Bellomo, R., Cappai, A. T., and Biassoni, R. (1997). *Int Immunol* **9**, 485–91.
Momot, T., Koch, S., Hunzelmann, N., Krieg, T., Ulbricht, K., Schmidt, R. E., and Witte, T. (2004). *Arthritis Rheum* **50**, 1561–5.
Moretta, L., and Moretta, A. (2004). *EMBO J* **23**, 255–9.
Moser, J. M., Gibbs, J., Jensen, P. E., and Lukacher, A. E. (2002). *Nat Immunol* **22**, 22.
Namekawa, T., Snyder, M. R., Yen, J. H., Goehring, B. E., Leibson, P. J., Weyand, C. M., and Goronzy, J. J. (2000). *J Immunol* **165**, 1138–45.
Neely, G. G., Robbins, S. M., Amankwah, E. K., Epelman, S., Wong, H., Spurrell, J. C., Jandu, K. K., Zhu, W., Fogg, D. K., Brown, C. B., and Mody, C. H. (2001). *J Immunol* **167**, 5011–7.
Norris, S., Doherty, D. G., Curry, M., McEntee, G., Traynor, O., Hegarty, J. E., and O'Farrelly, C. (2003). *Cancer Immunol Immunother* **52**, 53–8.
Ogasawara, K., Hamerman, J. A., Ehrlich, L. R., Bour-Jordan, H., Santamaria, P., Bluestone, J. A., and Lanier, L. L. (2004). *Immunity* **20**, 757–67.
Olcese, L., Cambiaggi, A., Semenzato, G., Bottino, C., Moretta, A., and Vivier, E. (1997). *J Immunol* **158**, 5083–6.
Ortega, C., Romero, P., Palma, A., Orta, T., Pena, J., Garcia-Vinuesa, A., Molina, I. J., and Santamaria, M. (2004). *Immunol Cell Biol* **82**, 587–95.
Perrin, G., Speiser, D., Porret, A., Quiquerez, A. L., Walker, P. R., and Dietrich, P. Y. (2002). *Immunol Lett* **81**, 125–32.
Pessino, A., Sivori, S., Bottino, C., Malaspina, A., Morelli, L., Moretta, L., Biassoni, R., and Moretta, A. (1998). *J Exp Med* **188**, 953–60.

Pietra, G., Romagnani, C., Falco, M., Vitale, M., Castriconi, R., Pende, D., Millo, E., Anfossi, S., Biassoni, R., Moretta, L., and Mingari, M. C. (2001). *Eur J Immunol* **31,** 3687–93.

Plougastel, B., and Trowsdale, J. (1997). *Eur J Immunol* **27,** 2835–9.

Radosavljevic, M., Cuillerier, B., Wilson, M. J., Clement, O., Wicker, S., Gilfillan, S., Beck, S., Trowsdale, J., and Bahram, S. (2002). *Genomics* **79,** 114–23.

Raulet, D. H. (2003). *Nat Rev Immunol* **3,** 781–90.

Renedo, M., Arce, I., Rodriguez, A., Carretero, M., Lanier, L. L., Lopez-Botet, M., and Fernandez-Ruiz, E. (1997). *Immunogenetics* **46,** 307–11.

Roberts, A. I., Lee, L., Schwarz, E., Groh, V., Spies, T., Ebert, E. C., and Jabri, B. (2001). *J Immunol* **167,** 5527–30.

Romagnani, C., Pietra, G., Falco, M., Mazzarino, P., Moretta, L., and Mingari, M. C. (2004). *Hum Immunol* **65,** 437–45.

Rosen, D. B., Araki, M., Hamerman, J. A., Chen, T., Yamamura, T., and Lanier, L. L. (2004). *J Immunol* **173,** 2470–8.

Ruckert, R., Asadullah, K., Seifert, M., Budagian, V. M., Arnold, R., Trombotto, C., Paus, R., and Bulfone-Paus, S. (2000). *J Immunol* **165,** 2240–50.

Saruhan-Direskeneli, G., Uyar, F. A., Cefle, A., Onder, S. C., Eksioglu-Demiralp, E., Kamali, S., Inanc, M., Ocal, L., and Gul, A. (2004). *Rheumatology (Oxford)* **43,** 423–7.

Shum, B. P., Flodin, L. R., Muir, D. G., Rajalingam, R., Khakoo, S. I., Cleland, S., Guethlein, L. A., Uhrberg, M., and Parham, P. (2002). *J Immunol* **168,** 240–52.

Snyder, M. R., Lucas, M., Vivier, E., Weyand, C. M., and Goronzy, J. J. (2003). *J Exp Med* **197,** 437–49.

Speiser, D. E., Pittet, M. J., Valmori, D., Dunbar, R., Rimoldi, D., Lienard, D., MacDonald, H. R., Cerottini, J. C., Cerundolo, V., and Romero, P. (1999). *J Exp Med* **190,** 775–82.

Ugolini, S., Arpin, C., Anfossi, N., Walzer, T., Cambiaggi, A., Forster, R., Lipp, M., Toes, R. E., Melief, C. J., Marvel, J., and Vivier, E. (2001). *Nat Immunol* **2,** 430–5.

Uhrberg, M. (2005). *Mol Immunol* **42,** 471–5.

Uhrberg, M., Valiante, N. M., Young, N. T., Lanier, L. L., Phillips, J. H., and Parham, P. (2001). *J Immunol* **166,** 3923–32.

Vales-Gomez, M., Reyburn, H. T., Erskine, R. A., Lopez-Botet, M., and Strominger, J. L. (1999). *EMBO J* **18,** 4250–60.

Vance, R. E., Jamieson, A. M., and Raulet, D. H. (1999). *J Exp Med* **190,** 1801–12.

Vely, F., Peyrat, M., Couedel, C., Morcet, J., Halary, F., Davodeau, F., Romagne, F., Scotet, E., Saulquin, X., Houssaint, E., Schleinitz, N., Moretta, A., Vivier, E., and Bonneville, M. (2001). *J Immunol* **166,** 2487–94.

Verneris, M. R., Karami, M., Baker, J., Jayaswal, A., and Negrin, R. S. (2004). *Blood* 103, 3065–72.

Vitale, M., Bottino, C., Sivori, S., Sanseverino, L., Castriconi, R., Marcenaro, E., Augugliaro, R., Moretta, L., and Moretta, A. (1998). *J Exp Med* **187,** 2065–72.

Vivier, E., and Anfossi, N. (2004). *Nat Rev Immunol* **4,** 190–8.

Wu, J., Groh, V., and Spies, T. (2002). *J Immunol* **169,** 1236–40.

Wu, J., Song, Y., Bakker, A. B., Bauer, S., Spies, T., Lanier, L. L., and Phillips, J. H. (1999). *Science* **285,** 730–2.

Yen, J. H., Moore, B. E., Nakajima, T., Scholl, D., Schaid, D. J., Weyand, C. M., and Goronzy, J. J. (2001). *J Exp Med* **193,** 1159–67.

Dendritic Cell–NK Cell Cross-Talk: Regulation and Physiopathology

L. Zitvogel[1] (✉) · M. Terme[1] · C. Borg[1] · G. Trinchieri[2]

[1]Immunology Unit, ERM0208 INSERM, Institut Gustave Roussy, 39 rue Camille Desmoulins, 94805 Villejuif, France
zitvogel@igr.fr

[2]Schering Plough, Dardilly, France

1	Introduction on Dendritic Cells	158
2	Why Is the Interaction of Antigen-Presenting Cells with NK Cells of High Interest?	159
3	Regulation of NK Cell Activation by DC	160
4	NK Cell Priming by DC in Lymph Nodes	162
5	The DC–NK Cell Interplay in the Periphery	164
6	Reciprocal Activation of DC by NK Cells	164
7	DC–NK Cell Cross-Talk During Infectious Diseases	165
8	DC–NK Cell Cross-Talk in Cancer	167
9	Concluding Remarks	169
	References	170

Abstract Dendritic cells (DC) are key players at the interface between innate resistance and cognate immunity. Recent evidence highlighted that innate effector cells can induce DC maturation, a checkpoint for the triggering of primary T cell responses in vivo. Moreover, mature DC also promote NK cell effector functions, necessary and sufficient, in some cases, for Th1 polarization. The site of the DC–NK cell interplay likely determines its relevance in physiopathology and the outcome on the ongoing immune response. This review focuses on the current knowledge of the regulation of NK cell priming by DC and, reciprocally, on the consequences of NK cell activation on DC functions. The relevance of DC–NK cell cross-talk in the control of infectious diseases and tumor growth is discussed, highlighting the impact of this dialogue on the design of immunotherapy protocols.

1
Introduction on Dendritic Cells

This chapter discusses the interaction of NK cells with the professional antigen-presenting cells of the immune system, the dendritic cells (DC), in regulating both innate resistance and adaptive immunity. DC are antigen-presenting cells, cornerstones between pathogen entry and lymph nodes that quickly respond to foreign antigens. Located in peripheral organs, skin, and mucosal surfaces, DC sample the environment for self and foreign material [1]. However, after antigen uptake DC, in order to process and present the antigen within MHC class I and II molecules, must undergo a complex maturation program that is triggered by exposure to stress signals. Such stress signals can be ligands for Toll-like receptors (TLR) (such as conserved molecules expressed by pathogens, double- or single-stranded RNA, CpG DNA [2–4]), proinflammatory cytokines, and/or T cell-derived-stimuli (such as CD40L). After DC maturation, DC migrate, upregulate the expression of MHC class I and II and costimulatory molecules, and become very efficient at priming naive T cells.

The best-characterized human blood DC subsets are the myeloid DC (mDC) and the plasmacytoid precursor DC (pDC). $CD11c^+/CD1a^+/CD14^-$ mDC can be purified from blood or lymphoid organs. DC with similar characteristics can be differentiated in culture from bone marrow or cord blood $CD34^+$ cells in the presence of GM-CSF and TNFα or IL-4 [5] or from monocytes in the presence of GM-CSF and IL-4 [6]. pDC are isolated from blood or lymphoid organs, exhibit a $CD11c^-/CD123^+/BDCA2^+/CD45RA^+$ phenotype, and produce large amounts of type I interferon (IFN) on exposure to viruses or CpG oligonucleotides [7]. mDC and pDC differentially express TLR: TLR3, -4, and -8 are found in mDC but not in pDC, and TLR7 and -9 are found in pDC but not in mDC [8–10]. Both DC subsets can elicit Th1/Th2 polarization [11–13]. The current prevailing view is that a functional DC specificity is not imparted during DC ontogeny but that plasticity enables appropriate responses to various pathogens [14].

Three major mouse DC subsets have been identified in secondary lymphoid organs [15]. Two of these subsets express high levels of CD11c. The $CD11c^{bright}/CD11b^+/CD8\alpha^-$ DC subset localizes in the spleen marginal zone bridging channels, whereas the $CD11c^{bright}/CD11b^-/CD8\alpha^+$ DC subset bearing DEC205 (interdigitating DC) is mostly localized in T cell areas of the spleen, where it efficiently primes naive T cells. The $CD11c^{bright}/CD11b^-/CD8\alpha^+$ DC subset is electively endowed with the ability to cross-present exogenous antigen [16]. Plasmacytoid precursor DC (pDC), the third subset, are $CD11c^{dim}/B220^+/Ly6C^+/CD45RA^+/120G8^+/PDCA-1^+$ cells that are broadly distributed in lymphoid and nonlymphoid organs. In the spleen, pDC are dispersed in the T cell zone and the red pulp [15]. $CD11c^{bright}/CD11b^+$ DC and pDC can be propagated from bone marrow precursors in GM-CSF (with or without TNFα or IL-4) [17, 18] and Flt3-L [19], respectively. Likewise, DC can be propagated from mouse splenocytes in Flt3-L, GM-CSF, and IL-6 [20]. Mouse pDC express higher levels of TLR7 and -9 than $CD11c^{bright}$ DC, which express more abundant levels of TLR4 [8]. Whereas pDC produce large amounts of type I IFN when exposed to viruses [21], $CD11c^{bright}$ DC infected by viruses can also produce type I IFN [22]. All mouse DC subsets can produce IL-12 and induce Th1 polarization [14, 23].

2
Why Is the Interaction of Antigen-Presenting Cells with NK Cells of High Interest?

IFN-γ is produced during incubation of blood mononuclear cells (PBMC) with some TLR ligands (such as polyI:C for TLR3 or R848 for TLR7–8). The main source of IFN-γ is the NK cell pool together with NKT cells and unconventional T cells. However, in the absence of HLA-DR$^+$ antigen-presenting cells, IFN-γ is no longer produced by NK cells. Except for TLR2 ligands (KpOmpA) or TLR3 ligands that have been described to directly trigger NK cell production of defensins or chemokines, antigen-presenting cells are needed to promote NK cell reactivity in vitro [24, 25]. These HLA-DR$^+$ cells required for induction of IFN-γ production by NK cells in response to stimulation via TLR3 or TLR7–8 are mDC, whereas pDC or $CD14^+/CD16^{+/-}$ monocytes are mostly inactive. However, as few as 0.2% of pDC preexposed to influenza virus or CpG ODN (TLR9 ligands) can trigger NK cell lytic activity against the NK cell-resistant Daudi target cells [26]. The regulation of NK cell activation by DC is being slowly unraveled in the mouse and human settings, for both cytolytic and secretory activities as a function of the stimuli received by DC. Indeed, in the absence of stimulation, immature DC cannot promote NK cell effector functions. In Sect. 8.8, we will, however, describe pathophysiological stimuli leading to NK cell triggering in the absence of DC maturation (i.e., DC inhibition of c-kit tyrosine kinase and expression of the BCR/ABL protooncogene).

3
Regulation of NK Cell Activation by DC

Pioneering studies by Fernandez et al. showed that the DC growth factor Flt3-L, which promotes both DC and NK cell expansion, was also capable of promoting in nude mice a NK cell-dependent antitumor effect that could be significantly abrogated by treatment with an anti-CD8α mAb [27]. These experiments suggested a direct role for CD8α$^+$ DC in NK cell triggering in vivo. This role was directly demonstrated by the adoptive transfer of the mouse DC cell line D1 into AK7 mesothelioma tumors, leading to tumor eradication except in nude mice in which NK cells were depleted by concomitant administration of neutralizing anti-NK1.1 Ab. Furthermore, it was demonstrated that in vitro bone marrow-derived DC (BM-DC) or D1 cells stimulated by TNFα could stimulate NK cell effector functions. Neither macrophages nor NK cell targets could promote NK cell lytic activity in vitro to the levels induced by mature DC. However, the molecular mechanisms by which TNFα–stimulated DC mediate NK cell activation remain unknown [27]. Afterwards, most of the murine studies used BM-DC stimulated with TLR4 ligands such as LPS or *Escherichia coli* bacteria. After TLR4 triggering, BM-DC propagated in the absence of IL-4, transiently produced IL-2 [28, 29], and induced IL-2-dependent IFNγ secretion by mouse NK cells in vitro [30] (Fig. 1a). In this setting, low-level type I IFN produced by BM-DC stimulated by *E. coli* promoted NK cell cytotoxicity [30]. In this setting, NK cell activation was dependent on cell-to-cell contact but independent of IL-12 and IL-18. In vivo, inoculation of *E. coli* promoted NK cell IFNγ production and DC represented a source of IL-2 contributing to NK cell activation [30].

However, IL-2 was not produced by BM-DC propagated in the presence of IL-4 and stimulated with LPS [31]. Rather, IL-15 and IL-15Rα were upregulated and play a critical role to promote NK cell cytotoxicity and IFN-γ secretion in vitro [32] (Fig. 1b). Borg et al. [33] by using cells from IL-12 genetically deficient mice, revealed a critical role for IL-12 in NK cell IFN-γ secretion promoted by mature mouse DC. In the absence of LPS stimulation, BM-DC generated in the presence of IL-4 were able to activate NK cells, unlike BM-DC generated in the absence of IL-4. The triggering receptor expressed on myeloid cells-2 (TREM2) associated with KARAP/DAP12 adaptor molecule was upregulated on BM-DC by IL-4 and was involved in DC-mediated NK cell activation [34] (Fig. 1c).

The molecular mechanisms involved in NK cell triggering by human DC start to be unraveled. Mature DC or immature DC in the presence of maturation stimuli, such as LPS or *Mycobacterium tuberculosis* or IFNα, are able to activate NK cells [35–38]. The crucial role of IL-12 in IFN-γ secretion by

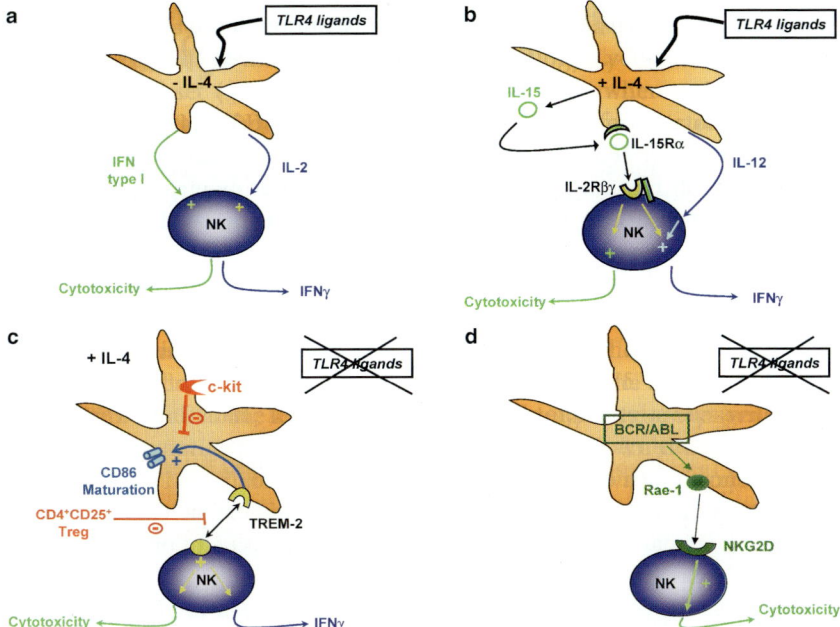

Fig. 1a–d Regulation of the DC-mediated NK cell activation in mouse models. TLR ligands, protooncogenes BCR/ABL and c-kit, and Treg can modulate the DC–NK cell dialogue. TLR4 ligands promote IL-2 and IFNα production when triggering a DC differentiated in the absence of IL-4 (**a**). In the presence of IL-4, TLR4 ligands promote IL-15Rα and IL-15 expression required for NK cell activation (**b**). In DC propagated in GM-CSF and IL-4, but not stimulated with TLR4 ligands, the TREM2/KARAPDAP12 signaling pathway is critical for the bidirectional activation (**c**). The BCR/ABL tyrosine kinase endows DC with NK cell stimulatory capacities in a NKG2D-dependent manner by upregulating Rae-1 expression (**d**). The c-kit receptor and CD4$^+$CD25$^+$ T reg inhibit the bidirectional DC–NK cell interaction (**c**)

human NK cells stimulated by monocyte- or CD34$^+$-derived DC and LPS or by peripheral blood mDC in response to TLR3 or TLR8 ligands has been formally demonstrated. Other cytokines, such as IL-18, and/or cellular contacts are also involved [26, 33, 36] (S. Burg, F. Briere, G. Trinchieri, C. Caux, P. Garrone, unpublished results). However, NK cell activation by DC also requires direct cell-to-cell contacts and depends on the adhesion molecule LFA-1 [39]. The formation of DC/NK cell conjugates was found to depend on cytoskeleton remodeling and lipid raft mobilization in DC. BM-DC derived from mice with loss of function of the Wiskott Aldrich syndrome protein, a major cytoskeletal regulator expressed in hematopoietic cells, fail to promote NK cell lytic activity and IFN-γ secretion [33]. Moreover, disruption of the DC cytoskeleton with pharmacological agents abolished the DC-mediated NK cell activation. Synapse formation promoted the polarized secretion of preassembled stores of IL-12 by DC toward the NK cell. Synaptic delivery of IL-12 by DC was found to be required for IFN-γ secretion by NK cells, as assessed with inhibitors of cytoskeleton rearrangements and Transwell experiments. Therefore, the cross-talk between LPS-activated DC and NK cells is dictated by functional synapses [33].

Upon IFNα stimulation, MHC-class I-related chain-A and -B (MICA/B), ligands for NKG2D receptor are induced on monocyte-derived DC and are responsible for NK cell activation [40]. MICA/B expression on DC is modulated not only by type I IFN but also by DC derived IL-15 [41].

Myeloid DC stimulated by TLR3 ligands and plasmacytoid DC after exposure to viruses or TLR9 ligands promote NK cell lytic activity in a type I IFN-dependent fashion [26].

Mature monocyte-derived DC and, to a much lesser extent, $CD34^+$-derived interstitial dermal-like DC induce human NK activation and proliferation by a mechanism requiring IL-15 and IL-12. Langerhans cells (LC), in contrast, fail to induce NK cell activation, probably because of their impaired ability to produce IL-12 and IL-15Rα. They require exogenous IL-2 or IL-12 to activate NK cells in vitro [42]. However, LC can maintain NK cell survival in vitro after a proliferation phase induced by interstitial dermal DC [42].

4
NK Cell Priming by DC in Lymph Nodes

Unlike in peripheral blood and spleen, the presence of NK cells in lymph nodes (LN) has been controversial. However, recent data have shown that numerous NK cells are located in LN around B cell follicles in the T cell area in close vicinity with $DEC205^+$ DC [43]. Most of NK cells in LN are $CD56^{bright}/CD94/NKG2A^+/NKG2D^+$ [44, 45], but unlike circulating NK cells they are noncytotoxic and perforin negative and do not express KIRs, CD16, and other NCRs (NKp30 and NKp46) [43]. The total number of LN NK cells in humans is, in the absence of infection or inflammation, ten times higher than circulating NK cells. LN NK cells have the potential to react to incoming DC to secrete cytokines regulating Th differentiation or to develop into cytotoxic NK cells [43, 44]. Indeed, recent studies have shown that in culture DC derived from secondary lymphoid organs and activated with LPS induced IFN-γ production from $CD56^{bright}$ NK cells within 6 h [43]. In this scenario, DC could activate resident LN NK cells and would contribute to the regulation of LN resident $CD56^{bright}$ NK cell cytokine secretion (IFN-γ but also TNF, GM-CSF, IL-10, and IL-13). However, an alternative scenario could be that on migration and arrival in LN, DC recruit NK cells from blood through high endothelial venules (HEV). In the periphery $CD56^{bright}$ NK cells, which are preferentially activated by interaction with DC in vitro, express CCR7 and CD62L, and thus could be selectively recruited into the LN [46, 47], but $CD56^{dim}$ NK cells could be also recruited to LN by other chemokines secreted by DC. Adoptive transfer studies of labeled NK cells in mouse demonstrated that circulating NK cells can be found in draining LN after inoculation of mature DC or *Leishmania major* promastigotes [48, 49]. Using two-photon intravital microscopy with a fluorescent tracker specific for NK cell monitoring (anti-CD49b), Bajenoff et al. [49] characterized NK cell behavior in mouse LN in the steady state and on infection with *L. major*. In the steady state, NK cells resided in the LN outer paracortex in close vicinity with DC near the HEV. Unlike T cells, which moved rapidly, NK cells were slow motile-cells. After infection with the parasite, NK cells rapidly accumulated in the LN outer paracortex in close interaction with DC and T cells and secreted IFN-γ but did not acquire higher motility [49].

Terme et al. [34] were the first to show that adoptively transferred DC (footpad inoculation) can prime NK cells in the LN in vivo. Only BM-DC differentiated in the presence of IL-4 or matured with LPS could promote NK cell activation in LN. In experiments in which BM-DC differentiated in the presence of IL-4 were injected in nude mice, the number of $DX5^+$ or $NK1.1^+$ NK cells expressing CD69 was increased twofold by 24 h, whereas in immunocompetent C57Bl/6 mice, the number of $CD69^+$ NK cells was increased three- to fourfold, suggesting a potential role for IL-2 produced by $CD4^+$ T cells in this NK cell activation [34]. However, an 11-fold increase of $CD69^+$ NK cells was observed in draining lymph nodes when mice were pretreated at metronomic dosing with cyclophosphamide (CTX) that suppresses $CD4^+CD25^+$ T regulatory functions (Ghiringhelli et al., J Exp Med in press). We confirmed that $CD4^+CD25^+$ T cells (Treg) regulate DC–NK cell cross-talk in vitro by inhibiting both the DC-mediated induction of NK cell IFNγ secretion and the NK cell-mediated DC activation (Terme et al., in preparation) (Fig. 1c). In the CTX-treated mice, IL-4-propagated BM-DC producing high amounts of fractalkine promoted NK cell recruitment in LN in a CX3CR1- and CCR5-dependent manner (Terme et al., in preparation).

After the pioneering studies by Scharton and Scott [50] that demonstrated that IFN-γ production by NK cells in draining LN was necessary for the protective Th1 response to *L. major* infection, more recent data have highlighted the role of NK cell recruitment in LN in the induction of Th1 polarization [48]. LN NK cell recruitment was shown to be triggered by footpad injection of LPS-activated DC or adjuvants such as R848 or Ribi (but not by CpG1826 or CFA) and was dependent on CXCR3 rather than on CCR7 [48]. NK cell depletion leads to defective Th1 polarization after LPS-matured OVA-pulsed DC injection. IFN-γ produced by migrating NK cells was necessary for Th1 polarization. However, it remains to be determined whether IFN-γ produced by NK cells is necessary at the level of naive T cells or at the level of DC presenting the MHC class II/OVA complexes [48].

5
The DC–NK Cell Interplay in the Periphery

Other sites of DC–NK cell interactions could be inflamed tissues. The chemokine receptor repertoire of $CD56^{dim}CD16^+$ blood NK cells (expressing CXCR1 and CX3CR1) suggests that they could migrate in response to IL-8 and soluble fractalkine [51]. A direct contact between DC and NK cells was first shown in *Malassezia*-induced atopic skin lesions [52] and later highlighted in imatinib mesylate (Gleevec/STI571)-induced lichenoid dermatitis [53]. We recently observed aberrant $PEN5^+$ NK cell infiltrates in tissues infiltrated with malignant Langerhans cell histiocytosis (C. Borg, unpublished data), suggesting that a dysregulation of the LC-NK cell cross-talk could participate in chronic inflammation.

6
Reciprocal Activation of DC by NK Cells

Communication between DC and NK cells is not unidirectional but bidirectional [36, 54–56]. Indeed, activated NK cells can induce or augment not only maturation of DC but also their lysis. Pioneering reports highlighted that in low NK-to-DC cell ratios, activated NK cells would favor DC maturation in in vitro human studies [36, 54]. Soluble factors such as TNF and IFN-γ, as well as cell-to-cell contacts, are required for NK cell-mediated DC activation [36, 54]. DC activation in response to activated NK cells results in DC maturation, upregulation of costimulatory and MHC class II molecules, enhanced antigen-presenting ability, and production of IL-12 [36, 54]. Strikingly, activated NK cells induce type I IFN and TNF production from plasmacytoid DC in the presence of suboptimal stimuli, for example, CpG [26]. We have reported in a mouse model that BM-DC generated in the presence of IL-4 are able to activate NK cells and in turn activated NK cells promote maturation of DC characterized by upregulation of CD80 and CD86. This maturation is in part due to the TREM2/KARAP/DAP12 pathway, at least for upregulation of CD86 [34].

NK cell activation could be a critical checkpoint for T cell responses considering that, in some circumstances, NK cell triggering promotes DC activation. Maillard et al. have shown that activated human NK cells (stimulated by tumor targets and type I IFN) induce DC maturation and that mature DC could promote Th1 response by producing large amounts of IL-12 [57]. DC activation by NK cells that had encountered target cells in the presence of type I IFN was dependent on soluble factors. In a mouse tumor model, Mocikat et al. highlighted the role of an appropriate threshold for NK cell triggering by tumor cells to induce DC activation, IL-12 production, and T cell priming in vivo [58].

A more intriguing aspect of the NK-DC interaction pertains to the capacity of activated NK cells to kill immature DC. Unlike most healthy cells, immature DC are uniquely susceptible to NK cell-mediated cytolysis [55, 59, 60]. The NK-to-DC ratio determines the outcome of DC: As previously discussed a low ratio (1 NK/5 DC) favors DC maturation, whereas a high ratio (5 NK/1 DC) results in DC lysis [54]. Signals delivered by NKp30 are critical to account for lysis of immature monocyte-derived DC [55]. A recent observation described that NK cell TRAIL can eliminate immature DC in vivo, limiting the efficacy of vaccination [61]. Indeed, elimination of NK cells or neutralization of TRAIL function during immunization with immature DC loaded with tumor antigens significantly enhanced cognate T cell responses [61]. Only immature DC are susceptible to NK cell lysis [59, 60, 62]. The resistance to NK cells is at least in part related to the upregulation of MHC class I molecules observed on DC during maturation [63]. The capacity of NK cells to lyse DC is confined to a small NK cell subset expressing the inhibitory receptor CD94/NKG2A and is inversely proportional to the density of this receptor [64]. However, a small CD94/NKG2A^{low} NK cell subset is capable of killing mature DC [64]. The physiological relevance of the phenomenon, however, remains unclear. In particular, unlike monocyte-derived immature DC, freshly isolated human peripheral blood myeloid and plasmacytoid DC have been shown to be resistant to NK cell killing [26].

7
DC–NK Cell Cross-Talk During Infectious Diseases

NK cells have been widely proposed to play a role in the resistance to viral infection in both patients and experimental animals, in particular those induced by herpesviruses, hepatitis viruses, and HIV [65, 66]. A critical role for NK cells in mice in the defense against MCMV infection has been clearly demonstrated [67]. The NK cell-mediated cytolytic functions against infected cells are essential in the spleen, and a critical role for cytokine and chemokine released by NK cells has been demonstrated in the liver [68]. Viral replication in the spleen is controlled genetically by the *Cmv1* locus [69, 70] encoding the Ly49H NK cell-activating receptor [71] that is present on a subset of NK cells and recognizes the MCMV m157 glycoprotein [72, 73]. The protective Ly49H$^+$ NK cell subset is expanded late in infection [74]. Andrews et al. [75] have demonstrated a functional interaction between Ly49H$^+$ NK cells and CD8α^+ DC whereby the expansion of Ly49H$^+$ NK cells favors the survival of spleen CD8α^+ DC during acute infection by MCMV, which, per se, impairs DC functions [76]. Reciprocally, CD8α^+ DC are essential for the expansion of Ly49H$^+$ NK cells via IL-12 and IL-18 [75]. The importance for NK cell expansion of additional signals such as those involving recognition by the NK cell Ly49H receptor of m157 on infected cells is unclear. Whether the DC–NK cell interaction during MCMV infection is determinant for the generation of an adaptive memory T cell response is still questionable.

The role of pDC and of the TLR9/MyD88 signaling pathways in MCMV viral clearance has been studied [77–79]. CpG motifs are abundant in the genomes of alpha and beta herpesviruses such as HSV and MCMV. Because these genomes are not highly methylated, the immunostimulatory capacities of CpG motifs are preserved. Both pDC and DC recognize MCMV through TLR9 [79]. TLR9-mediated type I IFN and IL-12 cytokine secretion promotes viral clearance by NK cells expressing Ly49H [79]. The depletion of pDC by mAb led to drastic reduction of type I IFN secretion but allowed other cell types to compensate and secrete high levels of IL-12, ensuring enhanced levels of IFN-γ and normal NK cell responses to MCMV [77–79]. Therefore, the TLR9/MyD88 pathway mediated a coordinated antiviral cytokine response promoted by pDC, DC, and macrophages allowing effective NK cell function and MCMV clearance [78, 79].

The functional relevance of DC-derived IL-2 in activation of NK cell bactericidal activity was recently reported [30]. The authors investigated whether the clearance of i.v. injected bacteria was different in RAG2$^{-/-}$ mice reconstituted with WT BM-DC that strongly induced NK cell IFNγ production or IL-2$^{-/-}$ BM-DC that were inefficient in promoting NK cell functions. At early time points after bacterial inoculation, the predominant source in vivo of IFN-γ was represented by NK cells. The number of bacteria in the spleen of mice reconstituted with IL-2$^{-/-}$ BM-DC was significantly higher than in the spleen of mice treated with WT DC [30].

8
DC–NK Cell Cross-Talk in Cancer

It is assumed that tumor cells are poorly immunogenic and not recognized by the immune system because proinflammatory signals required for DC activation are missing in vivo. However, NK cell activation, either spontaneously induced by the characteristics of the tumor cell transplanted (e.g., MHC class I low, TAP deficient) [80–82] or forced by overexpression on the tumor cells of NKG2D ligands [83, 84], CD27 [85], or gp96 [86], has been shown to promote the elicitation of cognate and protective immune responses to the tumor [57, 58, 85, 86]. IFN-γ secreted during NK cell-mediated tumor rejection is critical for CTL generation, particularly when tumors express CD70 or CD80 and CD86. However, tumor rejection following recognition of NKG2D ligands by NK cells led to CTL development in the absence of IFN-γ but required $CD4^+$ T cell help [87].

Following the studies of Fernandez et al. [27] demonstrating the relevance of DC-mediated NK cell activation in tumor rejection in a model of MHC class I low mesothelioma, we [53] showed that modulation of the c-kit tyrosine kinase signaling pathway in DC by imatinib mesylate (STI571/Gleevec) led to marked NK cell activation in various strains of mice. Indeed, 10- to 21-day oral therapy with STI571 promoted the selective expansion of $CD69^+$ NK cells and NK cell-dependent antitumor effects in tumor transplantation models using cells that were resistant to STI571 in vitro. This antitumor effect was augmented by pretreatment of mice with the DC growth factor Flt3-L. In vitro studies in which BM-DC propagated in the presence of GM-CSF and IL-4 were incubated in the presence of increasing doses of STI571 highlighted that nanomolar concentrations of STI571 were sufficient to endow DC with the ability to stimulate NK cells in vitro but did not promote DC maturation (Fig. 1c). The activation of NK cell IFNγ secretion by STI571-stimulated DC was not dependent on IL-12 but required cell-to-cell contacts. STI571 likely acted by inhibiting the c-kit pathway in DC because identical results were obtained by utilizing the pharmacological agent or DC from c-kit loss-of-function mutant W/W^v mice. The ability of STI571 to endow DC with NK cell stimulatory capacities was also achieved in a human setting using $CD34^+$ progenitors propagated in GM-CSF and TNF. Importantly, we could show that up to 50% of patients bearing a gastrointestinal sarcoma (GIST) and treated with STI571 acquired enhanced NK cell effector functions. Specifically, the levels of NK cell IFN-γ secretion promoted by ex vivo stimulation with mature DC were significantly enhanced 3- to 50-fold in patients treated for 2 months with STI571. The relevance of NK cell activation was suggested by a significant positive correlation between early NK cell triggering at 2 months and the objective clinical response at 1 year in a cohort of 42 patients, and importantly, the time to progression is significantly longer in patients exhibiting NK cell activation during the first 2 months of therapy. GIST cells display many of the typical features of NK cell sensitivity (TAP1 deficiency, overexpression of MIC and ULBP at mRNA and protein levels, loss of MHC class I molecules) and are lysed by NK cells derived from normal volunteers as efficiently as the prototypic highly NK susceptible K562 cells [53]. NK cells from 50% of GIST patients at diagnosis displayed downregulation of NKG2D expression that was not restored by STI571 despite clinical responses. The study of circulating DC in these patients may highlight some interesting findings pertaining to the DC/NK cell dialogue in vivo.

With groundbreaking data from clinical trials, Ruggeri et al. highlighted that mismatch of NK cell receptors and ligands during haploidentical bone marrow transplantation may be used to enhance engraftment and to prevent leukemia relapse by boosting graft-versus-leukemia effects without augmenting the risk of developing graft-versus-host disease [88]. However, HLA-C/KIR mismatches between residual recipient leukemic cells and donor NK cells might not fully account for NK cell activation in vivo, and host DC might play a critical role for NK cell triggering in this setting [88, 89]. Indeed, the cytokine storm associated with graft conditioning and/or concomitant infectious agents could promote DC maturation and NK cell activation. Nevertheless, the success of donor lymphocyte infusion in controlling residual disease in chronic myeloid leukemia (CML) patients with the BCR/ABL translocation remains poorly understood. We hypothesized [90] that the BCR/ABL translocation in myeloid DC might confer to DC selective NK cell stimulatory capacities in the absence of danger signals. We [90] have shown that monocyte-derived DC from CML patients were selectively endowed with NK cell stimulatory capacity. Using a gene transfer approach in mouse bone marrow progenitors, we demonstrated that BCR/ABL promoted DC-mediated NK cell activation. The DC–NK cell cross-talk promoted by the BCR/ABL translocation appears unique because JunB or interferon consensus sequence binding protein (ICSBP) loss of functions, which are also associated with other myeloproliferative disorders, did not promote DC-mediated NK cell activation. NK cell activation by BCR/ABL-expressing DC involved enhancement of expression of NKG2D activating receptors, and both NK cell activation and NKG2D enhancement were blocked by STI571 (Fig. 1d). Moreover, although NK cells from CML-developing mice did not secret IFNγ in response to IL-2, they responded to autologous BCR/ABL DC. We confirmed in CML patients that CML DC overexpressed NKG2D ligands and that CML DC-induced NK cell killing activity is partially inhibited by either STI571 or anti-NKG2D neutralizing antibody (Fig. 1d). However, CML DC were not mature and displayed only poor allostimulatory activities [90].

Therefore, the clonal BCR/ABL DC displayed the unique and selective ability to activate NK cells, suggesting that they may participate in the NK cell control of CML. Thus the treatment of CML patients with STI571, although critical at the early stage for its direct antileukemic effects reducing the tumor burden, might have at later stages a deleterious effect on the host DC–NK cell interaction.

9
Concluding Remarks

The emerging data on the regulation and mechanisms of DC–NK cell interaction are not yet shedding full light on the precise relevance of this interaction to the course of infectious diseases, tumor progression, and autoimmune disorders. However, the role of NK cells in these pathophysiological settings clearly needs to be readdressed in light of the new data. DC-mediated NK cell activation might be critical for the outcome of T cell responses, but it remains to be defined whether the surrounding antigen-presenting cells or the T cell themselves are the target of NK cell-derived cytokines. To fully appreciate the physiological role of NK cells in the immune response, it is essential to gain a deeper understanding of the differential regulation of various NK cell subsets by DC subsets and of the coordinated interaction between pDC, mDC, and NK cells. NK-DC interaction can lead to DC activation and may represent a critical link between innate resistance and cognate immunity, but the significance of a potential amplification loop of NK-DC cross-talk to NK or T cell activation is still questionable. Also, the biological relevance of the NK cell-mediated DC killing is unclear, and our recent results showing that Treg interfere in DC–NK cell cross-talk might contribute to the interpretation of this phenomenon. Some clues of the NK-DC interplay could be provided by dynamic studies in two-photon microscopy. Nevertheless, from our present understanding of DC–NK cross-talk realistic therapeutic possibilities are emerging, such as adoptive cell therapy and/or manipulation of bone marrow grafts to enhance NK cell activity with DC and the use of small molecules such as tyrosine kinase inhibitors to modulate NK cell functions in vivo.

References

1. Steinman RM. (2003) Some interfaces of dendritic cell biology. Apmis 111:675–697
2. Rescigno M et al. (1999) Coordinated events during bacteria-induced DC maturation. Immunol Today 20:200–203
3. Hartmann G et al. (1999) CpG DNA: a potent signal for growth, activation, and maturation of human dendritic cells. Proc Natl Acad Sci USA 96:9305–9310
4. Cella M et al. (1999) Maturation, activation, and protection of dendritic cells induced by double-stranded RNA. J Exp Med 189:821–829
5. Caux C et al. (1996) CD34+ hematopoietic progenitors from human cord blood differentiate along two independent dendritic cell pathways in response to GM-CSF+TNFα. J Exp Med 184:695–706
6. Sallusto F and Lanzavecchia A. (1994) Efficient presentation of soluble antigen by cultured human dendritic cells is maintained by granulocyte/macrophage colony-stimulating factor plus interleukin 4 and downregulated by tumor necrosis factor α. J Exp Med 179:1109–1118
7. Hochrein H et al. (2002) Human and mouse plasmacytoid dendritic cells. Hum Immunol 63:1103–1110
8. Reis e Sousa C. (2004) Toll-like receptors and dendritic cells: for whom the bug tolls. Semin Immunol 16:27–34
9. Krug A et al. (2001) Toll-like receptor expression reveals CpG DNA as a unique microbial stimulus for plasmacytoid dendritic cells which synergizes with CD40 ligand to induce high amounts of IL-12. Eur J Immunol 31:3026–3037
10. Jarrossay D et al. (2001) Specialization and complementarity in microbial molecule recognition by human myeloid and plasmacytoid dendritic cells. Eur J Immunol 31:3388–3393
11. Kalinski P et al. (1999) Final maturation of dendritic cells is associated with impaired responsiveness to IFN- and to bacterial IL-12 inducers: Decreased ability of mature dendritic cells to produce IL-12 during the interaction with Th cells. J Immunol 162
12. Vieira PL et al. (2000) Development of Th1-inducing capacity in myeloid dendritic cells requires environmental instruction. J Immunol 164:4507–4512
13. Tanaka H et al. (2000) Human monocyte-derived dendritic cells induce naive T cell differentiation into T helper cell type 2 (Th2) or Th1/Th2 effectors: Role of stimulator/responder ratio. J Exp Med 192:405–411
14. Boonstra A et al. (2003) Flexibility of mouse classical and plasmacytoid-derived dendritic cells in directing T helper type 1 and 2 cell development: dependency on antigen dose and differential toll-like receptor ligation. J Exp Med 197:101–109
15. Shortman K and Liu YJ. (2002) Mouse and human dendritic cell subtypes. Nat Rev Immunol 2:151–161
16. den Haan JM et al. (2001) CD8+ but not CD8− dendritic cells cross-prime cytotoxic T cells in vivo. J Exp Med 192:1685–1695
17. Inaba K et al. (1992) Generation of large numbers of dendritic cells from mouse bone marrow cultures supplemented with granulocyte/macrophage colony-stimulating factor. J Exp Med 176:1693–1702
18. Mayordomo JI et al. (1996) Therapy of murine tumors with p53 wild-type and mutant sequence peptide-based vaccines. J Exp Med 183:1357–1365

19. Gilliet M et al. (2002) The development of murine plasmacytoid dendritic cell precursors differentially regulated by Flt3-ligand and granulocyte/macrophage colony-stimulating factor. J Exp Med 195:953–958
20. Berthier R et al. (2000) A two-step culture method starting with early growth factors permits enhanced production of functional dendritic cells from murine splenocytes. J Immunol Methods 239:95–107
21. Asselin-Paturel C et al. (2001) Mouse type I IFN-producing cells are immature APCs with plasmacytoid morphology. Nat Immunol 2:1144–1150
22. Diebold SS et al. (2003) Viral infection switches non-plasmacytoid dendritic cells into high interferon producers. Nature 424:324–328
23. Cella M et al. (2000) Plasmacytoid dendritic cells activated by influenza virus and CD40L drive a potent TH1 polarization. Nat Immunol 1:305–310
24. Chalifour A et al. (2004) Direct bacterial protein PAMP recognition by human NK cells involves TLRs and triggers α-defensin production. Blood 104:1778–1783
25. Sivori S et al. (2004) CpG and double-stranded RNA trigger human NK cells by Toll-like receptors: induction of cytokine release and cytotoxicity against tumors and dendritic cells. Proc Natl Acad Sci USA 101:10116–10121
26. Gerosa F et al. (2005) The reciprocal interaction of NK cells with plasmacytoid or myeloid dendritic cells profoundly affects innate resistance functions. J Immunol 174:727–734
27. Fernandez NC et al. (1999) Dendritic cells directly trigger NK cell functions: cross-talk relevant in innate anti-tumor immune responses in vivo. Nat Med 5:405–411
28. Granucci F et al. (2001) Inducible IL-2 production by dendritic cells revealed by global gene expression analysis. Nat Immunol 2:882–888
29. Granucci F et al. (2003) Early IL-2 production by mouse dendritic cells is the result of microbial-induced priming. J Immunol 170:5075–5081
30. Granucci F et al. (2004) A contribution of mouse dendritic cell-derived IL-2 for NK cell activation. J Exp Med 200:287–295
31. Sauma D et al. (2004) Interleukin-4 selectively inhibits interleukin-2 secretion by lipopolysaccharide-activated dendritic cells. Scand J Immunol 59:183–189
32. Koka R et al. (2004) Cutting edge: murine dendritic cells require IL-15Rα to prime NK cells. J Immunol 173:3594–3598
33. Borg C et al. (2004) NK cell activation by dendritic cells (DCs) requires the formation of a synapse leading to IL-12 polarization in DCs. Blood 104:3267–3275
34. Terme M et al. (2004) IL-4 confers NK stimulatory capacity to murine dendritic cells: a signaling pathway involving KARAP/DAP12-triggering receptor expressed on myeloid cell 2 molecules. J Immunol 172:5957–5966
35. Fernandez NC et al. (2002) Dendritic cells (DC) promote natural killer (NK) cell functions: dynamics of the human DC/NK cell cross talk. Eur Cytokine Netw 13:17–27
36. Gerosa F et al. (2002) Reciprocal activating interaction between natural killer cells and dendritic cells. J Exp Med 195:327–333
37. Amakata Y et al. (2001) Mechanism of NK cell activation induced by coculture with dendritic cells derived from peripheral blood monocytes. Clin Exp Immunol 124:214–222

38. Yu Y et al. (2001) Enhancement of human cord blood CD34+ cell-derived NK cell cytotoxicity by dendritic cells. J Immunol 166:1590–1600
39. Poggi A et al. (2002) NK cell activation by dendritic cells is dependent on LFA-1-mediated induction of calcium-calmodulin kinase II: inhibition by HIV-1 Tat C-terminal domain. J Immunol 168:95–101
40. Jinushi M et al. (2003) Critical role of MHC class I-related chain A and B expression on IFN-α-stimulated dendritic cells in NK cell activation: impairment in chronic hepatitis C virus infection. J Immunol 170:1249–1256
41. Jinushi M et al. (2003) Autocrine/paracrine IL-15 that is required for type I IFN-mediated dendritic cell expression of MHC class I-related chain A and B is impaired in hepatitis C virus infection. J Immunol 171:5423–5429
42. Munz C et al. (2005) Mature myeloid dendritic cell subsets have distinct roles for activation and viability of circulating human natural killer cells. Blood 105:266–273
43. Ferlazzo G et al. (2004) Distinct roles of IL-12 and IL-15 in human natural killer cell activation by dendritic cells from secondary lymphoid organs. Proc Natl Acad Sci USA 101:16606–16611
44. Ferlazzo G et al. (2004) The abundant NK cells in human secondary lymphoid tissues require activation to express killer cell Ig-like receptors and become cytolytic. J Immunol 172:1455–1462
45. Ferlazzo G and Munz C. (2004) NK cell compartments and their activation by dendritic cells. J Immunol 172:1333–1339
46. Vitale M et al. (2004) The small subset of CD56brightCD16− natural killer cells is selectively responsible for both cell proliferation and interferon-γ production upon interaction with dendritic cells. Eur J Immunol 34:1715–1722
47. Frey M et al. (1998) Differential expression and function of L-selectin on CD56bright and CD56dim natural killer cell subsets. J Immunol 161:400–408
48. Martin-Fontecha A et al. (2004) Induced recruitment of NK cells to lymph nodes provides IFN-γgamma for T_H1 priming. Nat Immunol 5:1260–1265
49. Bajenoff M et al. (2004) NK cells are slow motile cells localized in the lymph node outer paracortex where they make contacts with dendritic cells. (Pasteur, I., ed.)
50. Scharton TM and Scott P. (1993) Natural killer cells are a source of interferon γ that drives differentiation of CD4+ T cell subsets and induces early resistance to *Leishmania major* in mice. J Exp Med 178:567–577
51. Cooper MA et al. (2001) The biology of human natural killer-cell subsets. Trends Immunol 22:633–640
52. Buentke E et al. (2002) Natural killer and dendritic cell contact in lesional atopic dermatitis skin—*Malassezia*-influenced cell interaction. J Invest Dermatol 119:850–857
53. Borg C et al. (2004) Novel mode of action of c-kit tyrosine kinase inhibitors leading to NK cell-dependent antitumor effects. J Clin Invest 114:379–388
54. Piccioli D et al. (2002) Contact-dependent stimulation and inhibition of dendritic cells by natural killer cells. J Exp Med 195:335–341
55. Ferlazzo G et al. (2002) Human dendritic cells activate resting natural killer (NK) cells and are recognized via the NKp30 receptor by activated NK cells. J Exp Med 195:343–351

56. Zitvogel L. (2002) Dendritic and natural killer cells cooperate in the control/switch of innate immunity. J Exp Med 195: F9–14
57. Mailliard RB et al. (2003) Dendritic cells mediate NK cell help for Th1 and CTL responses: two-signal requirement for the induction of NK cell helper function. J Immunol 171:2366–2373
58. Mocikat R et al. (2003) Natural killer cells activated by MHC class I(low) targets prime dendritic cells to induce protective CD8 T cell responses. Immunity 19:561–569
59. Wilson JL et al. (1999) Targeting of human dendritic cells by autologous NK cells. J Immunol 163:6365–6370
60. Carbone E et al. (1999) Recognition of autologous dendritic cells by human NK cells. Eur J Immunol 29:4022–4029
61. Hayakawa Y et al. (2004) NK cell TRAIL eliminates immature dendritic cells in vivo and limits dendritic cell vaccination efficacy. J Immunol 172:123–129
62. Ferlazzo G et al. (2003) The interaction between NK cells and dendritic cells in bacterial infections results in rapid induction of NK cell activation and in the lysis of uninfected dendritic cells. Eur J Immunol 33:306–313
63. Ferlazzo G et al. (2001) HLA class I molecule expression is up-regulated during maturation of dendritic cells, protecting them from natural killer cell-mediated lysis. Immunol Lett 76:37–41
64. Chiesa MD et al. (2003) The natural killer cell-mediated killing of autologous dendritic cells is confined to a cell subset expressing CD94/NKG2A, but lacking inhibitory killer Ig-like receptors. Eur J Immunol 33:1657–1666
65. Biron CA et al. (1989) Severe herpesvirus infections in an adolescent without natural killer cells. N Engl J Med 320:1731–1735
66. Biron CA. (1999) Initial and innate responses to viral infections—pattern setting in immunity or disease. Curr Opin Microbiol 2:374–381
67. Bancroft GJ et al. (1981) Genetic influences on the augmentation of natural killer (NK) cells during murine cytomegalovirus infection: correlation with patterns of resistance. J Immunol 126:988–994
68. Tay CH and Welsh RM. (1997) Distinct organ-dependent mechanisms for the control of murine cytomegalovirus infection by natural killer cells. J Virol 71:267–275
69. Scalzo AA et al. (1990) Cmv-1, a genetic locus that controls murine cytomegalovirus replication in the spleen. J Exp Med 171:1469–1483
70. Scalzo AA et al. (1992) The effect of the Cmv-1 resistance gene, which is linked to the natural killer cell gene complex, is mediated by natural killer cells. J Immunol 149:581–589
71. Brown MG et al. (2001) Vital involvement of a natural killer cell activation receptor in resistance to viral infection. Science 292:934–937
72. Arase H et al. (2002) Direct recognition of cytomegalovirus by activating and inhibitory NK cell receptors. Science 296:1323–1326
73. Smith HR et al. (2002) Recognition of a virus-encoded ligand by a natural killer cell activation receptor. Proc Natl Acad Sci USA 99:8826–8831
74. Dokun AO et al. (2001) Specific and nonspecific NK cell activation during virus infection. Nat Immunol 2:951–956

75. Andrews DM et al. (2003) Functional interactions between dendritic cells and NK cells during viral infection. Nat Immunol 4:175–181
76. Andrews DM et al. (2001) Infection of dendritic cells by murine cytomegalovirus induces functional paralysis. Nat Immunol 2:1077–1084
77. Dalod M et al. (2002) Interferon α/βand interleukin 12 responses to viral infections : pathways regulating dendritic cell cytokine expression in vivo. J Exp Med 195:517–528
78. Dalod M et al. (2003) Dendritic cell responses to early murine cytomegalovirus infection: subset functional specialization and differential regulation by interferon α/β. J Exp Med 197:885–898
79. Krug A et al. (2004) TLR9-dependent recognition of MCMV by IPC and DC generates coordinated cytokine responses that activate antiviral NK cell function. Immunity 21:107–119
80. Karre K et al. (1986) Selective rejection of H-2-deficient lymphoma variants suggests alternative immune defence strategy. Nature 319:675–678
81. Ljunggren HG and Karre K. (1985) Host resistance directed selectively against H-2-deficient lymphoma variants. Analysis of the mechanism. J Exp Med 162:1745–1759
82. Glas R et al. (2000) Recruitment and activation of natural killer (NK) cells in vivo determined by the target cell phenotype. An adaptive component of NK cell-mediated responses. J Exp Med 191:129–138
83. Cerwenka A et al. (2000) Retinoic acid early inducible genes define a ligand family for the activating NKG2D receptor in mice. Immunity 12:721–727
84. Diefenbach A et al. (2000) Ligands for the murine NKG2D receptor: expression by tumor cells and activation of NK cells and macrophages. Nat Immunol 1:119–126
85. Kelly JM et al. (2002) Induction of tumor-specific T cell memory by NK cell-mediated tumor rejection. Nat Immunol 3:83–90
86. Strbo N et al. (2003) Perforin is required for innate and adaptive immunity induced by heat shock protein gp96. Immunity 18:381–390
87. Hayakawa Y et al. (2002) Cutting edge: tumor rejection mediated by NKG2D receptor-ligand interaction is dependent upon perforin. J Immunol 169:5377–5381
88. Ruggeri L et al. (2002) Effectiveness of donor natural killer cell alloreactivity in mismatched hematopoietic transplants. Science 295:2097–2100
89. Ruggeri L et al. (1999) Role of natural killer cell alloreactivity in HLA-mismatched hematopoietic stem cell transplantation. Blood 94:333–339
90. Terme et al. (2005) BCR/ABL promotes dendritic cell-mediated natural killer cell activation. Cancer res 65:6409–6417

NK Cell Activating Receptors and Tumor Recognition in Humans

C. Bottino[1] · L. Moretta[1,2] · A. Moretta[2] (✉)

[1] Istituto Giannina Gaslini, Largo G. Gaslini 5, 16147 Genova, Italy

[2] Dipartimento di Medicina Sperimentale, Università degli Studi di Genova, Via L.B. Alberti 2, 16132 Italy
alemoret@unige.it

1	The NK Receptor Complex	175
2	Receptors	177
3	Coreceptors	177
4	Receptors or Coreceptors?	179
5	Concluding Remarks	180
References		181

Abstract Natural killer (NK) cells have been known for many years as the lymphocyte subset characterized by the highest cytolytic potential against virus-infected and tumor-transformed cells. A surprisingly high number of surface molecules have been recognized that regulate human NK cell function. These include MHC-specific inhibitory receptors, which impair NK cells' ability to attack normal self-tissues, and activating receptors and coreceptors that allow them to recognize and kill transformed cells. The recent identification of some of the cellular ligands specifically recognized by these receptors/coreceptors contributes to elucidation of the mystery of the role played by NK cells in immune responses.

1
The NK Receptor Complex

Natural killer (NK) lymphocytes are potent effector cells that, unlike T lymphocytes, are able to lyse targets in the absence of a priori stimulation. Notably, NK cells do not represent indistinct killers because they are equipped with a large array of surface molecules that allow them to discriminate between normal cells and potentially dangerous targets. NK cells express MHC class I (MHC I)-specific receptors that after recognition of ligands on surrounding normal cells inhibit the NK-mediated cytolytic activity [1–4]. In the case of virus infection or tumor transformation, cells can downregulate MHC I expression [5, 6] while upregulating ligands for NK activating molecules. Thus, in the absence of an efficient inhibition, engagement of activating molecules results in the enchainment of the NK-mediated cytotoxicity and target cell lysis [7–9]. Various activating molecules have been identified whose expression is either restricted to NK cells or shared by other cell types. Moreover, some of these molecules appear to function as main receptors, whereas others play a coactivator role. Thus a modern concept could be that, similar to T lymphocytes, NK cells recognize targets via a "NK receptor complex" formed by private receptors whose activity is sustained by public coreceptor molecules (Fig. 1).

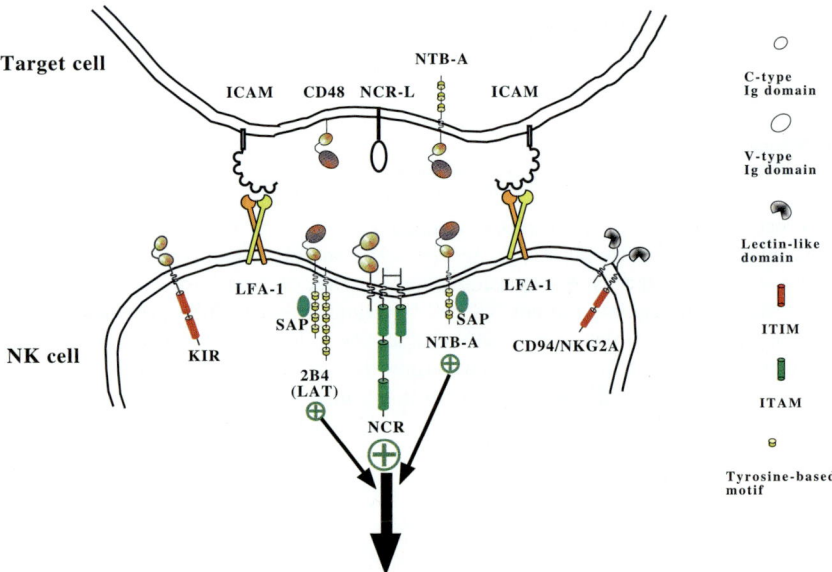

Fig. 1 NK receptor complex-ligand interactions. Natural killer (NK) cells express surface molecules that exert either inhibitory or activating function. Tumor targets downregulate HLA class I expression while expressing different ligands for activating NK molecules. In the absence of engagement of MHC class I-specific receptors (KIR and CD94/NKG2A), the interaction of receptors (NCR) and coreceptors (2B4 and NTB-A) with the specific ligands (NCR-L, CD48, and NTB-A) results in strong activation of NK-mediated cytolytic activity. Note that also the LFA-1-ICAM interactions are a common requirement for efficient target cell lysis being involved in the organization of immune synapses [38]

2
Receptors

The Natural cytotoxicity receptors (NCR) family includes three Ig-like molecules termed NKp46 (CD335), NKp44 (CD336), and NKp30 (CD337) [10] selectively expressed by all NK cells. In particular, NKp46 and NKp30 are present on both resting and activated NK cells, whereas NKp44 is acquired only on activation, its expression at the cell surface correlating with the acquisition of optimal cytolytic activity by activated NK cells. NCR associate with ITAM-containing polypeptides such as CD3ζ and Fcγ (NKp46 and NKp30) or DAP12 (NKp44) [9], which after receptor engagement become tyrosine phosphorylated via Src family kinases, recruit Syk family kinases [11], and transduce signals leading to activation of NK cell functions. Interestingly, NCR, instead of representing individual receptors, appear to form a molecular complex because both their expression and functions are coordinated. Indeed, NCR are present either at high or at low surface densities on NK cells (referred as NCR^{bright} or NCR^{dull}, respectively) and appear to functionally cooperate because the engagement of a particular NCR results in activation of downstream signaling events from the other NCR [9, 11]. Although the cellular ligands (NCR-L) recognized by NCR are still unknown, functional data suggest that NCR recognize surface molecules that are expressed on tumor- or virus-infected cells but not on the majority of normal nonactivated cells. Indeed, NCR involvement has been demonstrated in NK-mediated killing of PHA T cell blasts, melanomas, carcinomas, Epstein-Barr virus (EBV)-transformed B cell lines, as well as ex vivo-derived neuroblastomas and myeloid or lymphoblastic leukemias [12–15]. This would suggest that, similar to NKG2D-specific ligands, NCR-L might be represented by stress-induced molecules, that is, molecules that are either expressed de novo or upregulated by events such as cellular activation, tumor transformation, or viral infection. It should be noted that dendritic cells (DC) represent a remarkable case among normal cells. Indeed, both immature and mature DC appear to express the NKp30-L, because susceptibility to NK-mediated lysis is highly dependent on the engagement of NKp30 [16].

3
Coreceptors

The function of NCR is supported and enhanced by the simultaneous engagement of different coreceptors, that is, molecules whose ability to induce

NK cell activation depends on the engagement of main triggering receptors such as NCR (Fig. 1). These include non-NK-restricted surface molecules such as 2B4 (CD144) [17], NTB-A [18], NKp80 [19], and CD59 [20]. 2B4 and NTB-A are members of the CD2 subfamily of the immunoglobulin superfamily (Ig-SF), which are also expressed by subsets of all T cells as well as, in the case of NTB-A, by B cells. 2B4 specifically recognizes CD48 [21], a broadly distributed surface molecule, whereas NTB-A mediates homophilic recognition [22]. Interestingly, their cytoplasmic tails contain ITSMs (immunoreceptor tyrosine-based switch motifs) that undergo phosphorylation and recruit several signaling molecules such as SAP (also termed SH2D1A) and SH2-containing phosphatases (SHP) [18, 23, 24]. Whereas in normal NK cells engagement of both coreceptors results in triggering of cytotoxicity, they transduce inhibitory signals in NK cells derived from patients affected by X-linked lymphoproliferative disease (XLP). XLP is a severe inherited primary immune deficiency (PID) that, at variance with most forms of PID, in which there is a broad susceptibility to various infectious agents, is characterized by a unique proclivity to severe complications after infection by EBV. XLP are characterized by the absence or lack of function of SAP molecules due to critical mutations in the encoding gene located on human chromosome X at q25. As a consequence, in XLP-NK cells 2B4 and NTB-A fail to associate with SAP but associate with SHP and mediate inhibitory signals capable of blocking the NCR-mediated activation [18, 23]. Thus the engagement of 2B4 and NTB-A by the specific ligands expressed on EBV-infected cells results in a sharp inhibition of the NK [18, 23]- and T [25]-mediated cytotoxicity that likely explains the inability of XLP patients to control EBV infection that results in fulminant mononucleosis or B cell lymphomas.

Interestingly, the inhibitory function of these molecules appears to have a role in physiological conditions. Indeed, it has been shown that in early steps of NK maturation the expression of triggering receptors such as NKp46 and NKp30 precedes the expression of HLA-class I-specific inhibitory receptors. This might allow NK cells to attack the surrounding hematopoietic precursors at the site of NK cell maturation. Notably, at this stage SAP is absent and 2B4 and NTB-A have inhibitory function [26]. The inhibitory function of the coreceptors might be a fail-safe device that inhibits the cytolytic activity during the earliest stages of NK cell maturation.

Regarding the molecular bases of the 2B4 and NTB-A dual functions (i.e., activation vs. inhibition), it has been shown recently that different ITSM may have different functions. Whereas all four ITSM in the 2B4 cytoplasmic tail bind SAP, the third can additionally recruit SHP [24]. Thus in normal cells SAP could contribute to 2B4 (and NTB-A)-mediated NK cell activation by blocking the interaction of the coreceptors with SHP negative-regulatory molecules.

Notably, 2B4 (but not NTB-A) is constitutively associated with the linker for activation of T cells (LAT) [27], a transmembrane molecule characterized by a long cytoplasmic tail containing tyrosine-based motifs that is known to play a crucial role in the molecular events leading to TCR-mediated T cell activation. Thus 2B4 engagement not only results in tyrosine phosphorylation of the 2B4 itself but also in that of LAT, which is followed by recruitment of intracytoplasmic signaling molecules including PLCγ and Grb2 [27].

4
Receptors or Coreceptors?

In vitro and in vivo experimental evidence underscores the central role of NK receptor complex-ligands interactions described above in NK-mediated recognition and lysis of most tumors. However, other molecules participate in the process for which the question of whether they can fully activate or cooperate in the activation of NK cell function is still open. These are represented by NKG2D and DNAM-1, two activating molecules whose expression is not restricted to NK cells.

NKG2D (CD314) is a lectinlike homodimeric molecule that in humans recognizes MICA, MICB, and ULBPs [28–30], stress-induced molecules characterized by α domains with MHC class I folds. Whereas in mice, two NKG2D forms (mNKG2D-S and mNKG2D-S) have been characterized that associate with DAP10 and/or DAP12 [31, 32], in humans a single NKG2D exists that associates with DAP10 [33], a transmembrane signaling adaptor characterized by a cytoplasmic tyrosine-based YxxM motif coupling it to the PI-3K-dependent pathway. NKG2D is involved in NK-mediated killing of different tumors such as carcinoma and melanoma and T cell leukemia cell lines. On the contrary, NK-mediated killing of AML or freshly isolated neuroblastomas is NKG2D independent because these tumors are characterized by the MICA$^-$ ULBP$^-$ phenotype [13–15].

DNAM-1 (CD226) is an activating molecule that recognizes poliovirus receptor (PVR, CD155) and Nectin-2 (CD112) [34], two closely related molecules belonging to the Nectin family, which are highly expressed by tumors of different histotype. Accordingly, DNAM-1-ligand interactions play a relevant role in NK-mediated cytotoxicity against carcinoma and melanoma cell lines, as well as ex vivo-derived neuroblastomas and myeloid (but not lymphoid) leukemic cells [13, 14]. Importantly, the susceptibility to lysis of tumor cells strictly correlates with the expression and surface densities of the two ligands. Note that in humans, DNAM-1 is present not only on NK cells but also on T cells, monocytes, platelets, and a B cell subset. Moreover, nectins are widely expressed on normal cells including neuronal, epithelial, endothelial, and fibroblastic cells. On the basis of these observations, a DNAM-1 function has been proposed during platelet aggregation [35] and, through interactions with PVR on endothelium, in the diapedesis phase of leukocyte transmigration [36]. Finally, beside the role in DNAM-1-mediated tumor cell recognition, nectins mediate homophilic and heterophilic trans-interactions that participate in the regulation of intercellular junctions [36] and cell-matrix adhesion. In the latter case, it has been demonstrated that stimulation of PVR inhibits cell adhesion and enhances cell motility, suggesting a role for this molecule in tumor cell biology [37].

5
Concluding Remarks

The mechanisms that regulate NK cell activation are complex because they depend on the expression of inhibitory and triggering receptors as well as on the distribution and surface density of the receptor's cellular ligands. Coreceptor molecules in most instances recognize ligands that are expressed on normal tissues. Thus this type of interaction may require a continuous regulation by inhibitory receptors in order to avoid autoimmune reactions. As coreceptors are also expressed by cytolytic T cells it is possible that a similar mechanism of control may also apply to CTL. On the other hand, the ligands recognized by primary receptors such as NCR and NKG2D are likely expressed only by tissues undergoing different kinds of cellular stress. In contrast to coreceptors the engagement of NCR or NKG2D by their cellular ligands results in potent NK cell activation that in some instances might even overrule the inhibition induced by inhibitory MHC-specific receptors. This, however, may require either overexpression of the specific cellular ligands or simultaneous signaling by coreceptors. Finally, coreceptors may acquire the ability to act as primary receptors if their ligands are overexpressed and MHC class I is downregulated.

Acknowledgements This work was supported by grants awarded by Associazione Italiana per la Ricerca sul Cancro (A.I.R.C.), Istituto Superiore di Sanità (I.S.S.), Ministero della Sanità, Ministero dell'Università e della Ricerca Scientifica e Tecnologica (M.I.U.R.) and European Union FP6, LSHB-CT-2004-503319-AlloStem (the European Commission is not liable for any use that may be made of the information contained). Also the financial support of Fondazione Compagnia di San Paolo, Torino, Italy, is gratefully acknowledged.

References

1. Biron, C.A. et al. (1999) Natural killer cells in antiviral defense: function and regulation by innate cytokines. Annu. Rev. Immunol. 17, 189–220.
2. Parham, P. (2003) Immunogenetics of killer-cell immunoglobulin-like receptors. Tissue Antigens 62, 194–200.
3. Moretta, L. and Moretta, A. (2004) Killer immunoglobulin-like receptors. Curr. Opin. Immunol. 16, 626–633.
4. Lopez-Botet, M. et al. (2000) NK cell recognition of non-classical HLA class I molecules. Semin. Immunol. 12, 109–119.
5. Algarra, I. et al. (2004) The selection of tumor variants with altered expression of classical and nonclassical MHC class I molecules: implications for tumor immune escape. Cancer Immunol. Immunother. 53, 904–910.
6. Alcami, A. and Koszinowski, U.H. (2000) Viral mechanisms of immune evasion. Immunol. Today 21, 447–455.
7. Moretta, A. et al. (2001) Activating receptors and coreceptors involved in human natural killer cell-mediated cytolysis. Annu. Rev. Immunol. 19, 197–223.
8. Lanier, L.L. (2003) Natural killer cell receptor signaling. Curr. Opin. Immunol. 15, 308–314.
9. Bottino C. et al. (2005) Cellular ligands of activating NK receptors. Trends Immunol. 26, 221–226.
10. Moretta, A. et al. (2000) Natural cytotoxicity receptors that trigger human NK-mediated cytolysis. Immunol. Today 21, 228–234.
11. Augugliaro, R. et al. (2003) Selective cross-talk among natural cytotoxicity receptors in human natural killer cells. Eur. J. Immunol. 33, 1235–1241.
12. Sivori, S. et al. (2000) Involvement of natural cytotoxicity receptors in human natural killer cell mediated lysis of neuroblastoma and glyoblastoma cell lines. J. Neuroimmunol. 107, 220–225.
13. Castriconi, R. et al. (2004) Natural killer cell-mediated killing of freshly isolated neuroblastoma cells: critical role of DNAM-1/PVR interaction. Cancer Res. 64, 9180–9184.
14. Pende, D. et al. (2005) Analysis of the receptor-ligand interactions in the natural killer-mediated lysis of freshly isolated myeloid or lymphoblastic leukemias: evidence for the involvement of the Poliovirus receptor (CD155) and Nectin-2 (CD112). Blood 105, 2066–2073.
15. Nowbakht, P. et al. (2005) Ligands for natural killer cell-activating receptors are expressed upon the maturation of normal myelomonocytic cells but at low levels in acute myeloid leukemias. Blood 105, 3615–3622.
16. Moretta, A. (2002) Natural killer cells and dendritic cells: rendezvous in abused tissues. Nat. Rev. Immunol. 2, 957–964.
17. Sivori, S. et al. (2000) 2B4 functions as a co-receptor in human natural killer cell activation. Eur. J. Immunol. 30, 787–793.
18. Bottino, C. et al. (2001) NTB-A, a novel SH2D1A-associated surface molecule contributing to the inability of natural killer cells to kill Epstein-Barr virus-infected B cells in X-linked lymphoproliferative diseases. J. Exp. Med. 194, 235–246.
19. Vitale, M. et al. (2001) Identification of NKp80, a novel triggering molecule expressed by human natural killer cells. Eur. J. Immunol. 31, 233–242,

20. Marcenaro, E. et al. (2003) CD59 is physically and functionally associated with natural cytotoxicity receptors and activates human NK cell-mediated cytotoxicity. Eur. J. Immunol. 33, 3367–3376.
21. Nakajima, H. et al. (1999) Activating interactions in human NK cell recognition: the role of 2B4-CD48. Eur J Immunol. 29, 1676–1683.
22. Falco, M. et al. (2004) Homophilic interaction of NTBA, a member of the CD2 molecular family: induction of cytotoxicity and cytokine release in human NK cells. Eur J Immunol. 34, 1663–1672.
23. Parolini, S. et al. (2000) X-linked lymphoproliferative disease: 2B4 molecules displaying inhibitory rather than activating function are responsible for the inability of NK cells to kill EBV-infected cells. J. Exp. Med. 192, 337–346.
24. Eissmann, P. et al. (2005) Molecular basis for positive and negative signaling by the natural killer cell receptor 2B4 (CD244). Blood 105, 4722–4729.
25. Loic, D. et al. (2005) SAP controls the cytolytic activity of CD8+ T cells against EBV-infected cells. DOI 10.1182/blood-2004-08-3269
26. Sivori S. et al. (2002) Early expression of triggering receptors and regulatory role of 2B4 in human NK cell precursors undergoing in vitro differentiation. P. Natl. Acad. Sci. USA 99, 4526–4531.
27. Bottino C, et al. (2000) Analysis of the molecular mechanism involved in 2B4-mediated NK cell activation: evidence that human 2B4 is physically and functionally associated with the linker for activation of T cells (LAT). Eur. J. Immunol. 30, 3718–3722.
28. Li, P., et al., 2001. Complex structure of the activating immunoreceptor NKG2D and its MHC class I-like ligand MICA. Nat. Immunol. 2, 443–451.
29. Cosman, D., et al., 2001. ULBPs, novel MHC class I-related molecules, bind to CMV glycoprotein UL16 and stimulate NK cytotoxicity through the NKG2D receptor. Immunity 14, 123–133.
30. Cerwenka, A. and Lanier, L.L. (2003) NKG2D ligands: unconventional MHC class I-like molecules exploited by viruses and cancer. Tissue Antigens 61, 335–343.
31. Diefenbach, A. et al. (2002) Selective associations with signaling proteins determine stimulatory versus costimulatory activity of NKG2D. Nat Immunol. 3, 1142–1149.
32. Zompi, S. et al. (2003) NKG2D triggers cytotoxicity in mouse NK cells lacking DAP12 or Syk family kinases. Nat Immunol. 4, 565–572
33. Andre, P. et al. (2004) Comparative analysis of human NK cell activation induced by NKG2D and natural cytotoxicity receptors. Eur. J. Immunol. 34, 961–971.
34. Bottino, C. et al. (2003) Identification of PVR (CD155) and Nectin-2 (CD112) as cell surface ligands for the human DNAM-1 (CD226) activating molecule. J. Exp. Med. 198, 557–567.
35. Kojima, H., et al (2003) CD226 mediates platelet and megakaryocytic cell adhesion to vascular endothelial cells. J. Biol .Chem. 278:36748–36753.
36. Reymond, N. et al. (2004) DNAM-1 and PVR regulate monocyte migration through endothelial junctions. J. Exp. Med. 199, 1331–1341.
37. Oda T. et al. (2004) Ligand stimulation of CD155a inhibits cell adhesion and enhances migration of fibroblasts. Biochem. Biophys. Res. Commun. 319, 1253–1264.
38. Barber, D.F. et al. (2004) LFA-1 contributes an early signal for NK cell cytotoxicity. J. Immunol. 173, 3653–3659.

NK Cell Recognition of Mouse Cytomegalovirus-Infected Cells

S. M. Vidal[1] · L. L. Lanier[2] (✉)

[1]McGill Center for Host Resistance, and Department of Microbiology and Immunology, McGill University, 3775 University St., Montreal Quebec, H3A 2B4, Canada

[2]Department of Microbiology and Immunology, The Biomedical Sciences Graduate Program, The Cancer Research Institute, University of California San Francisco, 513 Parnassus Avenue, Box 0414, San Francisco, CA 94143-0414, USA
lanier@itsa.ucsf.edu

1	Introduction	184
2	The Virus—an Evolutionary Perspective	184
2.1	The Virus—Immune Evasion genes and Strategies	186
2.1.1	Downregulation of MHC Class I	186
2.1.2	MHC Class I Mimicry	187
3	Host NK Cells Play a Central Role in Host Defense Against Cytomegalovirus	189
3.1	The Host NK Cell Receptors of MHC Class I	189
3.1.1	CD94 and the NKG2 Receptor Family	191
3.1.2	The NKG2D Receptor and its Ligands	191
3.1.3	The Ly49 Receptor Family	194
4	Conclusions—The Battle Continues	198
	References	198

Abstract Natural killer (NK) cells and cytomegalovirus have been locked in an evolutionary arms race for millions of years in an attempt to overwhelm each other. Cytomegaloviruses deploy cunning disguises to avoid detection by NK cells. Studies of the mouse model of infection have shown that NK cells deploy multiple mechanisms to deal with mouse cytomegalovirus (MCMV) infection, which involve receptors of the C-lectin type superfamily. Remarkably, these receptors have two additional common features: They map to the same genetic region, known as the NK cell gene complex; and they recognize MHC class I-related structures. While reviewing these attack-counterattack measures, this chapter points to the central role that recognition of the MCMV-infected cells by NK cells plays in host resistance to infection.

1
Introduction

The special relationship between NK cells and cytomegaloviruses (CMV) has been appreciated ever since it was reported that both humans and mice lacking functional NK cells are particularly susceptible to infection with CMV [7, 12, 18, 19, 94, 105]. Early studies of innate immunity to mouse CMV (MCMV) showed that resistance or susceptibility to viral infection is controlled by host genetic factors [7]. By using classic genetic methods, Scalzo and colleagues reported that MCMV resistance in C57BL/6 mice demonstrated a simple dominant Mendelian mode of inheritance, a trait attributed to the *Cmv1* locus [91]. Subsequently, these investigators reported that NK cells were required to mediate early protection against MCMV, and the *Cmv1* locus was mapped to a region on mouse chromosome 6 that contained a cluster of genes encoding NK cell receptors (referred to as the NK cell complex or NKC) [92, 93]. In response to a vigorous host defense, MCMV has evolved mechanisms to counter NK cell recognition and responses. In this chapter, we first provide the background on MCMV and some of its evasion mechanisms, including major histocompatibility (MHC) class I downregulation and mimicry, then discuss the role of NK cells in MCMV infection, and finally review the current understanding of this intriguing host-pathogen interaction.

2
The Virus—an Evolutionary Perspective

With its 230-kb double-stranded DNA genome, wide tissue tropism, strict species specificity, and ability to establish latency, MCMV is a typical member of the betaherpes subfamily of the *Herpesviridae* [85] (Fig. 1a). Herpesviruses are considered an evolutionary success in terms of their occurrence in the animal kingdom because of their modest pathogenicity in the natural settings and their ability to establish latency. Part of this success can be attributed to the ability of herpesviruses to escape or modulate host immune responses through a complex array of virus-encoded mechanisms thought to result from an exquisite adaptation to their hosts. Many of these mechanisms are mediated by proteins encoded by families of related genes, which arose via gene duplication, and are localized in the extremities of the CMV genome [28, 85] (Fig. 1a). It appears that several of these viral genes have been captured from their host's genome during their evolution [73]. Betaherpesviruses are characterized by numerous and virus-specific mechanisms of immune evasion strategy [84], likely caused by their strict host tropism [73]. Although there is a substantial evolutionary divergence in the genomes of mouse and human CMV, infection of mice with MCMV has proven exceptionally useful for studying the complex host-pathogen interactions that occur during human CMV (HCMV) infection. This is in part because human and mouse CMV share 68 predicted proteins with significant amino acid identity [85] (Fig. 1a), as well as many similarities in their biological properties and clinical man-

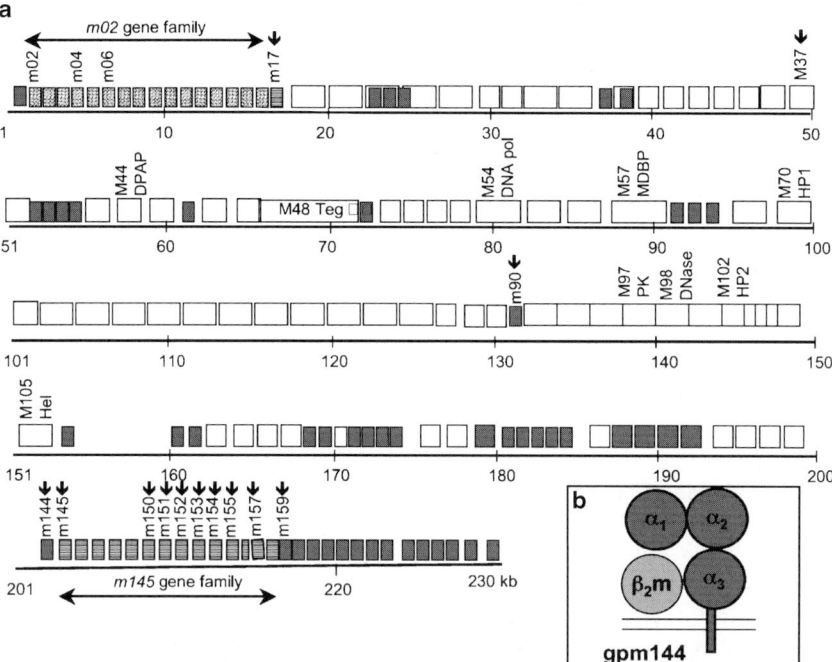

Fig. 1 a Schematic representation of MCMV genome. Rawlinson et al. (1996) predicted 170 open reading frames (ORF) in the MCMV genome represented by *rectangles*. *White rectangles* correspond to the predicted localization of 78 ORF with significant amino acid sequence similarity with ORF encoded in human CMV. We have indicated the localization of essential genes for origin-dependent replication, including *DPAP* (DNA polymerase accessory protein), *DNApol* (DNA polymerase), *MDBP* (single-stranded DNA binding protein), and the three components of the helicase complex (*HP1*, *HP2*, and *Hel*). Predicted ORF specific to MCMV are depicted in *gray*. The localization of the *m02* and *m145* gene at each of the extremities of the genomes is indicated. *Vertical arrows* point to the localization of ORF with predicted structural homology to mouse MHC class I. **b** Evasion molecules. Predicted structure of virus-encoded MHC class I-like molecules is characterized by the presence of three immunoglobin domains (α_1–α_3). m144 has been shown to bind host encoded β_2-immunoglobulin ($\beta_2 m$) but not peptide

ifestations [56]. Moreover, a common set of host responses are targeted by all CMVs, albeit through diverse mechanisms. As a result, it is frequently observed that evolutionarily distinct viral gene products have evolved to encode proteins with analogous activities and target similar pathways in a manner that suggests convergent evolution. Of note, nomenclature of animal CMV genes follows that set in place for HCMV, with uppercase letters (e.g., M44) for mouse MCMV genes that retain sequence similarity to HCMV and lowercase letters (m144) for those not conserved.

2.1
The Virus—Immune Evasion genes and Strategies

A characteristic feature of CMV infection in the normal host is the persistence of productive infection, viremia, and virus excretion for months or even years in the presence of the host immune response. This ability of the virus to avoid elimination or termination of active infection by the host's immune system is mediated by CMV gene products that have the potential to interfere with the immune response [46], as recently reviewed [1, 73, 74, 100]. Below we discuss the mechanisms of CMV-mediated MHC class I and MHC class I-like downregulation, as well as MHC class I mimicry, critical to the encounter between the CMV-infected cell and the NK cell.

2.1.1
Downregulation of MHC Class I

Several HCMV and MCMV gene products prevent the translocation of MHC class I proteins to the cell surface [8]. Four HCMV-encoded glycoproteins are involved in this process: US2, US3, US6, and US11 [46]. They are all single transmembrane (TM)-spanning (type I), immunoglobulin domain-bearing proteins of the US6 family, which probably arose by duplication of an ancestral gene. Binding of the US3 protein to MHC class I molecules causes their arrest in the endoplasmic reticulum (ER) [51]. On the other hand, binding of US6 to the transporter-associated peptide (TAP) proteins prevents peptide loading of MHC class I molecules [65]. Finally, US2 and US11 cause proteosomal degradation of MHC class I by redirecting them from the ER to the cytosol [108, 109].

In mice, three MCMV products expressed by the *m04*, *m06*, and *m152* genes in the early phase of viral gene expression also interfere with MHC class I presentation [45, 57, 112] (Fig. 1a). Remarkably, they are structurally and functionally unrelated to HCMV US2, US3, US6, or US11, a feature that might be explained by the fact that human and mouse MHC class I have evolved independently since their speciation [5]. The m04 and m06 products attach tightly to mature β2-microglobulin-associated MHC class I molecules in the ER [55, 86]. Protein m04 does not downregulate MHC class I at the plasma membrane; however, it forms complexes with ternary MHC class I molecules in the ER, which are then expressed on the cell surface [55]. The m06 protein binds to MHC class I complexes and redirects their transport into the endocytic pathway for rapid proteolytic destruction [86]. The gp40 protein encoded by *m152* accounts for the arrest and accumulation of MHC class I molecules in the ER-Golgi intermediate compartment [29, 114]. Consistent with the high level of variation of MHC class I proteins, MCMV proteins downregulating class I interact differentially with various MHC class I molecules [54, 59, 104]; thus their potency varies in a host-dependent manner.

These immune evasion genes belong to two gene families unique to MCMV: *m02* and *m145*. The *m04* and *m06* genes are among the 16 members of the *m02* family, whereas *m152* is one of the 11 members of the *m145* family [85] (Fig. 1a). Recent studies indicate additional immunoregulatory functions for *m152* and other *m145* family members. In particular, as discussed later, the *m152*, *m155*, and *m145* gene products retain intracellularly the MHC class I-like ligands of the activating NK cell receptor NKG2D [58, 66, 67]. Analogous mechanisms operate in HCMV infection; the human NKG2D ligands are targeted by the UL16 gene product [25], providing another example of the commonality of function through diverse immune evasion mechanisms used by mouse and human CMVs. Although studies of MCMV and HCMV clearly demonstrate their ability to downregulate expression of MHC class I on the surface of infected cells, it has been shown that NK cells in β2-microglobulin-deficient C57BL/6 mice are able to eliminate MCMV with the same efficiency as wild-type mice [98].

2.1.2
MHC Class I Mimicry

A number of CMV genes encoding homologs of cellular gene products are thought to play a role in subverting the host immune response. A comparison of the complete MCMV genome sequence with published host sequences demonstrated the presence of gene products similar to cellular proteins, such as MHC class I proteins, T cell receptor delta chain, and G protein-coupled chemokine receptors [1, 73, 85]. Viral homologs of MHC class I molecules have been found in mouse, rat, and human and other primate CMVs [38, 73]. The MHC class I homologs present in human and mouse CMVs, UL18 and m144, respectively, are evolutionarily distinct and are more similar to host MHC class I than they are to each other, suggesting a coevolutionary relationship with the host species [85]. UL18 and m144 are 348- and 383-residue type I transmembrane glycoproteins whose extracellular regions share about 25% amino acid sequence identity with the extracellular regions of their respective host's MHC class I molecules [10, 37, 85] (Fig. 1b).

As NK cells have the ability to spontaneously kill target cells with impaired MHC class I expression, viral MHC class I homologs have been proposed to function as a decoy interfering with NK cell-mediated killing of virus-infected cells [87]. However, this hypothesis remains controversial [24, 38]. Moreover, structural differences indicate distinct physiological functions of the mouse and human CMV MHC class I homologs. For instance, HCMV-encoded UL18 complexes with host β2-microglobulin and presents a peptide [36]. This molecule is recognized by the human LIR-1 (also named LILRB1 or ILT2) receptor expressed on myelomonocytic cells, some T cells, and a few NK cells [24], which does not seem to favor a unique role of UL18 on NK cell activity. LIR-1, however, is a member of a gene family genetically linked and structurally related to the killer-immunoglobulin-like receptors (KIR), which are preferentially expressed on NK cells [24]. The MCMV MHC class I homolog, 144, binds β2-microglobulin but does not present a peptide [37]. Although a receptor of m144 remains to be identified, infection of mice with a virus carrying a deletion at m144 results in a reduced viral titer in susceptible mice [37]. On the basis of this finding, Farrell and colleagues have proposed that this MHC class I homolog interferes with NK cell cytotoxic activity in mice. In addition, in vivo NK cell-mediated rejection of the m144-transfected RMA-S cell line lacking MHC class I expression is reduced compared to rejection of nontransfected RMA-S cells, further supporting a role of m144 in the control NK cell-mediated responses [26].

More recently, a bioinformatics approach based on the use of a position-sensitive substitution matrices program (3D-PSSM; http://www.sbg.bio.ic. ac.uk/~3dpssm/) has identified 11 additional MCMV genes encoding molecules with putative MHC class I folds [96] (m17, m37, m90, m144, m145, m150, m151, m152, m153, m155, m157, m159), as determined by predicted structural homology, despite the lack of significant similarity at the sequence level. With the exception of m37 and m90, the MHC class I structural homologs belong to the *m145* gene family. Among them, m157 was identified as a ligand for Ly49 molecules[6, 96], which are the classic MHC class I receptors present on mouse NK cells. Similarly, m145, m152, and m157 have been implicated in disruption of the function of another NK receptor, NKG2D (see below). The functions of other viral MHC class I-like proteins in MCMV infection remain to be identified, but a role in immunomodulation is also suspected.

3
Host NK Cells Play a Central Role in Host Defense Against Cytomegalovirus

A complex network of cells, soluble factors, cellular receptors, and intracellular signaling pathways organize the innate response against MCMV infection [15, 62, 76, 81, 95]. NK cells have a unique and nonredundant role in combating viral disease, particularly during the very early stages of infection [11]. In certain mouse strains relatively resistant to MCMV infection, depletion of NK cells results in an increase of viral titers by approximately one thousand-fold in certain tissues [92, 105]. Moreover, the identification of spontaneous mutations, as well as the characterization of models of targeted mutagenesis, helped to define NK cells as a major participant in host defense against herpesviruses. For example, a link between resistance to MCMV infection and NK cell function was established by studies showing that *beige* mice (whose NK cells have defective cytolytic granule formation) have increased susceptibility to MCMV [94]. Similarly, mice carrying targeted mutations within genes involved in the cytolytic function of NK cells, for example, perforin [39, 88] and granzyme A/B [88], are highly susceptibility to the early stages of MCMV infection. Correspondingly, herpesvirus infections have been reported to be more severe in humans lacking NK cells [12].

3.1
The Host NK Cell Receptors of MHC Class I

The primary effector mechanisms [11, 44, 60, 78] of NK cells are cell-mediated cytotoxicity and cytokine (in particular IFNγ) secretion [11, 44, 68, 78]. For target recognition, NK cells express multiple germ line-encoded cell surface activating or inhibitory receptors, which provide a fine balance of signals governing NK cell function and serve as detectors of abnormal cells [60]. NK cell inhibitory receptors survey tissues for expression of MHC class I molecules, which under normal conditions are ubiquitously expressed. When MHC class I molecules are downregulated, as a consequence of transformation or viral infection, this inhibitory signal is absent, potentially resulting in destruction of infected target cells [53]. It has been proposed that this is a result of target cells expressing ligands that can engage one or more of the NK activating receptors [60], as seems to be the case during MCMV infection. MHC class I-like molecules can also regulate the NK cell response. In mice there are at least three receptor systems, namely, CD94/NKG2, NKG2D, and Ly49 [113], that recognize MHC class I or MHC class I-like molecules, which may participate in the recognition of the MCMV-infected cell and determine the host's response to infection (Fig. 2a). These receptors are all type II transmembrane-spanning C-type lectin-like glycoproteins, encoded by a family of related genes in a region known as the NK cell receptor gene complex (NKC), including the *Cd94/Nkg2a, c-e, Nkg2d,* and *Ly49* genes (Fig. 2b). The NKC is located on the distal region of mouse chromosome 6, which is syntenic with regions on rat chromosome 4 and human chromosome 12p13 [60, 113] (Fig. 2a). In contrast to the rodent species, the *Ly49* gene cluster is absent in humans (a single copy of the *Ly49L* pseudogene has been identified in the human genome) [107]. Ly49 receptors are the functional analogs of human KIRs, which are encoded by genes located on human chromosome 19q26 [79]. Ly49 and KIR provide the largest genetic and functional diversity to the mouse and human NK cell receptor repertoires.

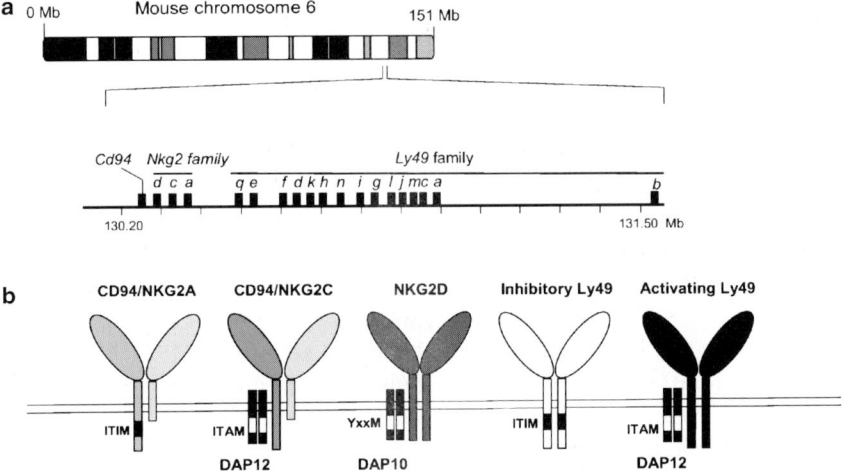

Fig. 2 Mouse C-type lectin-like MHC class I NK cell receptors map to distal chromosome 6. **a** Chromosomal and physical map of the distal portion of the NKC encoding showing the clustering of *Cd94, Nkg2,* and *Ly49* genes. **b** Schematic representation of C-type lectin-like MHC class I receptors. As discussed in the text, receptors are heterodimers (CD94/NKG2A) or homodimers (NKG2D or Ly49). Inhibitory receptors have immunoreceptor tyrosine-based inhibitory motifs (ITIMs) in their cytoplasmic tail, which are capable of recruiting SHP-1 phosphatase to initiate the attenuation of intracellular signals. Activating receptors lack cytoplasmic ITIMs but contain an arginine residue in their transmembrane domain, which mediates their association with DAP12, a signaling protein containing a single immunoreceptor tyrosine-based activation motif (ITAM). In mice, NKG2D can associate either with DAP12 or DAP10 (an adapter protein capable of recruiting the p85 subunit of PI3 kinase)

3.1.1
CD94 and the NKG2 Receptor Family

Whereas a single gene encodes CD94 [23, 103], NKG2 is comprised of a multigene family, including the *Nkg2A, C, E* genes in human [48], and *Nkg2a, c, e* in mice [47, 69]. The CD94 protein has a short cytoplasmic domain with no apparent functional motifs. Mouse NKG2A has a single immunoreceptor tyrosine-based inhibition motif (ITIM) in its intracellular region [47, 69], which recruits tyrosine phosphatases such as SHP-1, providing inhibitory function to the heterodimer. By contrast, when NKG2C is disulfide-linked to CD94, the heterodimer can function as an activating receptor by associating with the immunoreceptor tyrosine-based activation motif (ITAM)-bearing DAP12 adapter protein through its charged transmembrane residue [61, 79, 101] (Fig. 2b).

The human CD94/NKG2A and CD94/NKG2C heterodimers recognize the nonpolymorphic MHC class I molecule HLA-E [14]. In mice, heterodimers between CD94 and NKG2A, NKG2C, or NKG2E recognize Qa-1^b [101, 102]. The HLA-E and Qa-1^b molecules predominantly display peptides that are derived from the signal peptides of other classic MHC class I molecules (i.e., human HLA-A, -B, -C and mouse H-2K and H-2D, respectively) [14, 102]. Therefore, interactions between CD94/NKG2 and these nonclassic MHC class I molecules allow NK cells to monitor indirectly the expression of the classic MHC class I molecules [14]. Although having a common ligand, the inhibitory CD94/NKG2A heterodimers have stronger affinity for Qa-1^b or HLA-E than the activating CD94/NKG2C heterodimers [52, 101]. A reasonable expectation from these observations is that the inhibitory signals emanating from CD94/NKG2A should be prevented during CMV infection as a result of MHC class I loss in the target. This, however, might not be the case because the leader segment of the UL40 HCMV gene product contains a peptide that is identical to the peptide present in HLA class I leader segments [99]. The UL40 leader peptide can bind HLA-E and be presented to CD94NKG2A, thereby inhibiting NK cell-mediated responses [99]. Although this has been demonstrated in vitro, it is uncertain whether it contributes to HCMV virulence. Leader peptides of MCMV proteins do not contain sequences that are predicted to bind to Qa-1^b.

3.1.2
The NKG2D Receptor and its Ligands

NKG2D is another receptor of the C-type lectin-like superfamily encoded by a single, nonpolymorphic gene in the NKC of both humans and mice [47, 48]. *Nkg2d* is the most divergent member of the NKG2 family and encodes a protein that does not associate with CD94 but instead forms a disulfide-bonded homodimer (Fig. 2b). This receptor is expressed on essentially all NK cells, γδ-TcR+ T cells, and CD8$^+$ T cells [9, 49]. In mice, NKG2D associates noncovalently with the transmembrane-anchored DAP10 and DAP12 signaling adapter proteins [33, 42], whereas human NKG2D pairs exclusively with DAP10 [90, 110]. Engagement of this receptor on NK cells triggers potent cell-mediated cytotoxicity and the production of cytokines. Mouse NKG2D binds at least seven different ligands, which are cell surface glycoproteins with homology to the MHC class I proteins and are encoded by genes clustered on mouse chromosome 10. The mouse NKG2D ligands comprise five members of the RAE-1 family designated RAE-1α, β, γ, δ, ε, the H60 glycoprotein, and the MULT1 glycoprotein [20, 21, 32]. Although RAE-1 is expressed on embryonic tissues [77], generally the NKG2D ligands are expressed at low levels on healthy tissues of adult mice. The human orthologs of the RAE-1/H60/MULT1 molecules are referred to as the ULBP1, 2, 3, and 4 (or RAET-1) proteins [25, 50, 83]. In addition, humans possess two genes within the MHC on chromosome 12, *Mica* and *Micb*, which also encode ligands for NKG2D [9].

A connection between NKG2D and CMV was first revealed by the findings of Cosman and colleagues, who demonstrated that the HCMV UL16 protein specifically binds with high affinity to the ULBP-1 molecule (hence the name UL16-binding protein-1) [25]. The HCMV UL16 protein also binds to ULBP-2 and MICB but, curiously, not to MICA, ULBP-3, or ULBP-4 [25, 50] (therefore, the designation ULBP is a misnomer in the case of ULBP-3 and ULBP-4). In HCMV-infected cells, UL16 binds to MICB, ULBP-1, and ULBP-2 intracellularly and prevents transport of these NKG2D ligands to the cell surface, thereby preventing the infected cell from NKG2D-dependent recognition by NK cells [35, 89, 106, 110]. UL16 does not affect classic MHC class I proteins but appears to have evolved specifically to interfere with selected NKG2D ligands.

Although MCMV does not express a structural homolog of UL16, MCMV has devised its own mechanisms to deal with NKG2D-mediated immune surveillance. This is probably because the human ULBP and MIC proteins have very little homology to the mouse RAE-1, H60, and MULT1 proteins, as they share less than 20% identity in primary sequence [22]. Infection of cells with MCMV induces the transcription of mouse NKG2D ligand genes; however, mouse NKG2D ligand proteins are unable to reach the cell surface for display to the mouse immune system [57, 58, 66, 67].

Remarkably, MCMV has evolved three viral genes to prevent expression of NKG2D ligands on the surface of infected cells (Fig. 3). The *m152* gene encodes the gp40 MCMV protein, which efficiently disrupts expression of all five RAE-1 proteins [66]; the *m155* gene product prevents expression of H60 [67]; and

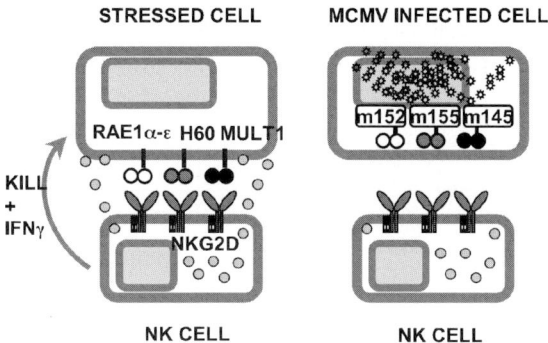

Fig. 3 NKG2D and its ligands in the recognition of MCMV-infected cell. Mouse NKG2D recognizes at least 7 ligands, which are upregulated in cells under stress (*top rectangle, right panel*), such as in tumor cells or virus-infected cells. NKG2D ligands RAE-1α–ε, H60, and MULT1 have a predicted MHC class I structure characterized by the presence of two extracellular domains with MHC class I folds. Engagement of NKG2D ligands activates NK cells (*bottom rectangles*), promoting release of perforin granules (*gray circles*) and IFN γ secretion. During infection (*left panel*), at least three MCMV proteins—m152, m155 and m145—prevent expression of NKG2D ligands on the cell surface as a means to evade NK cell-mediated destruction

the *m145* gene product blocks surface transport of MULT1 [58]. Although the mechanism used by gp40 to prevent RAE-1 expression has not been defined, m155 causes the proteosome-dependent degradation of H60 [67] and m145 prevents transport of MULT1 to the cell surface at a post-Golgi stage of protein maturation [58]. In addition to affecting RAE-1 expression, as previously mentioned, the *m152*-encoded gp40 protein can also inhibit expression of certain classic MHC class I proteins, which is unexpected given the very low degree of homology between RAE-1 and MHC class I. However, this suggests that gp40 has a dual role in immune evasion, by potentially preventing immune recognition of both RAE-1 and MHC class I. It is therefore surprising that mutant MCMV lacking *m152* shows only about a one log decrease in viral titer in the liver and spleen of infected mice, compared with mice infected with the wild-type Smith stain [66]. In addition, the T cell response against MCMV lacking *m152* is essentially identical to the response against wild-type virus [43]. By contrast, loss of the m145 viral protein (targeting MULT1) or m155 (targeting H60) has a more dramatic impact on viral replication early after infection. Nonetheless, m145, m152, and m155 all function as virulence factors in vivo, and together they serve to block cell surface expression of all the NKG2D ligand proteins in MCMV-infected cells. The fact that these viral proteins are primarily involved in evading an NK cell-mediated immune response has been established by showing that depletion of NK cells totally reverses the impaired replication of the *m152*-deficient, *m145*-deficient, and *m155*-deficient MCMV strain in vivo.

3.1.3
The Ly49 Receptor Family

The *Ly49* gene family encodes both activating and inhibitory receptors, which are expressed as disulfide-bonded homodimers on subsets of NK cells in an overlapping pattern. The inhibitory receptors contain ITIMs in their cytoplasmic domains, whereas the activating receptors lack ITIMs and associate with the ITAM-containing DAP12 adapter protein [97] (Fig. 2b).

To date, three distinct strain-specific *Ly49* haplotypes have been identified from the C57BL/6, 129Sv, and BALB/c mouse strains [63, 72, 82] (Fig. 4a). *Ly49* haplotypes are reminiscent of the genetic arrangement of human *KIR* genes, where framework genes encoding inhibitory receptors flank regions containing a variable number of genes encoding activating receptors [111]. Although there are distinct binding specificities for each Ly49 molecule, the specificities seem to be overlapping and promiscuous (Table 1). For example, the inhibitory Ly49A receptor from the B6 strain binds to $H-2D^b$, $H-2D^d$, $H-2D^k$, and $H-2D^p$, whereas Ly49I from the 129/J strain binds to $H-2D^k$, $H-2K^b$, $H-2K^d$, and $H-2K^k$ [71]. Inhibitory and activating isoforms of the Ly49 receptors share high similarity in their extracellular domains. In cases where related activating and inhibitory receptors have been shown to recognize the same MHC class I ligand, the activating receptors appear to bind with much lower affinity [75], which suggests a different physiological function for activating Ly49 receptors.

Table 1 Binding repertoire of inhibitory Ly49 receptors

Strain	Receptor	Ligand
C57BL/6	Ly49A	$H2-D^{b,d,k}$
	Ly49C	$H2-K^{b,d}$ $H2-D^{b,d,k}$
	Ly49G	$H2-D^d$
	Ly49I	$H2-D^{b,d}$, $H2-K^d$
129/J	Ly49G	$H2-D^d$, $H2-K^d$
	Ly49I	$H2-D^k$, $H2-K^{b,d,k}$, m157
	Ly49O	$H2-D^d$, $H2-L^d$
	Ly49V	$H2-D^{b,d,k}$, $H2-K^b$, $H2-L^d$

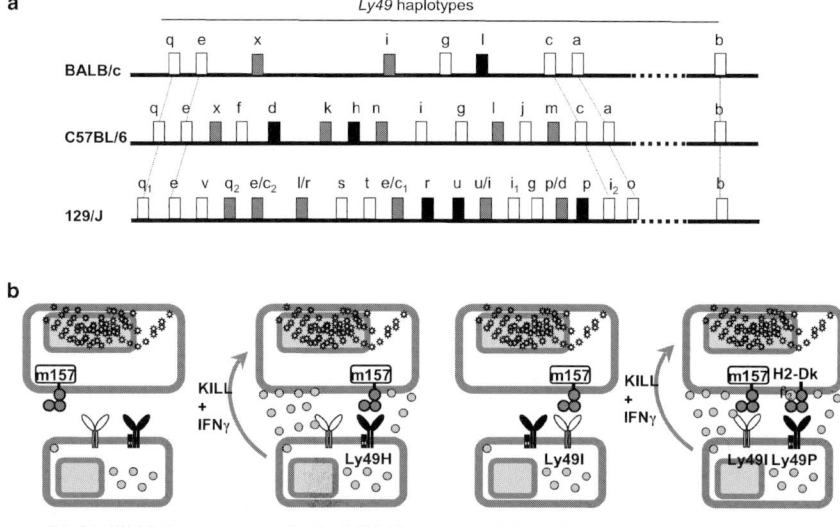

Fig. 4 a The *Ly49* haplotypes from strains 129/J, C57BL/6, and BALB/c. Genes encoding activating *Ly49* receptors are shown in *black*, inhibitory in *white*, and pseudogenes in *gray*. Framework genes in different strains are joined by a *dotted line*. b Recognition of the MCMV-infected cell by Ly49 receptors. MCMV-infected cells (*top rectangles*) express viral MHC class I-like molecules at the cell surface, such as m157. Host MHC class I molecules are retained intracellularly to varying degrees depending on the H2 haplotype of the host. For example, H2-D^k is expressed in MCMV-infected cells of MA/My origin. NK cells from different inbred strains (*bottom rectangles*) express a varied repertoire of activating (in *black*) and inhibitory (in *white*) Ly49 receptors. Appropriate engagement of activating Ly49 receptors induces release of perforin granules (*gray circles*) and secretion of cytokines, leading to the destruction of the MCMV-infected cells. As shown, the mechanisms of MCMV recognition vary in different inbred mouse strains and depend on the Ly49 and H2 haplotypes (see text for details)

A central role of activating Ly49 receptor genes in host response to infection, as well as in the specific recognition of the MCMV-infected cell, was appreciated after seminal studies by Grundy and Shellam of the natural variation in the host response against MCMV [91]. With the exception of a few inbred mouse strains, namely, C57BL/6 and MA/My, most strains of inbred mice studied to date are quite susceptible to MCMV infection as measured by organ-specific viral replication in the first days after infection, disease severity, and survival, indicating that host genetic factors control the susceptibility [2–4]. Through genetic analysis of progeny from MCMV-resistant and MCMV-susceptible parents, Scalzo et al. identified a single locus, *Cmv1*, as the major determinant of MCMV resistance in the C57BL/6 mouse strain [91–93].

Cmv1 is an autosomal dominant trait that restricts viral replication at the level of spleen viral titers, but less so in the liver, which are two major target organs during acute MCMV infection. *Cmv1* function is mediated by NK cells, which use both perforin and IFNγ secretion to control infection in the target organs [68]. This locus was found identical to the gene encoding an activating NK cell receptor Ly49H [15, 27, 62]. *Ly49h* is present in the MCMV-resistant strain C57BL/6 but is absent in susceptible strains such as BALB/c, DBA/2, and 129Sv [62]. In fact, a "clonal expansion" of Ly49H$^+$ NK cells is observed after MCMV infection in this mouse strain [34]. The crucial role of Ly49H-bearing NK cells in host defense against viral infection was validated by restoring MCMV resistance in genetically susceptible mice through transgenic expression of *Ly49h* [64]. The importance of the Ly49H/DAP12 receptor complex in MCMV resistance has also been supported by the generation of DAP12 (also named KARAP)-mutant mice bearing a nonfunctional ITAM. In these mice, a considerable increase in MCMV titers was observed in the spleen (30- to 40-fold) and in the liver (2- to 5-fold), showing a crucial role for DAP12 in the NK cell-mediated resistance to infection [95].

Ly49H specifically recognizes MCMV-infected cells via direct interaction with the *m157* MCMV gene product, which has structural homology to MHC class I molecules [6, 96] (Fig. 4b). Loss of the *m157* gene is associated with gain of virulence in Ly49H$^+$, but not in Ly49H$^-$ mouse strains, indicating that m157 is the only MCMV-encoded protein that activates Ly49H$^+$ NK cells [16]. Arase et al. demonstrated that m157 also binds to an inhibitory receptor, Ly49I, expressed on NK cells in 129 mice, suggesting that m157 may have evolved as a mechanism to escape NK cell killing by targeting inhibitory receptors in certain susceptible mice [6] (Fig. 4b). As mentioned before, *m157* is part of the MCMV *m145* gene family.

These observations predicted a dynamic interaction between Ly49 receptors and MCMV evasion genes, which has been recently confirmed. In fact, several MCMV strains isolated from wild mice had variants of the *m157* gene, many of which disrupted the open reading frame and inactivated the gene [17]. In addition, sequential passage of the commonly used Smith strain of MCMV in Ly49H$^+$ C57BL/6 mice resulted in loss-of-function mutations in the *m157* gene [41]. The phenomenon of m157 mutation was not observed in mice lacking Ly49H, indicating the strong selective pressure exerted by this NK cell-activating receptor on the virus. The emergence of MCMV variants that escaped innate immune control was also observed during infection of SCID mice, which have intact NK cell defenses but lack T and B cells [41].

Remarkably, the MCMV-resistant mouse strain MA/My lacks Ly49H and possesses a *Ly49* repertoire similar to that of the susceptible strain 129/J [31] (Fig. 4a). Nevertheless, genetic resistance in this strain is mediated by NK cells and depends on a specific allelic combination of *Ly49* and MHC class I genes [31]. Of the three activating Ly49 receptors cloned from MA/My NK cells, only Ly49P recognized MCMV-infected cells. The specificity of the Ly49P receptor for MCMV is supported by findings that Ly49P-bearing cells were unable to recognize $H2^k$-bearing cells not infected with MCMV or infected with another herpesvirus, HVγ68 [31]. Recognition of the MCMV-infected cells, however, is strictly dependent on the presence of the $H2^k$ haplotype in the MCMV-infected target cells (Fig. 4b). The interaction between Ly49P and the MCMV-infected cell was blocked completely by using anti-H2-D^k monoclonal antibodies [31]. These results support the existence of a novel NK cell mechanism implicated in MCMV resistance, which requires functional interactions between the Ly49P receptor and MHC class I molecule, H2-D^k, expressed on MCMV-infected cells. Although the exact nature of the interaction between Ly49P and H2-D^k in MCMV-infected cells remains to be defined, it is plausible that ligation of the H2-D^k molecule depends on the presence of a MCMV-specific peptide. Therefore, although the precise molecular machinery of target recognition is not yet known, an attractive explanation would be peptide-specific recognition of MCMV by the Ly49P receptor. A requirement for peptide selectivity was previously described for target-specific recognition by inhibitory MHC class I receptors [40, 80]. The observation that the activating Ly49P receptor may be necessary for peptide-dependent recognition of MCMV-infected cells suggests the existence of a highly specific mechanism of innate immunity mediated by NK cells, previously thought to be to the exclusive domain of cytotoxic T cells. These results also indicate that in addition to Ly49H there are mechanisms of defense against MCMV infection mediated by other Ly49 receptors. It is, however, remarkable that out of the few Ly49 activating receptors characterized to date two seem dedicated to protection against a single pathogen, MCMV. It is possible that activating Ly49 receptors might have additional undiscovered ligands that are encoded by other viruses.

A number of phenotypic traits associated with immune function or susceptibility to disease have been mapped to the NKC, including susceptibility to ectromelia virus [30], herpes simplex-1 [70], and cutaneous leishmaniasis [13]. The realization that Ly49H and Ly49P detect MCMV-infected cells by recognition of a virus-encoded class I homolog or an altered host MHC class I molecule, respectively, adds a new wrinkle to this evolutionary scheme and suggests that evolutionary pressures on these NK receptors for MHC class I extend beyond the ability to recognize "missing self." Consequently, the evidence resulting from the study of the interaction between NK cells and MCMV-infected cells is the revelation of remarkable specificity of these innate immune system receptors for viral determinants.

4
Conclusions—The Battle Continues

Host-pathogen interactions have been viewed as the battle of two genomes encoding gene products that display attack-counterattack strategies for survival. The model of MCMV illustrates how this depends on complex interactions between the NKC, MHC-related genes, and the MCMV genome. This may well anticipate the level of complexity of interactions between human NK cells and HCMV. The model of MCMV infection has advanced our fundamental understanding of the mechanisms of NK cell recognition of infection. In particular, the molecular interactions between the activating NKG2D and Ly49 receptors and MCMV-infected cells provide intriguing insights about the cat and mouse game under way between the pathogen and innate immunity. However, there are questions remaining to be answered: Are there other mechanisms of MCMV recognition? Are they shared by other pathogens? Are there definable motifs of recognition? What is the individual contribution of NK receptors to resistance? Undoubtedly, unanticipated findings will be discovered during the quest to uncover the nature of this special relationship between NK cells and CMV.

Acknowledgements L.L.L. is an American Cancer Society Research Professor and is supported by NIH Grants CA-89294, CA-89189, and CA-095137. S.M.V is a Canada Research Chair and is supported by grants from the Canadian Institutes of Health Research (CIHR) and the Canadian Genetic Diseases Network.

References

1. Alcami A: Viral mimicry of cytokines, chemokines and their receptors. *Nat. Rev. Immunol.* 2003, 3:36–50.
2. Allan JE, Shellam GR: Characterization of interferon induction in mice of resistant and susceptible strains during murine cytomegalovirus infection. *J. Gen. Virol.* 1985, 66(Pt 5):1105–1112.
3. Allan JE, Shellam GR: Genetic control of murine cytomegalovirus infection: virus titres in resistant and susceptible strains of mice. *Arch. Virol.* 1984, 81:139–150.
4. Allan JE, Shellam GR, Grundy JE: Effect of murine cytomegalovirus infection on mitogen responses in genetically resistant and susceptible mice. *Infect. Immun.* 1982, 36:235–242.
5. Allcock RJ, Martin AM, Price P: The mouse as a model for the effects of MHC genes on human disease. *Immunol. Today* 2000, 21:328–332.
6. Arase H, Mocarski ES, Campbell AE, Hill AB, Lanier LL: Direct recognition of cytomegalovirus by activating and inhibitory NK cell receptors. *Science* 2002, 296:1323–1326.

7. Bancroft GJ, Shellam GR, Chalmer JE: Genetic influences on the augmentation of natural killer (NK) cells during murine cytomegalovirus infection: correlation with patterns of resistance. *J. Immunol.* 1981, 126:988-994.
8. Basta S, Bennink JR: A survival game of hide and seek: cytomegaloviruses and MHC class I antigen presentation pathways. *Viral Immunol.* 2003, 16:231-242.
9. Bauer S, Groh V, Wu J, Steinle A, Phillips JH, Lanier LL, Spies T: Activation of NK cells and T cells by NKG2D, a receptor for stress-inducible MICA. *Science* 1999, 285:727-729.
10. Beck S, Barrell BG: Human cytomegalovirus encodes a glycoprotein homologous to MHC class-I antigens. *Nature* 1988, 331:269-272.
11. Biron CA, Brossay L: NK cells and NKT cells in innate defense against viral infections. *Curr. Opin. Immunol.* 2001, 13:458-464.
12. Biron CA, Byron KS, Sullivan JL: Severe herpesvirus infections in an adolescent without natural killer cells. *N. Engl. J. Med.* 1989, 320:1731-1735.
13. Blackwell JM: Genetic susceptibility to leishmanial infections: studies in mice and man. *Parasitology* 1996, 112 Suppl:S67-S74.
14. Braud VM, Allan DS, O'Callaghan CA, Soderstrom K, D'Andrea A, Ogg GS, Lazetic S, Young NT, Bell JI, Phillips JH, Lanier LL, McMichael AJ: HLA-E binds to natural killer cell receptors CD94/NKG2A, B and C. *Nature* 1998, 391:795-799.
15. Brown MG, Dokun AO, Heusel JW, Smith HR, Beckman DL, Blattenberger EA, Dubbelde CE, Stone LR, Scalzo AA, Yokoyama WM: Vital involvement of a natural killer cell activation receptor in resistance to viral infection. *Science* 2001, 292:934-937.
16. Bubi I, Wagner M, Krmpoti A, Saulig T, Kim S, Yokoyama WM, Jonji S, Koszinowski UH: Gain of virulence caused by loss of a gene in murine cytomegalovirus. *J. Virol.* 2004, 78:7536-7544.
17. Bubic I, Wagner M, Krmpotic A, Saulig T, Kim S, Yokoyama WM, Jonjic S, Koszinowski UH: Gain of virulence caused by loss of a gene in murine cytomegalovirus. *J. Virol.* 2004, 78:7536-7544.
18. Bukowski JF, Woda BA, Habu S, Okumura K, Welsh RM: Natural killer cell depletion enhances virus synthesis and virus-induced hepatitis in vivo. *J. Immunol.* 1983, 131:1531-1538.
19. Bukowski JF, Woda BA, Welsh RM: Pathogenesis of murine cytomegalovirus infection in natural killer cell-depleted mice. *J. Virol.* 1984, 52:119-128.
20. Carayannopoulos LN, Yokoyama WM: Recognition of infected cells by natural killer cells. *Curr. Opin. Immunol.* 2004, 16:26-33.
21. Cerwenka A, Bakker AB, McClanahan T, Wagner J, Wu J, Phillips JH, Lanier LL: Retinoic acid early inducible genes define a ligand family for the activating NKG2D receptor in mice. *Immunity* 2000, 12:721-727.
22. Cerwenka A, Lanier LL: NKG2D ligands: unconventional MHC class I-like molecules exploited by viruses and cancer. *Tissue Antigens* 2003, 61:335-343.
23. Chang C, Rodriguez A, Carretero M, Lopez-Botet M, Phillips JH, Lanier LL: Molecular characterization of human CD94: a type II membrane glycoprotein related to the C-type lectin superfamily. *Eur. J. Immunol.* 1995, 25:2433-2437.
24. Cosman D, Fanger N, Borges L: Human cytomegalovirus, MHC class I and inhibitory signalling receptors: more questions than answers. *Immunol. Rev.* 1999, 168:177-185.

25. Cosman D, Mullberg J, Sutherland CL, Chin W, Armitage R, Fanslow W, Kubin M, Chalupny NJ: ULBPs, novel MHC class I-related molecules, bind to CMV glycoprotein UL16 and stimulate NK cytotoxicity through the NKG2D receptor. *Immunity* 2001, 14:123–133.
26. Cretney E, Degli-Esposti MA, Densley EH, Farrell HE, Davis-Poynter NJ, Smyth MJ: m144, a murine cytomegalovirus (MCMV)-encoded major histocompatibility complex class I homologue, confers tumor resistance to natural killer cell-mediated rejection. *J. Exp. Med.* 1999, 190:435–444.
27. Daniels KA, Devora G, Lai WC, O'Donnell CL, Bennett M, Welsh RM: Murine cytomegalovirus is regulated by a discrete subset of natural killer cells reactive with monoclonal antibody to Ly49H. *J. Exp. Med.* 2001, 194:29–44.
28. Davison AJ: Evolution of the herpesviruses. *Vet. Microbiol.* 2002, 86:69–88.
29. del Val M, Hengel H, Hacker H, Hartlaub U, Ruppert T, Lucin P, Koszinowski UH: Cytomegalovirus prevents antigen presentation by blocking the transport of peptide-loaded major histocompatibility complex class I molecules into the medial-Golgi compartment. *J. Exp. Med.* 1992, 176:729–738.
30. Delano ML, Brownstein DG: Innate resistance to lethal mousepox is genetically linked to the NK gene complex on chromosome 6 and correlates with early restriction of virus replication by cells with an NK phenotype. *J. Virol.* 1995, 69:5875–5877.
31. Desrosiers M-P, Kielczewska A, Loredo-Osti J-C, Girard-Adam S, Makrigiannis A, Lemieux S, Pham T, Lodoen M, Lanier LL, Vidal SM: Epistasis between mouse *Ly49* and MHC class I loci is associated with a novel mechanism of NK cell mediated innate resistance to cytomegalovirus infection. *Nat. Genet.* 2005, In Press.
32. Diefenbach A, Jamieson AM, Liu SD, Shastri N, Raulet DH: Ligands for the murine NKG2D receptor: expression by tumor cells and activation of NK cells and macrophages. *Nat. Immunol.* 2000, 1:119–126.
33. Diefenbach A, Raulet DH: The innate immune response to tumors and its role in the induction of T-cell immunity. *Immunol. Rev.* 2002, 188:9–21.
34. Dokun AO, Kim S, Smith HR, Kang HS, Chu DT, Yokoyama WM: Specific and nonspecific NK cell activation during virus infection. *Nat. Immunol.* 2001, 2:951–956.
35. Dunn C, Chalupny NJ, Sutherland CL, Dosch S, Sivakumar PV, Johnson DC, Cosman D: Human cytomegalovirus glycoprotein UL16 causes intracellular sequestration of NKG2D ligands, protecting against natural killer cell cytotoxicity. *J. Exp. Med.* 2003, 197:1427–1439.
36. Fahnestock ML, Johnson JL, Feldman RM, Neveu JM, Lane WS, Bjorkman PJ: The MHC class I homolog encoded by human cytomegalovirus binds endogenous peptides. *Immunity* 1995, 3:583–590.
37. Farrell HE, Vally H, Lynch DM, Fleming P, Shellam GR, Scalzo AA, Davis-Poynter NJ: Inhibition of natural killer cells by a cytomegalovirus MHC class I homologue in vivo. *Nature* 1997, 386:510–514.
38. Farrell HE, Davis-Poynter NJ, Andrews DM, Degli-Esposti MA: Function of CMV-encoded MHC class I homologues. *Curr. Top. Microbiol. Immunol.* 2002, 269:131–151.

39. Fernandez JA, Rodrigues EG, Tsuji M: Multifactorial protective mechanisms to limit viral replication in the lung of mice during primary murine cytomegalovirus infection. *Viral Immunol.* 2000, 13:287–295.
40. Franksson L, Sundback J, Achour A, Bernlind J, Glas R, Karre K: Peptide dependency and selectivity of the NK cell inhibitory receptor Ly-49C. *Eur. J. Immunol.* 1999, 29:2748–2758.
41. French AR, Pingel JT, Wagner M, Bubic I, Yang L, Kim S, Koszinowski U, Jonjic S, Yokoyama WM: Escape of mutant double-stranded DNA virus from innate immune control. *Immunity* 2004, 20:747–756.
42. Gilfillan S, Ho EL, Cella M, Yokoyama WM, Colonna M: NKG2D recruits two distinct adapters to trigger NK cell activation and costimulation. *Nat. Immunol.* 2002, 3:1150–1155.
43. Gold MC, Munks MW, Wagner M, McMahon CW, Kelly A, Kavanagh DG, Slifka MK, Koszinowski UH, Raulet DH, Hill AB: Murine cytomegalovirus interference with antigen presentation has little effect on the size or the effector memory phenotype of the CD8 T cell response. *J. Immunol.* 2004, 172:6944–6953.
44. Grundy JE, Mackenzie JS, Stanley NF: Influence of H-2 and non-H-2 genes on resistance to murine cytomegalovirus infection. *Infect. Immun.* 1981, 32:277–286.
45. Gutermann A, Bubeck A, Wagner M, Reusch U, Menard C, Koszinowski UH: Strategies for the identification and analysis of viral immune-evasive genes—cytomegalovirus as an example. *Curr. Top. Microbiol. Immunol.* 2002, 269:1–22.
46. Hengel H, Brune W, Koszinowski UH: Immune evasion by cytomegalovirus—survival strategies of a highly adapted opportunist. *Trends Microbiol.* 1998, 6:190–197.
47. Ho EL, Heusel JW, Brown MG, Matsumoto K, Scalzo AA, Yokoyama WM: Murine Nkg2d and Cd94 are clustered within the natural killer complex and are expressed independently in natural killer cells. *Proc. Natl. Acad. Sci. USA* 1998, 95:6320–6325.
48. Houchins JP, Yabe T, McSherry C, Bach FH: DNA sequence analysis of NKG2, a family of related cDNA clones encoding type II integral membrane proteins on human natural killer cells. *J. Exp. Med.* 1991, 173:1017–1020.
49. Jamieson AM, Diefenbach A, McMahon CW, Xiong N, Carlyle JR, Raulet DH: The role of the NKG2D immunoreceptor in immune cell activation and natural killing. *Immunity* 2002, 17:19–29.
50. Jan CN, Sutherland CL, Lawrence WA, Rein-Weston A, Cosman D: ULBP4 is a novel ligand for human NKG2D. *Biochem. Biophys. Res. Commun.* 2003, 305:129–135.
51. Jones TR, Wiertz EJ, Sun L, Fish KN, Nelson JA, Ploegh HL: Human cytomegalovirus US3 impairs transport and maturation of major histocompatibility complex class I heavy chains. *Proc. Natl. Acad. Sci. USA* 1996, 93:11327–11333.
52. Kaiser BK, Barahmand-Pour F, Paulsene W, Medley S, Geraghty DE, Strong RK: Interactions between NKG2x immunoreceptors and HLA-E ligands display overlapping affinities and thermodynamics. *J. Immunol.* 2005, 174:2878–2884.
53. Karre K, Ljunggren HG, Piontek G, Kiessling R: Selective rejection of H-2-deficient lymphoma variants suggests alternative immune defence strategy. *Nature* 1986, 319:675–678.

54. Kavanagh DG, Gold MC, Wagner M, Koszinowski UH, Hill AB: The multiple immune-evasion genes of murine cytomegalovirus are not redundant: m4 and m152 inhibit antigen presentation in a complementary and cooperative fashion. *J. Exp. Med.* 2001, 194:967–978.
55. Kleijnen MF, Huppa JB, Lucin P, Mukherjee S, Farrell H, Campbell AE, Koszinowski UH, Hill AB, Ploegh HL: A mouse cytomegalovirus glycoprotein, gp34, forms a complex with folded class I MHC molecules in the ER which is not retained but is transported to the cell surface. *EMBO J.* 1997, 16:685–694.
56. Krmpotic A, Bubic I, Polic B, Lucin P, Jonjic S: Pathogenesis of murine cytomegalovirus infection. *Microbes Infect.* 2003, 5:1263–1277.
57. Krmpotic A, Busch DH, Bubic I, Gebhardt F, Hengel H, Hasan M, Scalzo AA, Koszinowski UH, Jonjic S: MCMV glycoprotein gp40 confers virus resistance to CD8+ T cells and NK cells in vivo. *Nat. Immunol.* 2002, 3:529–535.
58. Krmpotic A, Hasan M, Loewendorf A, Saulig T, Halenius A, Lenac T, Polic B, Bubic I, Kriegeskorte A, Pernjak-Pugel E, Messerle M, Hengel H, Busch DH, Koszinowski UH, Jonjic S: NK cell activation through the NKG2D ligand MULT-1 is selectively prevented by the glycoprotein encoded by mouse cytomegalovirus gene m145. *J. Exp. Med.* 2005, 201:211–220.
59. Krmpotic A, Messerle M, Crnkovic-Mertens I, Polic B, Jonjic S, Koszinowski UH: The immunoevasive function encoded by the mouse cytomegalovirus gene m152 protects the virus against T cell control in vivo. *J. Exp. Med.* 1999, 190:1285–1296.
60. Lanier LL: NK cell recognition. *Annu. Rev. Immunol.* 2005, 23:225–274.
61. Lanier LL, Corliss B, Wu J, Phillips JH: Association of DAP12 with activating CD94/NKG2C NK cell receptors. *Immunity* 1998, 8:693–701.
62. Lee SH, Girard S, Macina D, Busa M, Zafer A, Belouchi A, Gros P, Vidal SM: Susceptibility to mouse cytomegalovirus is associated with deletion of an activating natural killer cell receptor of the C-type lectin superfamily. *Nat. Genet.* 2001, 28:42–45.
63. Lee SH, Gitas J, Zafer A, Lepage P, Hudson TJ, Belouchi A, Vidal SM: Haplotype mapping indicates two independent origins for the Cmv1s susceptibility allele to cytomegalovirus infection and refines its localization within the Ly49 cluster. *Immunogenetics* 2001, 53:501–505.
64. Lee SH, Zafer A, de RY, Kothary R, Tremblay ML, Gros P, Duplay P, Webb JR, Vidal SM: Transgenic expression of the activating natural killer receptor Ly49H confers resistance to cytomegalovirus in genetically susceptible mice. *J. Exp. Med.* 2003, 197:515–526.
65. Lehner PJ, Karttunen JT, Wilkinson GW, Cresswell P: The human cytomegalovirus US6 glycoprotein inhibits transporter associated with antigen processing-dependent peptide translocation. *Proc. Natl. Acad. Sci. USA* 1997, 94:6904–6909.
66. Lodoen M, Ogasawara K, Hamerman JA, Arase H, Houchins JP, Mocarski ES, Lanier LL: NKG2D-mediated natural killer cell protection against cytomegalovirus is impaired by viral gp40 modulation of retinoic acid early inducible 1 gene molecules. *J. Exp. Med.* 2003, 197:1245–1253.

67. Lodoen MB, Abenes G, Umamoto S, Houchins JP, Liu F, Lanier LL: The cytomegalovirus m155 gene product subverts natural killer cell antiviral protection by disruption of H60-NKG2D interactions. *J. Exp. Med.* 2004, 200:1075–1081.
68. Loh J, Chu DT, O'Guin AK, Yokoyama WM, Virgin HW: Natural killer cells utilize both perforin and γinterferon to regulate murine cytomegalovirus infection in the spleen and liver. *J. Virol.* 2005, 79:661–667.
69. Lohwasser S, Hande P, Mager DL, Takei F: Cloning of murine NKG2A, B and C: second family of C-type lectin receptors on murine NK cells. *Eur. J. Immunol.* 1999, 29:755–761.
70. Lundberg P, Welander P, Openshaw H, Nalbandian C, Edwards C, Moldawer L, Cantin E: A locus on mouse chromosome 6 that determines resistance to herpes simplex virus also influences reactivation, while an unlinked locus augments resistance of female mice. *J. Virol.* 2003, 77:11661–11673.
71. Makrigiannis AP, Pau AT, Saleh A, Winkler-Pickett R, Ortaldo JR, Anderson SK: Class I MHC-binding characteristics of the 129/J Ly49 repertoire. *J. Immunol.* 2001, 166:5034–5043.
72. Makrigiannis AP, Pau AT, Schwartzberg PL, McVicar DW, Beck TW, Anderson SK: A BAC contig map of the Ly49 gene cluster in 129 mice reveals extensive differences in gene content relative to C57BL/6 mice. *Genomics* 2002, 79:437–444.
73. Mocarski ES, Jr.: Immune escape and exploitation strategies of cytomegaloviruses: impact on and imitation of the major histocompatibility system. *Cell Microbiol.* 2004, 6:707–717.
74. Mocarski ES, Jr.: Immunomodulation by cytomegaloviruses: manipulative strategies beyond evasion. *Trends Microbiol.* 2002, 10:332–339.
75. Nakamura MC, Linnemeyer PA, Niemi EC, Mason LH, Ortaldo JR, Ryan JC, Seaman WE: Mouse Ly-49D recognizes H-2Dd and activates natural killer cell cytotoxicity. *J. Exp. Med.* 1999, 189:493–500.
76. Nguyen KB, Watford WT, Salomon R, Hofmann SR, Pien GC, Morinobu A, Gadina M, O'Shea JJ, Biron CA: Critical role for STAT4 activation by type 1 interferons in the interferon-γ response to viral infection. *Science* 2002, 297:2063–2066.
77. Nomura M, Zou Z, Joh T, Takihara Y, Matsuda Y, Shimada K: Genomic structures and characterization of Rae1 family members encoding GPI-anchored cell surface proteins and expressed predominantly in embryonic mouse brain. *J. Biochem.(Tokyo)* 1996, 120:987–995.
78. Orange JS, Wang B, Terhorst C, Biron CA: Requirement for natural killer cell-produced interferon γ in defense against murine cytomegalovirus infection and enhancement of this defense pathway by interleukin 12 administration. *J. Exp. Med.* 1995, 182:1045–1056.
79. Parham P: MHC class I molecules and KIRs in human history, health and survival. *Nat. Rev. Immunol.* 2005, 5:201–214.
80. Peruzzi M, Wagtmann N, Long EO: A p70 killer cell inhibitory receptor specific for several HLA-B allotypes discriminates among peptides bound to HLA-B*2705. *J. Exp. Med.* 1996, 184:1585–1590.
81. Presti RM, Pollock JL, Dal Canto AJ, O'Guin AK, Virgin HW: Interferon γ regulates acute and latent murine cytomegalovirus infection and chronic disease of the great vessels. *J. Exp. Med.* 1998, 188:577–588.

82. Proteau MF, Rousselle E, Makrigiannis AP: Mapping of the BALB/c Ly49 cluster defines a minimal natural killer cell receptor gene repertoire. *Genomics* 2004, 84:669–677.
83. Radosavljevic M, Cuillerier B, Wilson MJ, Clement O, Wicker S, Gilfillan S, Beck S, Trowsdale J, Bahram S: A cluster of ten novel MHC class I related genes on human chromosome 6q24.2–q25.3. *Genomics* 2002, 79:114–123.
84. Raftery M, Muller A, Schonrich G: Herpesvirus homologues of cellular genes. *Virus Genes* 2000, 21:65–75.
85. Rawlinson WD, Farrell HE, Barrell BG: Analysis of the complete DNA sequence of murine cytomegalovirus. *J. Virol.* 1996, 70:8833–8849.
86. Reusch U, Muranyi W, Lucin P, Burgert HG, Hengel H, Koszinowski UH: A cytomegalovirus glycoprotein re-routes MHC class I complexes to lysosomes for degradation. *EMBO J.* 1999, 18:1081–1091.
87. Reyburn HT, Mandelboim O, Vales-Gomez M, Davis DM, Pazmany L, Strominger JL: The class I MHC homologue of human cytomegalovirus inhibits attack by natural killer cells. *Nature* 1997, 386:514–517.
88. Riera L, Gariglio M, Valente G, Mullbacher A, Museteanu C, Landolfo S, Simon MM: Murine cytomegalovirus replication in salivary glands is controlled by both perforin and granzymes during acute infection. *Eur. J. Immunol.* 2000, 30:1350–1355.
89. Rolle A, Mousavi-Jazi M, Eriksson M, Odeberg J, Soderberg-Naucler C, Cosman D, Karre K, Cerboni C: Effects of human cytomegalovirus infection on ligands for the activating NKG2D receptor of NK cells: up-regulation of UL16-binding protein (ULBP)1 and ULBP2 is counteracted by the viral UL16 protein. *J. Immunol.* 2003, 171:902–908.
90. Rosen DB, Araki M, Hamerman JA, Chen T, Yamamura T, Lanier LL: A Structural basis for the association of DAP12 with mouse, but not human, NKG2D. *J. Immunol.* 2004, 173:2470–2478.
91. Scalzo AA, Fitzgerald NA, Simmons A, La Vista AB, Shellam GR: Cmv-1, a genetic locus that controls murine cytomegalovirus replication in the spleen. *J. Exp. Med.* 1990, 171:1469–1483.
92. Scalzo AA, Fitzgerald NA, Wallace CR, Gibbons AE, Smart YC, Burton RC, Shellam GR: The effect of the Cmv-1 resistance gene, which is linked to the natural killer cell gene complex, is mediated by natural killer cells. *J. Immunol.* 1992, 149:581–589.
93. Scalzo AA, Lyons PA, Fitzgerald NA, Forbes CA, Yokoyama WM, Shellam GR: Genetic mapping of Cmv1 in the region of mouse chromosome 6 encoding the NK gene complex-associated loci Ly49 and musNKR-P1. *Genomics* 1995, 27:435–441.
94. Shellam GR, Allan JE, Papadimitriou JM, Bancroft GJ: Increased susceptibility to cytomegalovirus infection in beige mutant mice. *Proc. Natl. Acad. Sci. USA* 1981, 78:5104–5108.
95. Sjolin H, Tomasello E, Mousavi-Jazi M, Bartolazzi A, Karre K, Vivier E, Cerboni C: Pivotal role of KARAP/DAP12 adaptor molecule in the natural killer cell-mediated resistance to murine cytomegalovirus infection. *J. Exp. Med.* 2002, 195:825–834.

96. Smith HR, Heusel JW, Mehta IK, Kim S, Dorner BG, Naidenko OV, Iizuka K, Furukawa H, Beckman DL, Pingel JT, Scalzo AA, Fremont DH, Yokoyama WM: Recognition of a virus-encoded ligand by a natural killer cell activation receptor. *Proc. Natl. Acad. Sci. USA* 2002, 99:8826–8831.
97. Smith KM, Wu J, Bakker AB, Phillips JH, Lanier LL: Ly-49D and Ly-49H associate with mouse DAP12 and form activating receptors. *J. Immunol.* 1998, 161:7–10.
98. Tay CH, Welsh RM, Brutkiewicz RR: NK cell response to viral infections in β2-microglobulin-deficient mice. *J. Immunol.* 1995, 154:780–789.
99. Tomasec P, Braud VM, Rickards C, Powell MB, McSharry BP, Gadola S, Cerundolo V, Borysiewicz LK, McMichael AJ, Wilkinson GW: Surface expression of HLA-E, an inhibitor of natural killer cells, enhanced by human cytomegalovirus gpUL40. *Science* 2000, 287:1031.
100. Tortorella D, Gewurz B, Schust D, Furman M, Ploegh H: Down-regulation of MHC class I antigen presentation by HCMV; lessons for tumor immunology. *Immunol. Invest.* 2000, 29:97–100.
101. Vance RE, Jamieson AM, Raulet DH: Recognition of the class Ib molecule Qa-1^b by putative activating receptors CD94/NKG2C and CD94/NKG2E on mouse natural killer cells. *J. Exp. Med.* 1999, 190:1801–1812.
102. Vance RE, Kraft JR, Altman JD, Jensen PE, Raulet DH: Mouse CD94/NKG2A is a natural killer cell receptor for the nonclassical major histocompatibility complex (MHC) class I molecule Qa-1^b. *J.Exp.Med.* 1998, 188:1841–1848.
103. Vance RE, Tanamachi DM, Hanke T, Raulet DH: Cloning of a mouse homolog of CD94 extends the family of C-type lectins on murine natural killer cells. *Eur. J. Immunol.* 1997, 27:3236–3241.
104. Wagner M, Gutermann A, Podlech J, Reddehase MJ, Koszinowski UH: Major histocompatibility complex class I allele-specific cooperative and competitive interactions between immune evasion proteins of cytomegalovirus. *J. Exp. Med.* 2002, 196:805–816.
105. Welsh RM, Brubaker JO, Vargas-Cortes M, O'Donnell CL: Natural killer (NK) cell response to virus infections in mice with severe combined immunodeficiency. The stimulation of NK cells and the NK cell-dependent control of virus infections occur independently of T and B cell function. *J. Exp. Med.* 1991, 173:1053–1063.
106. Welte SA, Sinzger C, Lutz SZ, Singh-Jasuja H, Sampaio KL, Eknigk U, Rammensee HG, Steinle A: Selective intracellular retention of virally induced NKG2D ligands by the human cytomegalovirus UL16 glycoprotein. *Eur. J. Immunol.* 2003, 33:194–203.
107. Westgaard IH, Berg SF, Orstavik S, Fossum S, Dissen E: Identification of a human member of the Ly-49 multigene family. *Eur. J. Immunol.* 1998, 28:1839–1846.
108. Wiertz EJ, Jones TR, Sun L, Bogyo M, Geuze HJ, Ploegh HL: The human cytomegalovirus US11 gene product dislocates MHC class I heavy chains from the endoplasmic reticulum to the cytosol. *Cell* 1996, 84:769–779.
109. Wiertz EJ, Tortorella D, Bogyo M, Yu J, Mothes W, Jones TR, Rapoport TA, Ploegh HL: Sec61-mediated transfer of a membrane protein from the endoplasmic reticulum to the proteasome for destruction. *Nature* 1996, 384:432–438.
110. Wu J, Song Y, Bakker AB, Bauer S, Spies T, Lanier LL, Phillips JH: An activating immunoreceptor complex formed by NKG2D and DAP10. *Science* 1999, 285:730–732.

111. Yawata M, Yawata N, bi-Rached L, Parham P: Variation within the human killer cell immunoglobulin-like receptor (KIR) gene family. *Crit. Rev. Immunol.* 2002, 22:463–482.
112. Yewdell JW, Hill AB: Viral interference with antigen presentation. *Nat. Immunol.* 2002, 3:1019–1025.
113. Yokoyama WM, Plougastel BF: Immune functions encoded by the natural killer gene complex. *Nat. Rev. Immunol.* 2003, 3:304–316.
114. Ziegler H, Thale R, Lucin P, Muranyi W, Flohr T, Hengel H, Farrell H, Rawlinson W, Koszinowski UH: A mouse cytomegalovirus glycoprotein retains MHC class I complexes in the ERGIC/cis-Golgi compartments. *Immunity* 1997, 6:57–66.

NK Cell Receptors Involved in the Response to Human Cytomegalovirus Infection

M. Gumá[1] · A. Angulo[2] · M. López-Botet[1] (✉)

[1]Molecular Immunopathology Unit, DCEXS, Universitat Pompeu Fabra, Dr. Aiguader 80, 08003 Barcelona,Spain
miguel.lopez-botet@upf.edu

[2]Institut d'Investigacions Biomediques August Pi i Sunyer (IDIBAPS), Barcelona,Spain

1	Introduction	208
2	Involvement of Inhibitory NKR in the Response to HCMV	210
2.1	CD94/NKG2A	210
2.2	KIR	212
2.3	CD85j (ILT2, LIR-1)	213
3	Activating NK Cell Receptors in the Response to HCMV	214
3.1	NKG2D	214
3.2	Natural Cytotoxicity Receptors	215
3.3	CD94/NKG2C	215
4	Concluding Remarks	217
References		218

Abstract Human cytomegalovirus (HCMV) infection is a paradigm of the complexity reached by host-pathogen interactions. To avoid recognition by cytotoxic T lymphocytes (CTL) HCMV inhibits the expression of HLA class I molecules. As a consequence, engagement of inhibitory killer immunoglobulin-like receptors (KIR), CD94/NKG2A, and CD85j (ILT2 or LIR-1) natural killer cell receptors (NKR) specific for HLA class I molecules is impaired, and infected cells become vulnerable to an NK cell response driven by activating receptors. In addition to the well-defined role of the NKG2D lectin-like molecule, the involvement of other triggering receptors (i.e., activating KIR, CD94/NKG2C, NKp46, NKp44, and NKp30) in the response to HCMV is being explored. To escape from NK cell-mediated surveillance, HCMV interferes with the expression of NKG2D ligands in infected cells. In addition, the virus may keep NK inhibitory receptors engaged preserving HLA class I molecules with a limited role in antigen presentation (i.e., HLA-E) or, alternatively, displaying class I surrogates. Despite considerable progress in the field, a number of issues regarding the involvement of NKR in the innate immune response to HCMV remain uncertain.

1
Introduction

Human cytomegalovirus (HCMV) is a prototypic betaherpesvirus that infects with a high prevalence all human populations (Pass 2001). Primary infection in healthy immunocompetent individuals is usually mild or asymptomatic. Replicating HCMV is eventually cleared by the host immune response, but the virus remains in a lifelong latent state. Reactivation of HCMV, associated with unapparent shedding, can sporadically occur in seropositive carriers facilitating the spread of the virus to additional hosts. The long-term persistence after primary infection of circulating T cells specific for viral antigens presumably reflects the impact of this recurrent process on the immune system. In contrast, primary infection, reinfection, or reactivation of HCMV may cause a significant morbidity in individuals with immature or compromised immune systems. In transplant recipients, HCMV infection can lead to severe complications such as pneumonia, hepatitis, or graft failure. Retinitis is a common HCMV-induced pathology in human immunodeficiency virus (HIV)-infected patients. In addition, HCMV is the leading viral cause of congenital disorders such as hearing loss, chorioretinitis, or mental retardation. Several studies have also implicated HCMV infection as a cofactor contributing to atherosclerosis and coronary restenosis after angioplasty.

HCMV is a large enveloped double-stranded DNA virus; its 230-kb genome encodes for around 200 open reading frames, a vast number of which have not yet been related to any specific functional role during infection (Mocarski and Courcelle 2001). HCMV exhibits strict species specificity, a relatively slow replication cycle, and a narrow cell tropism in tissue culture. Despite the fact that HCMV infects different cell types in the host (i.e., fibroblasts, hepatocytes, and epithelial, endothelial, smooth muscle, stromal, neuronal, and hematopoietic cells), complete productive infection in vitro is mainly sustained in fibroblasts and, less efficiently, in endothelial and differentiated myelomonocytic cells. Expression of HCMV genes in fully permissive cells follows a temporally ordered cascade in which three phases, designated as immediate-early, early, and late, can be distinguished. Viral gene expression is limited in some cell types, where only a restricted/abortive HCMV infection takes place, thus representing potential sites of viral persistence in vivo. In particular, myelomonocytic cells harboring HCMV genomes are thought to serve as reservoirs of latent virus. Under specific stimuli, such as proinflammatory cytokines, monocytes may differentiate into mature macrophages, allowing productive HCMV replication and dissemination.

The majority of in vitro studies on HCMV have been performed with laboratory strains (i.e., AD169, Towne) that have been subjected to extensive passages on human fibroblast cell lines. This manipulation results in genetic deletions, and, in fact, at least an extra 15-kb region containing more than 19 ORFs is only present in freshly isolated clinical strains of HCMV (Cha et al. 1996). Genetic polymorphisms have also been reported in HCMV clinical isolates (Pignatelli et al. 2004); however, the relevance of HCMV genetic variability in the context of viral immunopathogenesis and disease outcome is still poorly understood (Cerboni et al. 2000). A powerful approach to study the function of individual CMV genes is the generation and analysis of viral mutants carrying specific genome deletions. The introduction of full-length CMV genomes into *Escherichia coli* as an artificial chromosome (BAC) clone (Adler et al. 2003) has facilitated efficient and reliable targeted mutagenesis.

Experimental animal models, mainly using murine CMV (MCMV), have been extensively employed to provide insights into HCMV biology and pathogenesis. Despite a significant divergence, MCMV shares many features with its human counterpart in terms of replication during acute infection, tissue tropism, establishment of latency, and reactivation (Ho 1991). In addition, human and murine viruses exhibit a similar genetic organization and encode homologous gene products (Chee et al. 1990; Rawlinson et al. 1996).

Early studies in animal models revealed that an effective defense against CMV requires the coordinated participation of the innate and adaptive immune responses, mainly involving NK cells and specific CTL (Biron and Brossay 2001; French and Yokoyama 2003; Scalzo 2002); reciprocally, CMV have adopted a variety of immune evasion strategies. Human CTL recognize peptide epitopes derived from different HCMV antigens such as the UL83 (pp65) and UL32 (pp150) structural proteins, as well as the immediate-early transactivator UL123 (IE-1; pp72) (Mocarski and Courcelle 2001). To interfere with antigen presentation, HCMV impairs the expression of HLA class I molecules, employing several proteins encoded by a gene cluster located in the unique short (US) region of the HCMV genome (Hengel et al. 1999; Tortorella et al. 2000). Among them, US2 and US11 are expressed at early-late stages of the viral replication cycle and translocate class I heavy chains from the ER to the cytosol, where they are degraded. US3 is an immediate-early protein that retains class I molecules at the endoplasmic reticulum (ER), whereas the late US6 protein impairs TAP-mediated peptide transport. Two additional genes in the US region, US8 and US10, encode glycoproteins that bind MHC class I heavy chains, although they do not appear to drastically alter processing and cell surface expression of the MHC class I molecules (Furman et al. 2002; Tirabassi and Ploegh 2002). Remarkably, US2 and US3 may also interfere with MHC class II antigen presentation (Hegde et al. 2003).

The redundant mechanisms for inhibition of HLA class I expression likely reflect the importance of this immune evasion strategy. As a consequence,

NK cells are released from the control exerted by inhibitory receptors specific for class I molecules and can mediate cytotoxicity and cytokine production against infected cells. To escape from NK cell-mediated surveillance, HCMV impairs the expression of ligands for activating receptors. Alternatively, the virus may keep NK inhibitory receptors engaged, either preserving ligands with a limited role in antigen presentation (i.e., HLA-E and HLA-C) or displaying class I surrogates in infected cells (Lopez-Botet et al. 2004).

2
Involvement of Inhibitory NKR in the Response to HCMV

NK cells express several inhibitory receptors such as KIR, the CD94/NKG2A killer lectin-like receptor (KLR) and CD85j (ILT2 or LIR-1) (Colonna et al. 1999; Lopez-Botet and Bellon 1999; Moretta and Moretta 2004), that are also expressed by some T lymphocytes (Vivier and Anfossi 2004). The spectra of class I HLA molecules covered by inhibitory KIR and, indirectly, by CD94/NKG2A are partially overlapping. Both receptor systems complement each other to monitor the surface expression of most class I molecules, which are also broadly recognized by CD85j. The heterogeneous distribution of NKR in distinct NK cell subsets enables the system to react against variable alterations of HLA class I expression, provided that activating signals overcome the inhibitory threshold.

2.1
CD94/NKG2A

CD94 and NKG2 are lectin-like membrane glycoproteins encoded at the NK gene complex (NKC) in human chromosome 12 (Chang et al. 1995; Houchins et al. 1991). The CD94/NKG2A heterodimer constitutes an inhibitory receptor that recruits the SHP-1 tyrosine phosphatase through the immunoreceptor tyrosine-based inhibition motif (ITIM)-bearing NKG2A subunit. By contrast, CD94/NKG2C forms a triggering receptor linked to KARAP/DAP12, an immunoreceptor tyrosine-based activation motif (ITAM)-bearing adapter molecule that connects these receptors to a protein tyrosine kinase (PTK) activation pathway (Lanier 2003; Lopez-Botet and Bellon 1999). The function of other putative activating molecules encoded by the NKG2E gene (Yabe et al. 1993) remains unknown. HLA-E was shown to be a specific ligand for both CD94/NKG2A and CD94/NKG2C receptors, presenting peptides derived from the signal sequences of other HLA class I molecules (Borrego et al. 1998; Braud et al. 1998; Lee et al. 1998). HLA-E is dimorphic at position 107, where the few allotypes identified display either an Arg (HLA-E^R) or a Gly (HLA-E^G) (Strong et al. 2003). Resolution of the crystal structure of HLA-E revealed the basis of its affinity for hydrophobic leader sequence-derived peptides (O'Callaghan et al. 1998).

Detection of HLA-E by CD94/NKG2A is currently viewed as a sensor mechanism that probes the status of HLA class I biosynthesis. Yet there is evidence supporting the idea that HLA-E may bind to hydrophobic peptides from other proteins; some of these sequences are very similar to those derived from HLA class I molecules, whereas others appear completely unrelated. Among the first group, a peptide from the HSP60 was shown to potentially compete with endogenous class I-derived nonamers for binding to HLA-E (Michaelsson et al. 2002); the complex was not recognized by CD94/NKG2A, rendering stressed cells vulnerable to an NK-mediated attack. The biological relevance of this observation in the context of the immune response against virus-infected targets is still uncertain.

On the other hand, a nonamer derived from the leader sequence of the UL40 HCMV protein was also reported to interact with HLA-E (Tomasec et al. 2000; Ulbrecht et al. 2000). Expression of the class Ib molecule was preserved in infected cells, conferring protection against a CD94/NKG2A+ NK cell line. Moreover, fibroblasts infected by a UL40-deletion mutant of the AD169 HCMV strain were killed by CD94/NKG2A+ primary NK cell lines more efficiently than cells infected by the wild-type virus (Wang et al. 2002). The possibility that HLA-E may be maintained during HCMV infection to effectively evade the NK response has been questioned by another study (Falk et al. 2002); some differences between experimental approaches may explain the discrepancy.

To be preserved in HCMV-infected cells, HLA-E should be refractory to the action of viral proteins that target class I molecules (i.e., US2, US3, US6, and US11). Indeed, HLA-E presentation of the UL40-derived nonamer was confirmed to be TAP independent and resistant to US6 (Tomasec et al. 2000). We compared the effect of US2, US6, or US11 on endogenous HLA-E and HLA class Ia expression in a human B cell lymphoma line, assessing in parallel their influence on target susceptibility to NK cell clones (Llano et al. 2003). In this system, US6 downregulated all class I molecules, whereas US11 selectively preserved HLA-E. This rendered US11+ cells sensitive to NK clones under the control of KIR2DL2 and/or CD85j receptors, maintaining resistance to CD94/NKG2A+ KIR2DL2− cells. US2 also spared HLA-E, although it selectively targeted class Ia molecules, inhibiting HLA-A and HLA-C but not HLA-B expression. Altogether these observations support the hypothesis that US6-resistant presentation of the UL40-derived peptide together with the restricted action of US2 and US11 may contribute to maintain HLA-E expression during the infection. In that way, the virus should be able to interfere with HLA class Ia antigen presentation to CD8+ lymphocytes, concomitantly protecting infected cells against CD94/NKG2A+ effectors.

Recent observations suggest that the immune system may counteract this evasion strategy. In this regard, it has been shown that some CTL may specifically recognize HLA-E (Garcia et al. 2002; Moretta et al. 2003; Pietra et al. 2001). We originally demonstrated binding of HLA-E tetramers to the TCR of a T cell clone, which specifically killed cells expressing the class Ib molecule associated to some HLA class I and virus-derived peptides (i.e., BZLF1 from EBV) (Garcia et al. 2002). Mingari et al. have extended these studies, proposing that CTL recognizing HLA-E bound to the UL40 nonamer might have a relevant role in the response against HCMV-infected cells (Pietra et al. 2003).

2.2
KIR

The KIR gene family is located in human chromosome 19q13.4; different KIR haplotypes that include partially overlapping sets of genes have been identified (Moretta and Moretta 2004; Vilches and Parham 2002). A group of KIRs (i.e., KIR2DL and KIR3DL) display cytoplasmic ITIM, which once phosphorylated become docking sites for the SHP-1 protein tyrosine phosphatase involved in inhibitory signaling. Other KIR bear shorter intracytoplasmic domains lacking ITIM (i.e., KIR2DS/3DS) and, similarly to NKG2C, contain a charged transmembrane residue (Lys) interacting with KARAP/DAP12. Some KIR specifically interact with sets of HLA class Ia allotypes that share structural features at the α1 domain, whereas the ligands for other KIR still remain unknown.

The possibility that HCMV-infected cells might preserve HLA-C to escape from KIR-mediated surveillance, as originally proposed for HIV (Cohen et al. 1999), remains unclear. On one hand, US2 was shown to bind HLA-A but not HLA-E, -B7, -B27, or HLA-Cw4 molecules (Gewurz et al. 2001); moreover, HLA-C appeared resistant to US2 and US11 when expressed in a trophoblast cell line (Schust et al. 1998). In contrast, endogenous HLA-Cw7 was downregulated in US2+ and US11+ transfected cells (Llano et al. 2003), and Huard and Fruh reported that US11+ targets were sensitive to KIR2DL+ NK cells, indirectly supporting the idea that HLA-C expression was inhibited (Huard and Fruh 2000). In the same line, Falk et al. reported that downregulation of HLA class I molecules, including HLA-C, did not occur in fibroblasts infected with a deletion mutant lacking the US2-US11 region (Falk et al. 2002).

2.3
CD85j (ILT2, LIR-1)

The Ig-like transcript (ILT) or leukocyte Ig-like receptor (LIR) gene family flanks the KIR locus at chromosome 19p13.4, encoding for molecules preferentially expressed by the myeloid lineage (Colonna et al. 1999). Some ILT (LIR, CD85) molecules contain cytoplasmic ITIM that recruit SHP phosphatases, whereas others display a charged transmembrane residue (Arg) and associate to the FcεR γ chain. Among the first group, ILT2 (LIR-1, CD85j) and ILT4 (LIR-2) broadly interact with HLA class I molecules (Colonna et al. 1997; Cosman et al. 1997). ILT2 is detected on NK and T cell subsets, as well as on B cells and monocytes/macrophages, whereas ILT4 expression is restricted to the latter.

Engagement of inhibitory receptors by HLA class I surrogates expressed in CMV-infected cells constitutes a potential way to subvert the NK cell response. In this regard, the ILT2 receptor was reported to bind the UL18 HCMV HLA class I-like molecule with an affinity higher than that for class I molecules (Chapman et al. 2000; Cosman et al. 1997). However, the hypothesis that UL18 may interfere with NK cell activity during HCMV infection has not received consistent experimental support. Moreover, a reduced susceptibility to NK cell-mediated lysis of HCMV-infected cells was shown to be independent of UL18 expression (Odeberg et al. 2002). The possibility that UL18 may act on other CD85j+ cell types (i.e., monocytes/macrophages) should be envisaged.

Remarkably, Leong et al. observed that, rather than conferring protection, UL18 increased susceptibility to NK-mediated lysis; however, ILT2 was not analyzed in that study (Leong et al. 1998). More recently, Ciccone and colleagues (Saverino et al. 2004) reported that CD8+ T lymphocytes killed UL18+ cells in an MHC-unrestricted and TCR-independent manner ; moreover, fibroblasts infected by an HCMV deletion mutant lacking UL18 were resistant to lysis. Strikingly, T cell-mediated cytotoxicity of HCMV+ fibroblasts was inhibited by UL18- and CD85j-specific mAbs, although only at very late stages of infection (i.e., 6 days). These functional data were interpreted as an indirect indication that a cognate UL18-CD85j interaction might trigger T cell effector functions. This hypothesis requires further experimental support to confirm the ability of CD85j to activate T lymphocytes and, eventually, to define the signaling pathway(s) involved. The identification of other triggering receptor(s) specific for UL18 might also contribute to explain the observations. It is of note that CD85j expression was shown to be increased in PBL from patients undergoing HCMV infection after lung transplantation (Berg et al. 2003); in the same line, we observed that the proportions of CD85j+ T lymphocytes were increased in HCMV+ individuals (Gumá et al.

2004). The mechanisms underlying the impact of HCMV infection on CD85j expression should be explored. UL18 polymorphisms have been reported to influence its interaction with ILT12 (Valés-Gómez et al. 2005).

Preliminary reports point out that HCMV may synthesize additional class I-like molecules to interfere with the NK-mediated response (Sissons et al. and Wang et al. reported at the 29th Annual International Herpesvirus Workshop, Reno, Nevada, July 2004); whether these proteins engage inhibitory NKR is as yet unknown. It is of note that the corresponding genes (i.e., UL141 and UL142) can be found in HCMV clinical isolates but are deleted in commonly used laboratory strains (i.e., AD169 and Towne). Recently, UL141 has been described to exert a blocking effect on the expression of CD155, a ligand for the DNAM-1 activating receptor (Tomasec et al. 2005).

3
Activating NK Cell Receptors in the Response to HCMV

The nature of the cellular ligands for triggering human NK cell receptors has been only partially unraveled. Some of them appear to be constitutively expressed by target cells (i.e., HLA class I molecules), others are inducible under stress conditions and can be detected in virus-infected and tumor cells (i.e., MICA/B), whereas a third category remains unknown. Although the possibility that MHC class I molecules bound to foreign peptides may be efficiently recognized by triggering NKR remains theoretical, studies in mice point out that some NK-activating receptors may recognize pathogen-derived molecules.

3.1
NKG2D

Human NKG2D (hNKG2D) is a lectin-like molecule expressed by NK and T cells that is coupled to a PI3K signaling pathway through the DAP10 adapter (Vivier et al. 2002; Wu et al. 1999). NKG2D has been reported to function either as a triggering receptor (Billadeau et al. 2003) or a costimulatory molecule in conjunction with other PTK-linked receptors (Groh et al. 2001; Wu et al. 2002). Like its murine homolog, hNKG2D interacts with stress-inducible molecules, which are also detected in some transformed and virus-infected cells. Several class I-related ligands have been defined for human NKG2D, including the polymorphic MICA/B molecules and a family of proteins termed "UL16-binding proteins" (ULBP) or retinoic acid early inducible-1 (RAE-1)-like (Bacon et al. 2004; Bauer et al. 1999; Chalupny et al. 2003; Cosman et al. 2001; Raulet 2003).

NKG2D ligands are expressed in CMV-infected cells and costimulate virus-specific CTL (Groh et al. 2001; Raulet 2003). The existence of viral escape mechanisms that target NKG2D function indirectly illustrates the importance of this mechanism of response to HCMV. In this regard, the UL16 glycoprotein inhibits surface expression of MICB, ULBP1, and ULBP2 (Valés-Gómez et al. 2003; Welte et al. 2003) and also interacts with RAET1G (Bacon et al. 2004), thus potentially interfering with the NKG2D-mediated response. On infection with a UL16 deletion mutant, all ULBP molecules were expressed at the cell surface, leading to an increase in NKG2D-mediated lysis (Rolle et al. 2003). On the other hand, Oderberg et al. have proposed that UL16 may also exert a direct protective effect against cytolytic mediators released by NK cells (Odeberg et al. 2003).

3.2
Natural Cytotoxicity Receptors

Several Ig-like natural cytotoxicity receptors (NCR) connected to PTK signaling pathways have been shown to trigger NK cell functions (Moretta et al. 2001). NKp46 is coupled to the ζ or γ adapters, activating cytotoxicity and cytokine production on recognition of still undefined cellular ligand(s). The nature of the molecules recognized by the DAP12-associated NKp44 and the ζ-linked NKp30 NCR also remain unknown. Although the role of NCR in the defense against HCMV remains uncertain, the putative expression of NCR ligands by different cell types suggests that these receptors might contribute to the response against virus-infected cells that have downregulated HLA class I molecules. On the other hand, the possibility that quantitative/qualitative changes in expression of NCR ligands may take place during HCMV infection cannot be excluded. The involvement of additional activating receptors (Moretta et al. 2004) in the response to HCMV should be also explored. Recently, pp65 has been shown to interact with NKp30, inhibiting NK cell function (Amon et al. 2005).

3.3
CD94/NKG2C

Most inhibitory receptor families include activating molecules whose physiological role remains unclear. It has been hypothesized that KIR2DS/3DS and CD94/NKG2C receptors may contribute to trigger cytotoxicity and cytokine production when the dominant control by inhibitory receptors falls beneath a critical threshold (Lopez-Botet et al. 2000). As the affinity of stimulatory NKR for class I molecules appears lower than that of the inhibitory counterparts, either a selective downmodulation of the inhibitory ligand and/or an increase of the activating NKR avidity for their ligands would be required. The first situation may take place in HCMV-infected cells, where HLA-E molecules appear to be selectively spared from the action of US proteins. With regard to the second possibility, there is no evidence for the existence of class I-peptide complexes or other ligands recognized with high affinity by the activating NKR. Nevertheless, the hypothesis that some activating NKR may directly interact with microbial products has gained experimental support. Ly49H associates to DAP12 and plays a pivotal role in the defense against MCMV-infected cells, triggering NK cell functions on its interaction with the m157 viral protein (Arase et al. 2002; Smith et al. 2002).

As observed for Ly49H expression during MCMV infection (Dokun et al. 2001), it is conceivable that HCMV might shape the NKR repertoire and the distribution of NK cell subsets. In this regard, increased proportions of CD94/NKG2C+ NK and T cells were detected in HCMV+ individuals (Gumá et al. 2004), presumably reflecting the challenge exerted by the virus on the innate immune system and suggesting that they might participate in the response to the pathogen. In contrast to the CD94/NKG2A+ subset, most CD94/NKG2C+ cells coexpressed KIR and CD85j, displaying lower levels of NCR. Detection of CD85j+ CD94/NKG2C− cells suggests that both phenotypic features are independently associated to HCMV infection.

CD94/NKG2C+ T lymphocytes populations generally displayed a TCRαβ+ CD8+ CD56+ CD28− phenotype and appear to be oligoclonal; however, NKG2C+ TCRγδ and rare NKG2C+ CD4+ cells were also detectable in some donors (Gumá M and López-Botet M, submitted). The antigen specificity of NKG2C+ cells is uncertain. It is of note that most HCMV-specific CTL identified with HLA-A*0201/pp65 tetramers did not express NKG2C (Gumá et al. 2004). Moreover, despite the fact that some CD94/NKG2C+ cells may correspond to HLA-E-specific CTL (Garcia et al. 2002), this association is not a general finding as NKG2C was reported to be undetectable in HLA-E-specific CTL (Pietra et al. 2003).

Comparably to the response induced in NK cells, specific engagement of the CD94/NKG2C lectin-like receptor was observed to trigger the proliferation and effector functions of a subset of CD94/NKG2C+ CD8+ T cells; moreover, the KARAP/DAP12 adapter protein was detected in CD94/NKG2C+ T cell clones (Gumá et al. 2005). Altogether these results support the idea that the KLR may potentially constitute an autonomous activation pathway alternative to the TCR, stimulating the response of NKG2C+ T lymphocytes against HCMV-infected cells.

Several mechanisms may account for the variable increase of CD94/NKG2C+ cells in HCMV+ individuals. First, changes in the NKR repertoire might result from alterations in the cytokine network secondary to the viral infection. IL-21 has been shown to promote the expression of NCR and NKR during the NK cell differentiation from CD34+ precursors (Sivori et al. 2003); moreover, TGFβ and IL-15 induce CD94/NKG2A expression in T cells (Mingari et al. 1998). On the other hand, as observed for Ly49H+ cells, CD94/NKG2C-mediated recognition of HCMV-infected cells could promote the expansion/survival of the corresponding NK and T cell subsets. As stressed above, this would require an increased avidity of the KLR-ligand interaction and/or a selective loss of ligands for inhibitory receptors coexpressed by CD94/NKG2C+ cells (i.e., KIR, ILT2). The preservation of HLA-E bound to the UL40-derived peptide in HCMV-infected cells could favor a response of CD94/NKG2C+ lymphocytes; studies are in progress to address these key questions.

Although HCMV and MCMV are quite disparate, CD94/NKG2 receptors are conserved in mice and specifically recognize $Qa1^b$, a functional homolog of HLA-E (Vance et al. 1999). Studies are required to evaluate whether MCMV infection may target the expression of Qa1 or have any impact on the expression of NKG2C.

4
Concluding Remarks

A number of questions regarding the involvement of NKR in the innate immune response to HCMV remain open. Among these, the existence of human triggering receptors capable of driving the NK cell response to HCMV on recognition of virus-encoded proteins or peptides is uncertain. The identification of NCR ligands becomes essential to define their putative participation in the response against HCMV. The analysis of CD94/NKG2C expression may become an additional useful parameter to explore the host-pathogen relationship, and studies of the NKR repertoire in clinical settings involving HCMV are warranted. On the other hand, further studies are required to understand the implications of the UL18-CD85j interaction in the response to HCMV, and the role in immune evasion of the other class I-like genes deserves attention.

Acknowledgements This work was supported by grants from Plan Nacional de I+D (SAF2004-07632; SAF2002-00270) and European Community (QLRT-2001-01112). MG is recipient of a fellowship from Instituto de Salud Carlos III (ISCIII), Ministry of Health. AA is a fellow from the Ramón y Cajal program.

References

Adler H, Messerle M, Koszinowski UH (2003) Cloning of herpesviral genomes as bacterial artificial chromosomes. Rev Med Virol 13:111–121

Arase H, Mocarski ES, Campbell AE, Hill AB, Lanier LL (2002) Direct recognition of cytomegalovirus by activating and inhibitory NK cell receptors. Science 296:1323–1326

Arrnon TI, Achdout H, Levi O, Markel G, Saleh N, Katz G, Gazit R, Gonen-Gross T, Hanna J, Nahari E, Porgador A, Honigman A, Placxhter B, Mevorach D, Wolf DG, Mandelboim O (2005) Inhibition of the NKp30 activating receptor by pp65 of human cytomegalovirus. Nat Immunol 6:515–523

Bacon L, Eagle RA, Meyer M, Easom N, Young NT, Trowsdale J (2004) Two human ULBP/RAET1 molecules with transmembrane regions are ligands for NKG2D. J Immunol 173:1078–1084

Bauer S, Gröh V, Wu J, Steinle A, Phillips JH, Lanier LL, Spies T (1999) Activation of NK cells and T cells by NKG2D, a receptor for stress- inducible MICA. Science 285:727–729

Berg L, Riise GC, Cosman D, Bergstrom T, Olofsson S, Kärre K, Carbone E (2003) LIR-1 expression on lymphocytes, and cytomegalovirus disease in lung-transplant recipients. Lancet 361:1099–1101

Billadeau DD, Upshaw JL, Schoon RA, Dick CJ, Leibson PJ (2003) NKG2D-DAP10 triggers human NK cell-mediated killing via a Syk-independent regulatory pathway. Nat Immunol 4:557–564

Biron CA, Brossay L (2001) NK cells and NKT cells in innate defense against viral infections. Curr Opin Immunol 13:458–464

Borrego F, Ulbrecht M, Weiss EH, Coligan JE, Brooks AG (1998) Recognition of human histocompatibility leukocyte antigen (HLA)-E complexed with HLA class I signal sequence-derived peptides by CD94/NKG2 confers protection from natural killer cell-mediated lysis. J Exp Med 187:813–818

Braud VM, Allan DS, O'Callaghan CA, Soderström K, D'Andrea A, Ogg GS, Lazetic S, Young NT, Bell JI, Phillips JH, Lanier LL, McMichael AJ (1998) HLA-E binds to natural killer cell receptors CD94/NKG2A, B and C. Nature 391:795–799

Cerboni C, Mousavi-Jazi M, Linde A, Soderströom K, Brytting M, Wahren B, Kärre K, Carbone E (2000) Human cytomegalovirus strain-dependent changes in NK cell recognition of infected fibroblasts. J Immunol 164:4775–4782

Cha TA, Tom E, Kemble GW, Duke GM, Mocarski ES, Spaete RR (1996) Human cytomegalovirus clinical isolates carry at least 19 genes not found in laboratory strains. J Virol 70:78–83

Chalupny NJ, Sutherland CL, Lawrence WA, Rein-Weston A, Cosman D (2003) ULBP4 is a novel ligand for human NKG2D. Biochem Biophys Res Commun 305:129–135

Chang C, Rodríguez A, Carretero M, López-Botet M, Phillips JH, Lanier LL (1995) Molecular characterization of human CD94: a type II membrane glycoprotein related to the C-type lectin superfamily. Eur J Immunol 25:2433–2437

Chapman TL, Heikema AP, West AP, Björkman PJ (2000) Crystal structure and ligand binding properties of the D1D2 region of the inhibitory receptor LIR-1 (ILT2). Immunity 13:727–736

Chee MS, Bankier AT, Beck S, Bohni R, Brown CM, Cerny R, Horsnell T, Hutchison CA, III, Kouzarides T, Martignetti JA. (1990) Analysis of the protein-coding content of the sequence of human cytomegalovirus strain AD169. Curr Top Microbiol Immunol 154:125–169

Cohen GB, Gandhi RT, Davis DM, Mandelboim O, Chen BK, Strominger JL, Baltimore D (1999) The selective downregulation of class I major histocompatibility complex proteins by HIV-1 protects HIV-infected cells from NK cells. Immunity 10:661–671

Colonna M, Nakajima H, Navarro F, López-Botet M (1999) A novel family of Ig-like receptors for HLA class I molecules that modulate function of lymphoid and myeloid cells. J Leukoc Biol 66:375–381

Colonna M, Navarro F, Bellón T, Llano M, García P, Samaridis J, Angman L, Cella M, López-Botet M (1997) A common inhibitory receptor for major histocompatibility complex class I molecules on human lymphoid and myelomonocytic cells. J Exp Med 186:1809–1818

Cosman D, Fanger N, Borges L, Kubin M, Chin W, Peterson L, Hsu ML (1997) A novel immunoglobulin superfamily receptor for cellular and viral MHC class I molecules. Immunity 7:273–282

Cosman D, Mullberg J, Sutherland CL, Chin W, Armitage R, Fanslow W, Kubin M, Chalupny NJ (2001) ULBPs, novel MHC class I-related molecules, bind to CMV glycoprotein UL16 and stimulate NK cytotoxicity through the NKG2D receptor. Immunity 14:123–133

Dokun AO, Kim S, Smith HR, Kang HS, Chu DT, Yokoyama WM (2001) Specific and nonspecific NK cell activation during virus infection. Nat Immunol 2:951–956

Falk CS, Mach M, Schendel DJ, Weiss EH, Hilgert I, Hahn G (2002) NK cell activity during human cytomegalovirus infection is dominated by US2–11-mediated HLA class I down-regulation. J Immunol 169:3257–3266

French AR, Yokoyama WM (2003) Natural killer cells and viral infections. Curr Opin Immunol 15:45–51

Furman MH, Dey N, Tortorella D, Ploegh HL (2002) The human cytomegalovirus US10 gene product delays trafficking of major histocompatibility complex class I molecules. J Virol 76:11753–11756

García P, Llano M, Beltrán de Heredia A, Willberg CB, Caparrós E, Aparicio P, Braud VM, López-Botet M (2002) Human T cell receptor-mediated recognition of HLA-E. Eur J Immunol 32:936–944

Gewurz BE, Wang EW, Tortorella D, Schust DJ, Ploegh HL (2001) Human cytomegalovirus US2 endoplasmic reticulum-lumenal domain dictates association with major histocompatibility complex class I in a locus- specific manner. J Virol 75:5197–5204

Gröh V, Rhinehart R, Randolph-Habecker J, Topp MS, Riddell SR, Spies T (2001) Costimulation of $CD8\alpha\beta$ T cells by NKG2D via engagement by MIC induced on virus-infected cells. Nat Immunol 2:255–260

Gumá M, Angulo A, Vilches C, Gomez-Lozano N, Malats N, López-Botet M (2004) Imprint of human cytomegalovirus infection on the NK cell receptor repertoire. Blood 104:3664–3671

Gumá M, Busch LK, Salazar-Fontana LI, Bellosillo B, Morte C, Garcia P, Lopez-Botet M (2005) The CD94/NKG2C killer lectin-like receptor constitutes an alternative activation pathway for a subset fo $CD8^+$ T cells. Eur J Immunol 35:2071–2080

Hegde NR, Chevalier MS, Johnson DC (2003) Viral inhibition of MHC class II antigen presentation. Trends Immunol 24:278–285

Hengel H, Reusch U, Gutermann A, Ziegler H, Jonjic S, Lucin P, Koszinowski UH (1999) Cytomegaloviral control of MHC class I function in the mouse. Immunol Rev 168:167–176

Ho M (1991) Cytomegaloviruses: biology and infection. Plenum Publishing Corp., New York

Houchins JP, Yabe T, McSherry C, Bach FH (1991) DNA sequence analysis of NKG2, a family of related cDNA clones encoding type II integral membrane proteins on human natural killer cells. J Exp Med 173:1017–1020

Huard B, Früh K (2000) A role for MHC class I down-regulation in NK cell lysis of herpes virus-infected cells. Eur J Immunol 30:509–515

Lanier LL (2003) Natural killer cell receptor signaling. Curr Opin Immunol 15:308–314

Lee N, Llano M, Carretero M, Ishitani A, Navarro F, López-Botet M, Geraghty D (1998) HLA-E is a major ligand for the natural killer inhibitory receptor CD94/NKG2A. Proc Natl Acad Sci USA 95:5199–5204

Leong CC, Chapman TL, Bjorkman PJ, Formankova D, Mocarski ES, Phillips JH, Lanier LL (1998) Modulation of natural killer cell cytotoxicity in human cytomegalovirus infection: the role of endogenous class I major histocompatibility complex and a viral class I homolog [published erratum appears in J Exp Med 1998 Aug 3;188(3):following 614]. J Exp Med 187:1681–1687

Llano M, Gumá M, Ortega M, Angulo A, López-Botet M (2003) Differential effects of US2, US6 and US11 human cytomegalovirus proteins on HLA class Ia and HLA-E expression: impact on target susceptibility to NK cell subsets. Eur J Immunol 33:2744–2754

López-Botet M, Angulo A, Gumá M (2004) Natural killer cell receptors for major histocompatibility complex class I and related molecules in cytomegalovirus infection. Tissue Antigens 63:195–203

López-Botet M, Bellón T (1999) Natural killer cell activation and inhibition by receptors for MHC class I. Curr Opin Immunol 11:301–307

López-Botet M, Bellón T, Llano M, Navarro F, García P, de Miguel M (2000) Paired inhibitory and triggering NK cell receptors for HLA class I molecules. Hum Immunol 61:7–17

Michaelsson J, Teixeira de Matos C, Achour A, Lanier LL, Kärre K, Söoderstrom K (2002) A signal peptide derived from hsp60 binds HLA-E and interferes with CD94/NKG2A recognition. J Exp Med 196:1403–1414

Mingari MC, Moretta A, Moretta L (1998) Regulation of KIR expression in human T cells: a safety mechanism that may impair protective T-cell responses. Immunol Today 19:153–157

Mocarski ES, Courcelle CT (2001) Cytomegaloviruses and their replication. In: Knipe DM, Howley PM, Griffin DE, Lamb RA (eds) Lippincott Williams & Wilkins, Philadelphia, pp 2629–2673

Moretta A, Bottino C, Vitale M, Pende D, Cantoni C, Mingari MC, Biassoni R, Moretta L (2001) Activating receptors and coreceptors involved in human natural killer cell-mediated cytolysis. Annu Rev Immunol 19:197–223

Moretta L, Bottino C, Pende D, Vitale M, Mingari MC, Moretta A (2004) Different checkpoints in human NK-cell activation. Trends Immunol 25:670–676

Moretta L, Moretta A (2004) Killer immunoglobulin-like receptors. Curr Opin Immunol 16:626–633
Moretta L, Romagnani C, Pietra G, Moretta A, Mingari MC (2003) NK-CTLs, a novel HLA-E-restricted T-cell subset. Trends Immunol 24:136–143
O'Callaghan CA, Tormo J, Willcox BE, Braud V, Jakobsen BK, Stuart DI, McMichael A, Green DR (1998) Structural features impose tight peptide binding specificity in the nonclassical MHC molecule HLA-E. Mol Cell 1:531–541
Odeberg J, Browne H, Metkar S, Froelich CJ, Branden L, Cosman D, Söderberg-Naucler C (2003) The human cytomegalovirus protein UL16 mediates increased resistance to natural killer cell cytotoxicity through resistance to cytolytic proteins. J Virol 77:4539–4545
Odeberg J, Cerboni C, Browne H, Karre K, Moller E, Carbone E, Soderberg-Naucler C (2002) Human cytomegalovirus (HCMV)-infected endothelial cells and macrophages are less susceptible to natural killer lysis independent of the downregulation of classical HLA class I molecules or expression of the HCMV class I homologue, UL18. Scand J Immunol 55:149–161
Pass RF (2001) Cytomegalovirus. In: Knipe DM, Howley PM, Griffin DE, Lamb RA (eds) Lippincott, Williams & Wilkins, Philadelphia, pp 2675–2705
Pietra G, Romagnani C, Falco M, Vitale M, Castriconi R, Pende D, Millo E, Anfossi S, Biassoni R, Moretta L, Mingari MC (2001) The analysis of the natural killer-like activity of human cytolytic T lymphocytes revealed HLA-E as a novel target for TCR α/β-mediated recognition. Eur J Immunol 31:3687–3693
Pietra G, Romagnani C, Mazzarino P, Falco M, Millo E, Moretta A, Moretta L, Mingari MC (2003) HLA-E-restricted recognition of cytomegalovirus-derived peptides by human CD8+ cytolytic T lymphocytes. Proc Natl Acad Sci USA 100:10896–10901
Pignatelli S, Dal Monte P, Rossini G, Landini MP (2004) Genetic polymorphisms among human cytomegalovirus (HCMV) wild-type strains. Rev Med Virol 14:383–410
Raulet DH (2003) Roles of the NKG2D immunoreceptor and its ligands. Nat Rev Immunol 3:781–790
Rawlinson WD, Farrell HE, Barrell BG (1996) Analysis of the complete DNA sequence of murine cytomegalovirus. J Virol 70:8833–8849
Rolle A, Mousavi-Jazi M, Eriksson M, Odeberg J, Söderberg-Naucler C, Cosman D, Kärre K, Cerboni C (2003) Effects of human cytomegalovirus infection on ligands for the activating NKG2D receptor of NK cells: up-regulation of UL16-binding protein (ULBP)1 and ULBP2 is counteracted by the viral UL16 protein. J Immunol 171:902–908
Saverino D, Ghiotto F, Merlo A, Bruno S, Battini L, Occhino M, Maffei M, Tenca C, Pileri S, Baldi L, Fabbi M, Bachi A, De Santanna A, Grossi CE, Ciccone E (2004) Specific recognition of the viral protein UL18 by CD85j/LIR-1/ILT2 on CD8+ T cells mediates the non-MHC-restricted lysis of human cytomegalovirus-infected cells. J Immunol 172:5629–5637
Scalzo AA (2002) Successful control of viruses by NK cells–a balance of opposing forces? Trends Microbiol 10:470–474
Schust DJ, Tortorella D, Seebach J, Phan C, Ploegh HL (1998) Trophoblast class I major histocompatibility complex (MHC) products are resistant to rapid degradation imposed by the human cytomegalovirus (HCMV) gene products US2 and US11. J Exp Med 188:497–503

Sivori S, Cantoni C, Parolini S, Marcenaro E, Conte R, Moretta L, Moretta A (2003) IL-21 induces both rapid maturation of human CD34+ cell precursors towards NK cells and acquisition of surface killer Ig-like receptors. Eur J Immunol 33:3439–3447

Smith HR, Heusel JW, Mehta IK, Kim S, Dorner BG, Naidenko OV, Iizuka K, Furukawa H, Beckman DL, Pingel JT, Scalzo AA, Fremont DH, Yokoyama WM (2002) Recognition of a virus-encoded ligand by a natural killer cell activation receptor. Proc Natl Acad Sci USA 99:8826–8831

Strong RK, Holmes MA, Li P, Braun L, Lee N, Geraghty DE (2003) HLA-E allelic variants. Correlating differential expression, peptide affinities, crystal structures and termal stabilities. J Biol Chem 278:5082–5090

Tirabassi RS, Ploegh HL (2002) The human cytomegalovirus US8 glycoprotein binds to major histocompatibility complex class I products. J Virol 76:6832–6835

Tomasec P, Braud VM, Rickards C, Powell MB, McSharry BP, Gadola S, Cerundolo V, Borysiewicz LK, McMichael AJ, Wilkinson GW (2000) Surface expression of HLA-E, an inhibitor of natural killer cells, enhanced by human cytomegalovirus gpUL40. Science 287:1031–1033

Tomasec P, Wang EC, Davison AJ, Vojtesek B, Armstrong M, Griffin C, McSharry BP, Morris RJ, Llewellyn-Lacey S, Rickards C, Nomoto A, Sinzger C, Wilkinson GW, (2005) Downregulation of natural killer cell-activating ligand CD155 by human cytomegalovirus UL141. Nat Immunol 6:181–188

Tortorella D, Gewurz BE, Furman MH, Schust DJ, Ploegh HL (2000) Viral subversion of the immune system. Annu Rev Immunol 18:861–926

Ulbrecht M, Martinozzi S, Grzeschik M, Hengel H, Ellwart JW, Pla M, Weiss EH (2000) Cutting edge: the human cytomegalovirus UL40 gene product contains a ligand for HLA-E and prevents NK cell-mediated lysis. J Immunol 164:5019–5022

Valés-Gómez M, Browne H, Reyburn HT (2003) Expression of the UL16 glycoprotein of human cytomegalovirus protects the virus-infected cell from attack by natural killer cells. BMC Immunol 4:4

Valés-Gómez M, Shiroishi M, Maenaka K, Reyburn HT (2005) Genetic variability of the major histocompatibility complex class I homologue encoded by human cytomegalovirus leads to differential binding to the inhibitor receptor ILT2. J Virol 79:2251–2260

Vance RE, Jamieson AM, Raulet DH (1999) Recognition of the class Ib molecule Qa-1^b by putative activating receptors CD94/NKG2C and CD94/NKG2E on mouse natural killer cells. J Exp Med 190:1801–1812

Vilches C, Parham P (2002) KIR: diverse, rapidly evolving receptors of innate and adaptive immunity. Annu Rev Immunol 20:217–251

Vivier E, Anfossi N (2004) Inhibitory NK-cell receptors on T cells: witness of the past, actors of the future. Nat Rev Immunol 4:190–198

Vivier E, Tomasello E, Paul P (2002) Lymphocyte activation via NKG2D: towards a new paradigm in immune recognition? Curr Opin Immunol 14:306–311

Wang EC, McSharry B, Retiere C, Tomasec P, Williams S, Borysiewicz LK, Braud VM, Wilkinson GW (2002) UL40-mediated NK evasion during productive infection with human cytomegalovirus. Proc Natl Acad Sci USA 99:7570–7575

Welte SA, Sinzger C, Lutz SZ, Singh-Jasuja H, Sampaio KL, Eknigk U, Rammensee HG, Steinle A (2003) Selective intracellular retention of virally induced NKG2D ligands by the human cytomegalovirus UL16 glycoprotein. Eur J Immunol 33:194–203

Wu J, Groh V, Spies T (2002) T cell antigen receptor engagement and specificity in the recognition of stress-inducible MHC class I-related chains by human epithelial γδ T cells. J Immunol 169:1236–1240

Wu J, Song Y, Bakker AB, Bauer S, Spies T, Lanier LL, Phillips JH (1999) An activating immunoreceptor complex formed by NKG2D and DAP10. Science 285:730–732

Yabe T, McSherry C, Bach FH, Fisch P, Schall RP, Sondel PM, Houchins JP (1993) A multigene family on human chromosome 12 encodes natural killer-cell lectins. Immunogenetics 37:455–460

The Impact of Variation at the *KIR* Gene Cluster on Human Disease

M. Carrington (✉) · M. P. Martin

Basic Research Program, SAIC-Frederick Inc., Laboratory of Genomic Diversity, National Cancer Institute, Bldg. 560 Rm. 21-89, P.O. Box B, Frederick, MD 21702, USA
carringt@ncifcrf.gov

1	Introduction	226
2	Superiority Complex of Inhibitory and Activating *KIR*	226
3	KIR Ligands and Their Need to Be Considered	229
4	Small Effects on Many Diseases	231
4.1	*KIR* Effects in Autoimmune and Inflammatory Diseases	232
4.2	*KIR* on Cancer	237
4.3	*KIR* Defense Against Microorganisms	238
4.4	*KIR* Contribution to Maternal–Fetal Bonding	241
5	Summary	244
References		248

Abstract Leukocyte behavior is controlled by a balance of inhibitory and stimulatory signals generated on ligand binding to a complex set of receptors located on the cell surface. The *killer cell immunoglobulin-like receptor (KIR)* genes encode one such family of receptors expressed by natural killer (NK) cells, key components of the innate immune system that participate in early responses against infected or transformed cells through production of cytokines and direct cytotoxicity. KIRs are also expressed on a subset of T cells, where they contribute to the intensity of acquired immune responses. Recognition of self HLA class I ligands by inhibitory KIR allows NK cells to identify normal cells, preventing an NK cell-mediated response against healthy autologous cells. Activation of NK cells through stimulatory receptors is directed toward cells with altered expression of class I, a situation characteristic of some virally infected cells and tumor cells. The "missing self" model for NK cell activation was proposed to explain killing of cells that express little or no class I, while cells expressing normal levels of class I are spared. Studies performed over the last several years have revealed extensive diversity at the *KIR* gene locus, which stems from both its polygenic (variable numbers of genes depending on *KIR* haplotype) and multiallelic polymorphism. Given the role of KIR in both arms of the immune response, their specificity for HLA class I allotypes, and their extensive genomic diversity, it is reasonable to imagine that *KIR* gene variation affects resistance and susceptibility to the pathogenesis of numerous diseases. Consequently, the evolution of *KIR* locus diversity within and across populations may be a function of disease morbidity and mortality. Here we review a growing body of evidence purporting the influence of *KIR* polymorphism in human disease.

1
Introduction

The *killer cell immunoglobulin-like receptor* (*KIR*) locus encompasses a segment of about 150 kb situated among a group of genetically and functionally related genes within the *leukocyte receptor complex* (*LRC*) on chromosome 19q13.4 (Fig. 1). *KIR* genes are tandemly arrayed, and their haplotypes display extensive diversity, both in terms of gene content and allelic diversity (Uhrberg et al. 1997; Witt et al. 1999; Wilson et al. 2000; Trowsdale et al. 2001; Hsu et al. 2002a,b; Vilches and Parham 2002), resulting in minimal probability that two randomly selected individuals will have precisely the same *KIR* genotype (Shilling et al. 2002). Over 37 *KIR* haplotypes differing in gene content have been identified by segregation analysis to date (Fig. 2), a number that is clearly underrepresentative of the total given the extensive number of *KIR* gene profiles (i.e., the set of *KIR* genes present in a given individual without knowing whether each gene is present on one or both haplotypes) observed in a limited set of distinct populations. Because the genes share high sequence similarity overall (85%–99%), nonallelic homologous recombination (NAHR) may occur frequently at this locus, as it does at other tandemly arrayed homologous sequences (Stankiewicz and Lupski 2002; Carrington and Cullen 2004) Indeed, inspection of *KIR* gene sequences (Shilling et al. 1998; Martin et al. 2003) and haplotype structure (Martin et al. 2003) strongly indicates that NAHR is a primary mechanism responsible for the expansion and contraction of the *KIR* locus.

A general overview of the *KIR* genes and their products can be found at http://web.ncbi.nlm.nih.gov:2441/books/bookres.fcgi/mono_003/ch1d1.pdf. Sequences of *KIR* alleles are provided at http://www.ebi.ac.uk/ipd/kir/.

2
Superiority Complex of Inhibitory and Activating *KIR*

The polygenic nature of the *KIR* locus is particularly consequential in a functional sense because *KIR* genes encode receptors that can either inhibit or

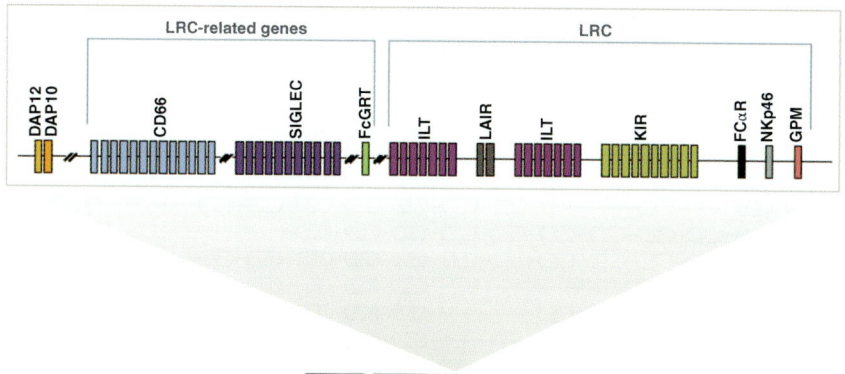

Fig. 1 Map of the *leukocyte receptor complex* (*LRC*). The *LRC* includes the *ILT*, *LAIR* and *KIR* genes, as well as genes encoding FcαR, NKp46 and GPV1. (From http://web.ncbi.nlm.nih.gov:2441/books/bookres.fcgi/mono_003/ch1d1.pdf)

activate NK cells, subpopulations of memory/effector αβ T cells (Ferrini et al. 1994; Mingari et al. 1995), γδ T cells (Nakajima et al. 1995; Battistini et al. 1997), and T cells in the liver (Norris et al. 1999). Much of the variability among *KIR* haplotypes in terms of gene content stems from the presence or absence of activating *KIR*, because most of the inhibitory *KIR* are present on all or nearly all haplotypes (Uhrberg et al. 1997). Activating KIR molecules that stimulate NK/CTL cytokine secretion and target cell cytolysis may be generally beneficial in response to microorganisms and tumor cells. However, both types of disorders (infectious and cancer) consist of diseases with very distinct etiologies, and immune activation is not necessarily beneficial at all stages of the disease process. In this regard, it is imaginable that *KIR* genotypes conferring strong activation could conceivably enhance the risk of developing tumors known to associate with localized inflammation, such as gastric cancer or colorectal cancer (Schottenfeld and Beebe-Dimmer 2004). Activating profiles may also be detrimental in autoimmune pathogenesis, potentially aggravating the disease process, although, again, this may be true for only certain autoimmune diseases and quite the opposite for others (Baxter and Smyth 2002; Flodstrom et al. 2002). Thus the diversity of *KIR* haplotypes, which likely imparts a continuum from relatively strong inhibition to strong activation, suggests the pleiotropic nature of *KIR* on different diseases in that a given *KIR* genotype affording protection against one disease may actually predispose to another unrelated disorder.

KIR haplotypes can be split into two basic types based on the presence of a single or multiple activating *KIR* genes (termed A or B haplotypes,

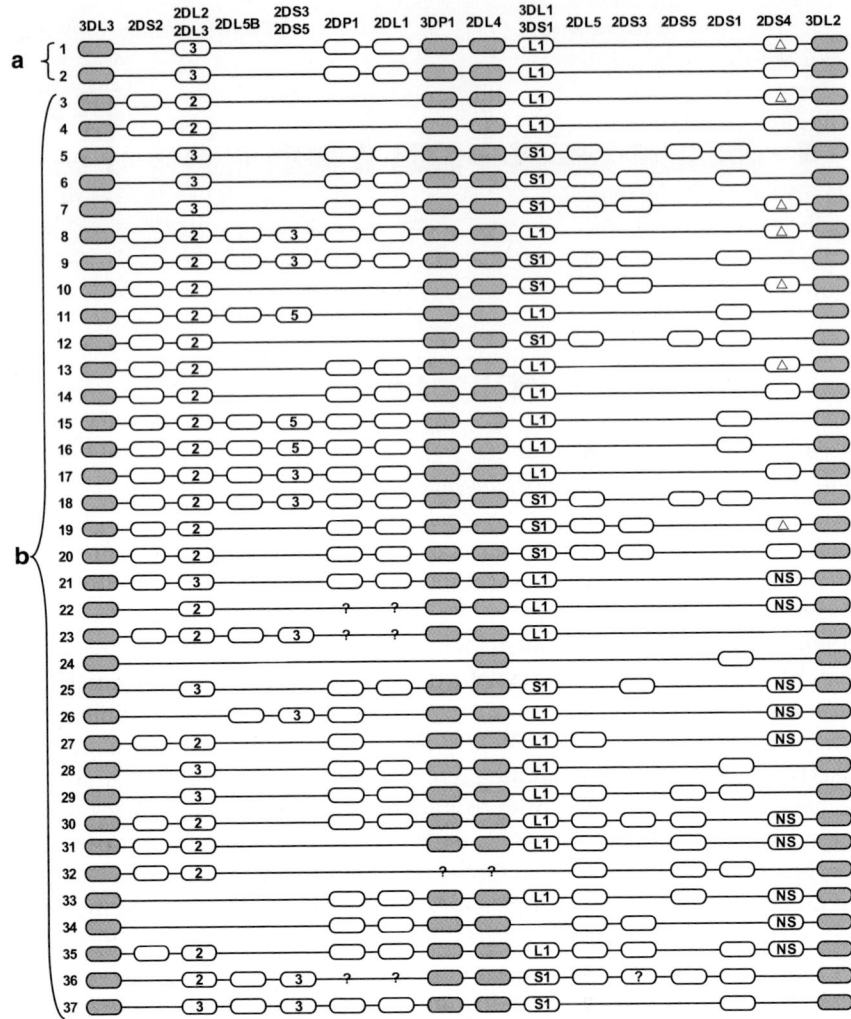

Fig. 2 *KIR* haplotypes identified by segregation analysis. Segregation analysis was used to determine these haplotypes, but many are not yet definitive, because it is not always possible to determine gene copy number precisely, even when using family material (Gomez-Lozano et al. 2002; Hsu et al. 2002b; Shilling et al. 2002; Uhrberg et al. 2002; unpublished observations, M.C.). Representatives of A vs. B haplotypes are coded as such on the *left* of the figure. KIR2DS4 alleles with the 21-bp deletion are depicted by △, and those that were not subtyped are marked *NS*. (From http://web.ncbi.nlm.nih.gov:2441/books/bookres.fcgi/mono_003/ch1d1.pdf)

respectively) (Uhrberg et al. 1997). *KIR2DS4*, which is the only activating *KIR* gene present on A haplotypes (Fig. 2), contains a null allele, due to a 21-base pair deletion in the transmembrane domain (Maxwell et al. 2002). The null allele has a frequency of about 80% in European Americans (Hsu et al. 2002b), so most A haplotypes do not encode any activating receptors present on the cell surface. The frequency of A haplotypes (which do not differ from one another in gene content but rather only in terms of allelic polymorphism) is roughly equivalent to that of B haplotypes (which differ from one another in terms of both gene content and allelic variability) among individuals of European descent (Hsu et al. 2002b), but this distribution varies radically across distinct populations (Toneva et al. 2001; Yawata et al. 2002). It is tempting to consider the A haplotype, with its paucity of activating *KIR* genes, as the inhibitory prototype. However, the level of KIR-mediated regulation of effector cells can be considered only in the context of whether the appropriate ligand is present on the target cell.

There are numerous activating and inhibitory receptors on NK cells (Lanier 2001a). Most inhibition of NK cells can be attributed to either inhibitory KIR or the relatively conserved C-type lectin inhibitory receptors, CD94/NKG2A (Long 1999). Furthermore, some inhibitory KIR have stronger affinity for their ligand than do others (Winter et al. 1998), fluctuating the strength of the inhibitory response. On the other hand, activation of NK cells is mediated by a number of different types of activating receptors and coreceptors (NKp46, NKp30, NKp44, NKG2D, 2B4, NTBA, DNAM-1, NKp80, CD59) (Moretta et al. 2001, 2004; Moretta and Moretta 2004), some of which are likely to play a central role in NK cell activation over and above that of the activating KIR. The relatively high frequency of healthy individuals expressing no activating KIR on their cell surface (i.e., those homozygous for the A haplotype carrying the null *KIR2DS4* allele; f=0.20 among unrelated individuals in 59 CEPH pedigrees; M.M., unpublished data) supports this assertion. Theoretically, KIR may participate in activation of effector cells directly through activating KIR or indirectly through weak inhibitory KIR signals that can be overcome by one or more of the various activating receptors expressed on the cells.

3
KIR Ligands and Their Need to Be Considered

Ligands for several of the inhibitory KIR have been conclusively identified (Table 1). KIR3DL1, KIR2DL1, KIR2DL2/2DL3, and KIR3DL2 each recognize a subset of allotypes encoded by the highly polymorphic classic *HLA* class I loci (Long and Rajagopalan 2000). *KIR2DL2* and *2DL3* segregate as alleles of a single locus, and they recognize the same set of HLA class I allotypes, although with different affinity (Winter et al. 1998). KIR3DL1 binds HLA-B allotypes that have the Bw4 motif (Gumperz et al. 1995) (determined by the sequence at position 77–83; Muller et al. 1989), whereas KIR2DL1 and KIR2DL2/2DL3 bind HLA-C allotypes with either asparagine (group 1 HLA-C allotypes specific for KIR2DL1) or lysine (group 2 HLA-C allotypes specific for KIR2DL2/2DL3) at position 80 (N80 and K80, respectively) (Colonna et al. 1992; Biassoni et al. 1995; Winter and Long 1997). However, these receptor-ligand relationships are generalities and are not always strictly observed (Winter et al. 1998). Furthermore, in some instances, peptides can affect KIR recognition of class I ligands (Peruzzi et al. 1996a,b; Mandelboim et al. 1997; Rajagopalan and Long 1997; Zappacosta et al. 1997; Hansasuta et al. 2004), although in general KIR recognition of HLA class I ligands appears to be rather impervious to the peptide residing in the binding groove (Lanier 1998). KIR3DL2 may represent an exception to this notion, however, because it was shown to bind HLA-A3 and -A11 tetramers only when they are refolded with one of several viral peptides tested (all of which were previously defined A3/A11 epitopes) (Hansasuta et al. 2004). The activating *KIR* genes, *KIR3DS1*, *KIR2DS1*, and *KIR2DS2*, share high sequence similarity in their extracellular domains with the inhibitory *KIR3DL1*, *KIR2DL1*, and *KIR2DL2/2DL3* genes, respectively (Trowsdale et al. 2001). Substantial data suggest that KIR2DS1 and KIR2DS2 bind the same or an overlapping set of HLA class I ligands as their inhibitory counterparts, but with much lower affinity (Moretta et al. 1995; Vales-Gomez et al. 1998). It is possible that the activating KIR may display

Table 1 KIR specificities for HLA class I

2DL1 and 2DS1	2DL2/3 & 2DS2	3DL1/S1	3DL2	2DL4
HLA-Cw grp 2	HLA-Cw grp 1	HLA-Bw4	HLA-A	HLA-G
Cw*02	Cw*01	B*08	A*3	
Cw*04	Cw*03	B*13	A*11	
Cw*05	Cw*07	B*27		
Cw*06	Cw*08	B*44		
		B*51		
		B*52		
		B*53		
		B*57		
		B*58		

Ligands for 2DL5, 2DS3, 2DS4, 2DS5, and 3DL3 remain undefined

high-affinity recognition of altered forms of class I, or other molecules such as stress proteins that resemble class I in structure and/or sequence, but none has yet been ascertained. Alternatively, high-affinity ligands for activating KIR may not exist because of possible adverse hyperimmune responses that may result from such an interaction.

Genetic diversity at unlinked loci encoding cell receptors and their ligands results in a situation in which the presence of one without the other should be the functional equivalent of having neither. *KIR2DL1, KIR2DL2/3, KIR3DL2,* and *KIR3DL1* are present in all or nearly all individuals of European descent, so analyses of *HLA* class I alleles grouped according to KIR recognition status (as defined to date) do provide preliminary data regarding the possible influence of HLA on disease outcome as a function of their role as ligands for KIR (Flores-Villanueva et al. 2001; Sharma et al. 2003). Nevertheless, strong linkage disequilibrium (LD) exists between the *HLA* class I genes (particularly between *HLA-B* and *-C,* the primary loci encoding ligands for KIR) and also between pairs of *KIR* genes, necessitating close scrutiny of all ligand and receptor genes to identify the most plausible "disease gene" in a given study. Studies have also begun to implicate functional differentiation of KIR on the basis of allelic variability in certain *KIR* genes (Gardiner et al. 2001; Pando et al. 2003), adding further complexity to the identification of variants directly influencing disease outcome. The extent of diversity at the *KIR* locus, particularly across populations, has not approached exhaustion. This, along with our rather restricted knowledge of the KIR ligands, limits our ability to conclusively pinpoint the *KIR* gene along with its ligand that confers resistance/susceptibility to disease. Still, a body of research has strongly implicated the *KIR* locus in several diseases, including those of tumorigenic, maternal-fetal, autoimmune, and infectious etiologies, suggesting ubiquitous effects of these genes on an abundance of human diseases and justifying further investigation.

4
Small Effects on Many Diseases

Rapid evolution of the *KIR* locus is supported by a number of observations (Vilches and Parham 2002). Comparisons of *KIR* sequences and haplotypes both within and across species have illustrated the substantial diversity of the *KIR* gene family, a salient characteristic that may be a function of species-/population-specific pathogenic organisms (Khakoo et al. 2000; Sambrook et al. 2004). Functional *KIR* genes are present in primate species (Khakoo et al. 2000; Hershberger et al. 2001; Mager et al. 2001; Guethlein et al. 2002;

Rajalingam et al. 2004), but only distantly related *KIR* homologs have been identified in other mammalian species (McQueen et al. 2002; Hoelsbrekken et al. 2003; Welch et al. 2003). The differences between the *KIR* loci among the common chimpanzee (our closest living relative) compared to humans are striking (only 3 of 14 chimp *KIR* genes and 1 of about 30 rhesus monkey gene sequences identified so far appear to be direct orthologs of human *KIR*; Khakoo et al. 2000; Sambrook et al. 2004) given the very similar genomes of these two species overall. *KIR* diversity within a single human population can be extensive, but perhaps more telling of the rapid evolution of *KIR* are the remarkable differences in *KIR* haplotype (and profile) frequencies across human populations (Toneva et al. 2001; Yawata et al. 2002). Such differences may not be so surprising when one considers the fact that frequencies of KIR ligands, the rapidly evolving *HLA* class I alleles, also vary significantly across populations; certainly the *KIR* and *HLA* loci must coevolve in order to maintain beneficial relationships (Khakoo et al. 2000).

The ability of immune response genes to evolve rapidly makes good sense from the standpoint of dealing with new or emerging pathogens. Rapid evolution of the *KIR* locus may represent a means for the innate immune system to maintain some level of fluidity, a characteristic that is essential for the acquired immune system. Like other gene families involved in innate immunity (e.g., chemokines and their receptors), the *KIR* genes encode molecules that are functionally redundant, an important feature for genes attempting to handle both new and old foes. The only *KIR* genes present on every *KIR* haplotype are *KIR3DL2* and *KIR3DL3*, which are located at the extreme ends of the *KIR* locus and are therefore less likely to be eliminated in a NAHR event. *KIR2DL4* is virtually always present as well, although healthy, reproductive individuals who are missing *KIR2DL4* have been reported (Gomez-Lozano et al. 2003). Thus it is conceivable that no individual *KIR* gene is required for a healthy existence. Nevertheless, specific *KIR* genes or combinations of genes may provide some protection against diseases afflicting a population, potentially explaining the remarkable differences in *KIR* haplotype (and profile) frequencies across distinct populations.

4.1
KIR Effects in Autoimmune and Inflammatory Diseases

Historically, the most robust disease associations with the highly polymorphic *HLA* class I/class II loci have been autoimmune in nature, and only very few infectious diseases have shown strong, consistent *HLA* associations (Cooke and Hill 2001; Gao et al. 2001). It would not be surprising if the strongest effects of *KIR* variation were also observed in autoimmune diseases. Some previously determined *HLA* associations with autoimmune diseases might actually be explained by synergistic interactions between *KIR* and alleles encoding their *HLA* class I ligands. An obvious hypothesis in this regard is that *KIR* genotypes expected to confer relatively strong activation to effector cells increase the risk of autoimmune disease. On the other hand, NK cell activation may be protective against some autoimmune disorders by suppressing or eliminating dendritic cells and monocytes (Shah et al. 1985; Gilbertson et al. 1986; Djeu and Blanchard 1988; Chambers et al. 1996; Geldhof et al. 1998; Carbone et al. 1999), cells known to stimulate the generation of cytotoxic T lymphocytes. NK cell activation may also confer protection by participating in clearance of the microorganisms that are instrumental in initiating autoimmunity. A rather substantial body of evidence has indicated deficiencies in NK cells (i.e., decreased numbers and activity) in several autoimmune diseases, including systemic lupus erythematosus (SLE), multiple sclerosis, and type 1 diabetes (reviewed in Baxter and Smyth 2002). It is not so clear whether the depressed NK cell activity observed among individuals with these autoimmune diseases is a cause or an effect of the disease, but given this phenotypic association, it will be of interest to test for potentially beneficial effects of activating KIR on these diseases.

A number of studies have investigated KIR expression in rheumatoid arthritis (RA). The frequency of CD8+ cells expressing CD158a (this specificity includes both KIR2DL1 and its activating counterpart, KIR2DS1) was decreased among patients with RA relative to healthy controls, and there was significantly less IL-2-induced upregulation of CD158a+ CD16+ cells from RA patients relative to healthy controls (Kogure et al. 2001). In another study of RA patients, KIR2DS2 expression in the absence of inhibitory KIR was observed on $CD4^+CD28^{null}$ T cells, expansion of which is characteristic in this disease (Namekawa et al. 2000). Antibodies to both KIR2DL1 and KIR2DL3 (which should also recognize KIR2DS1 and KIR2DS2) were identified in sera of some RA patients, as well as patients with SLE and Behçet disease (Matsui et al. 2001) but not in healthy donors, a situation that could disrupt an appropriate balance between effector cell inhibition and activation. Collectively, these studies raised the possibility that abnormal KIR expression may be involved in development of RA.

RA was also the first disease in which an effect of *KIR* genotype was observed. In a subset of RA patients with vascular complications, KIR2DS2 molecules were frequently observed on $CD4^+CD28^{null}$ T cells, a cell type thought to be involved in endothelial damage (Yen et al. 2001) and expansion of which is particularly high in RA vasculitis patients (Martens et al. 1997). These investigators went on to show a significant increase in the genomic presence of *KIR2DS2* among patients with RA vasculitis relative to either healthy controls or patients with RA in the absence of vasculitis. Because KIR2DS2 binds group 1 HLA-C alleles (those with N80), the association between *KIR2DS2* and RA vasculitis should theoretically increase with the additional presence of *HLA-C* group 1. Although the *HLA-C* group 1 allele *HLA-Cw*03* frequency was increased among RA vasculitis patients, this was not a general pattern for all group 1 alleles (indeed, *HLA-Cw*07*, another group 1 allele, showed borderline protection against vasculitis, and *HLA-Cw*05*, a group 2 allele that does not bind KIR2DS2, showed significant susceptibility to vasculitis) (Yen et al. 2001). Sample size limited the power of these analyses (n=30 for RA vasculitis), so an association between RA vasculitis and group 1 alleles as a whole cannot be ruled out, but the investigators alluded to the interesting possibility that KIR2DS2 may recognize HLA-Cw*03 in the context of a specific epitope generated in the disease process, rather than nonspecifically binding the entire set of group 1 allotypes. This is conceivable, given previous observations of peptide specificity in KIR binding to HLA class I ligand (Peruzzi et al. 1996a,b; Mandelboim et al. 1997; Rajagopalan and Long 1997; Zappacosta et al. 1997; Hansasuta et al. 2004).

The presence of $CD4^+CD28^{null}$ T cells in the inflammatory infiltrate of atherosclerotic plaques has implicated these cells in acute coronary syndromes (ACS) as well (Nakajima et al. 2003). As in RA vasculitis, $CD4^+CD28^{null}$ T cells from ACS patients express KIR2DS2, conveying the ability of these cells to kill in the absence of T cell receptor triggering. These studies, along with others, highlight the influence of KIR molecules expressed on T cell subsets in disease pathogenesis.

KIR2DS2 is in strong LD with *KIR2DL2* (and therefore negative LD with *KIR2DL3*) and is rarely found on a *KIR* haplotype in the absence of *KIR2DL2* (see Fig. 2) among individuals of European descent. Nevertheless, the unusual *KIR* profile, *KIR2DS2+/KIR2DL2−*, was observed at a frequency of nearly 12% among a group of German scleroderma patients (relative to 2% in controls) (Momot et al. 2004). All other activating *KIR* tested were also found at a higher frequency in the patient group compared to controls (although generally not significantly), except for *KIR2DS4*, which is always present on A haplotypes. *KIR2DS2* in combination with HLA-C group 1 alleles also appears to be more frequent among individuals with type 1 diabetes (van der Slik et al. 2003), putting this gene in contention for *the* autoimmune KIR variant, as has been described for the *HLA* haplotype *HLA-A1-B8-DR3*.

We previously reported increased susceptibility to developing psoriatic arthritis (PsA) in the presence of the activating *KIR2DS1* and/or *KIR2DS2*, most notably when ligands for the corresponding homologous inhibitory KIR were missing (Martin et al. 2002b). For example, individuals with *KIR2DS1* were most strongly associated with PsA when KIR2DL1 ligands, *HLA-C* group

2, were absent. The same situation was true for *KIR2DS2* in the absence of *HLA-C* group 1. This suggested that the absence of ligands for inhibitory KIR might lower the threshold for effector cell activation, increasing the risk of a potentially harmful activating signal (Fig. 3a). *Any* inhibitory KIR-HLA interaction, however, could potentially provide counteracting inhibition to an activating signal, including one that occurs through a heterologous inhibitory KIR relative to the activating KIR in question. Thus an activating KIR, such as KIR2DS1, might be detrimental in terms of developing PsA if the ligand for either KIR2DL1 or KIR2DL2/3 is missing (i.e., in homozygotes for either group of *HLA-Cw* ligands). NK cells are kept in check through constitutive dominant inhibitory receptors for class I ligands (Ljunggren and Karre 1990; Valiante et al. 1997), and effector functions occur only when activating signals outdo inhibitory signals (Cerwenka and Lanier 2001; Diefenbach and Raulet 2001; Lanier 2001a,b). This can be achieved either by enhanced activating receptor-ligand interactions, which are expected when activating KIR are present, or by weak inhibitory receptor-ligand interactions that impart a low threshold for activation, which are expected when ligand for inhibitory KIR are missing (unlike KIR2DS1 and KIR2DS2, inhibitory KIR2DL1 and KIR2DL2/3 are virtually always present) (Lanier 2001a). Based on this line of thought, we proposed a second model in which susceptibility to PsA increases progressively with increasing levels of KIR-mediated activation of NK cells as defined by the presence of KIR2DS1 and/or KIR2DS2 and homozygosity for *HLA-C* group 1 or 2 (Fig. 3b) (Nelson et al. 2004). The data showed a highly significant trend where compound activating *KIR/HLA* genotypes conferred the greatest level of susceptibility to PsA and, alternatively, genotypes associated with most inhibition were most protective. The PsA studies underscore the need to continually pursue credible models for the effects of *KIR/HLA* on disease, a process that will remain dynamic as long as KIR biology continues to unfold.

The involvement of *KIR* genotype in PsA, an inflammatory arthritis occurring in a subset of patients with psoriasis vulgaris (PV) (Gladman and Rahman 2001), raises the question as to whether *KIR* genotype specifically affects the development of arthritis in psoriasis patients or of psoriasis itself. Typing for the presence/absence of 14 *KIR* genes in a group of 96 Japanese PV patients revealed an increased frequency of *KIR2DS1*, a gene that was also associated with PsA (Suzuki et al. 2004). Other genes commonly found on B haplotypes were also found with increased frequency in these patients, a finding that is meaningful despite the small control sample studied ($n=50$) because the A haplotype frequency is exceptionally high in the Japanese population (Yawata et al. 2002). A strong association of *KIR2DS1* with PV was also reported in a Polish cohort (Luszczek et al. 2004). These data suggest that

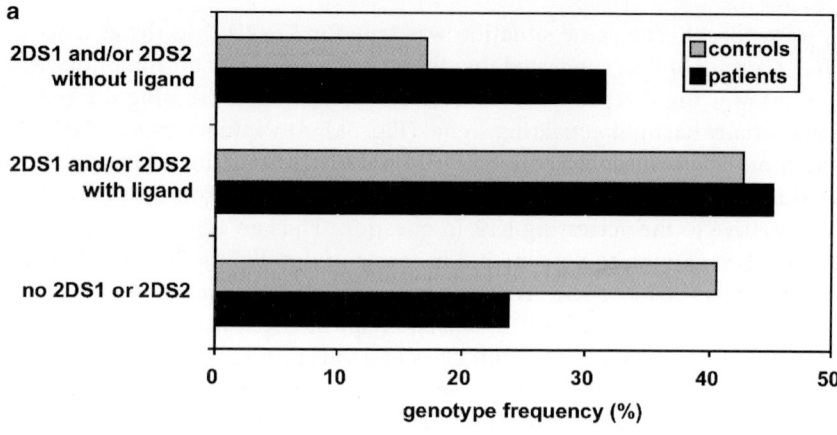

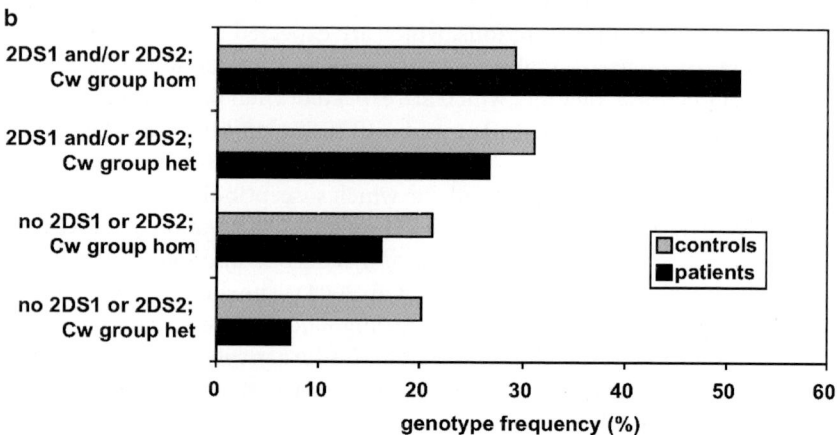

Fig. 3 Influence of *KIR2DS* and *HLA-Cw* group on PsA. **a** Old model: Frequency of individuals *i* with *2DS1* and/or *2DS2* who do not have ligand for the corresponding inhibitory KIR (*upper bars*), *ii* with *2DS1* and/or *2DS2* and ligand for the corresponding inhibitory *KIR* (*middle bars*), and *iii* missing both *2DS1* and *2DS2* (*lower bars*). (*P* for trend=2×10^{-5}). **b** New model: There is a trend toward decreasing susceptibility to PsA with genotypes conferring decreasing KIR-mediated NK cell activation (going from *upper bars* to *lower bars*). *C group hom* refers to individuals who have two copies of group 1 alleles or two copies of group 2 alleles. *C group het* refers to individuals who are heterozygous for a group 1 and a group 2 allele. (*P* for trend=2×10^{-7})

the *KIR* associations observed in PsA may be attributable to psoriasis overall, a possibility that should be pursued further by testing the *KIR*-PsA model described above (Nelson et al. 2004) in the Japanese and Polish data sets.

4.2
KIR on Cancer

Loss of HLA class I molecules on tumor cells may evolve during tumorigenesis as a mechanism of tumor cell escape from T cell-mediated elimination (Smith et al. 1989; Kaklamanis and Hill 1992). Under such circumstances, inhibitory receptors for HLA class I on NK cells will be disengaged and activating receptors will dictate, leading to NK cell killing of the tumor cell target. Involvement of activating KIR in this defense mechanism is suggested by a recent study in which KIR2DS4 was shown to interact with a non-MHC class I protein expressed on some melanoma cell lines and primary melanomas lacking MHC class I expression, resulting in killing of the tumor cells (Katz et al. 2004). These data suggest that novel, non-MHC class I ligands may be expressed on some tumor cells that are recognized by activating KIR, mediating effector cell killing of the tumor cell targets. However, that tumor cells displaying partial or total loss of class I molecules are observed in cancer patients implies that surveillance by NK cells for these targets is not flawless.

Tumor cell escape from effector cell killing through a mechanism that actually involves expression of HLA class I may occur in some instances. *KIR2DL2/2DL3* in combination with their group 1 *HLA-C* ligands were observed more frequently in a group of malignant melanoma (MM) patients compared to controls(Naumova et al. 2004), suggesting that tumor escape from immunosurveillance might be due to the prevalence of inhibitory over activating signals in MM patients. Such escape mechanisms may also involve expression of nonclassic class I molecules on tumor cells, such as HLA-E, which serves as a ligand for the inhibitory CD94/NKG2A molecule (Brooks et al. 1999), or HLA-G, a molecule that has been identified on some tumors (Fukushima et al. 1998; Paul et al. 1999; Lefebvre et al. 2002)and that binds the inhibitory receptor ILT-2 (Allan et al. 1999; Navarro et al. 1999) and KIR2DL4 (Rajagopalan and Long 1999; Faure and Long 2002). The generation of soluble MICA ligands for the activating receptor NKG2D by certain tumor cell types has been shown to block and downregulate NKG2D on CTL, resulting in defective CTL killing of tumor cell targets (Groh et al. 2002) (see chapter by Vidal and Lanier, this volume). A similar mechanism is conceivable for NK cells; an interaction between activating KIR expressed on NK cells and soluble HLA class I secreted by tumor cells devoid of HLA class I on their cell surface may lead to NK cell apoptosis (Spaggiari et al. 2002), a tumor escape mechanism that could be successful (for the tumor) if activating KIR are upregulated on effector cells in a given type of cancer (Melioli et al. 2003).

Diminished NK cell activity is well documented in chronic myelogenous leukemia (Fujimiya et al. 1986; Pierson and Miller 1996), and inhibitory KIR may contribute to the lack of NK or CTL antitumor responses in some cases (Bakker et al. 1998; Guerra et al. 2000; Gati et al. 2004). Distinct expression characteristics of KIR have also been observed in patients with some types of tumors as well as lymphoproliferative disease of granular lymphocytes (Bagot et al. 2001; Dorothee et al. 2003; Wechsler et al. 2003; Zambello et al. 2003; Poszepczynska-Guigne et al. 2004), and it will be important to determine whether such alterations in KIR expression contribute to disease progression. Genetic variability at the *KIR* locus could affect risk of developing certain types of cancer by any number of mechanisms, and not necessarily in a consistent pattern across cancer types. Only a few genetic association studies of *KIR* variation effects on malignancy have been reported to date. In one study, *KIR2DL2* and *KIR2DS2*, genes characteristic of the B haplotype that are in nearly complete LD, were observed at a significantly higher frequency among patients with various types of leukemia (Verheyden et al. 2004). Correspondingly, the frequency of AB genotypes, which would include *KIR2DL1*, *KIR2DL2*, and *KIR2DL3* along with the activating *KIR2DS2*, was also greater in this patient group. The authors concluded that the presence of the three inhibitory KIR results in major inhibitory capacity, favoring tumor cell escape from NK cell elimination. However, the data also support the possibility that KIR2DS2 increases the risk of malignancy somehow, highlighting the complexity of drawing conclusions regarding the effects of functionally related genes that are in strong LD with one another.

4.3
KIR Defense Against Microorganisms

CD8+ T cells serve a critical role in eliminating intracellular pathogens by detecting viral peptides in the context of MHC class I molecules on the surface of infected cells. Some viruses retaliate by disrupting cell surface expression of class I (Tortorella et al. 2000). But the competition ensues with the ability of NK cells to detect "missing self" (Karre et al. 1986) and kill cells that express little or no class I ligands for inhibitory receptors on the NK cell. Indeed, NK cell inhibition appears to correlate positively with level of MHC class I on target cells (Storkus et al. 1989). The skirmish continues with viral downregulation of some, but not all, ligands for inhibitory receptors on NK cells, but in general the species as a whole continues to thrive for now, in part because of the efforts of NK cells and their entourage of regulating receptors. The NK cell control of viral infections (especially herpesviruses, which seem to be the favorite adversaries of NK cells) has been the subject of excellent reviews (Biron et al. 1999), two of which are included in this volume (see chapters by MacFarlane and Campbell and Anderson, this volume).

Human NK cells express a number of activating receptors that have been implicated in resistance to viral disease (Parolini et al. 2000; Sivori et al. 2000; Mandelboim et al. 2001; Martin et al. 2002a), most of which are encoded by conserved genes. Specific *KIR* genes may be particularly aggressive in clearance of some microorganisms, and their presence in only a fraction of individuals (as well as their allelic polymorphism) could explain differences observed among individuals in their ability to control a given pathogen. Recent data from our lab suggest that an activating *KIR/HLA* genotype may result in protection from progression to AIDS in HIV-1-infected patients (Martin et al. 2002a). Individuals who carried at least one copy of both *KIR3DS1* and a subset of *HLA-B Bw4* alleles encoding isoleucine at position 80 (Bw4-80I) progressed to AIDS at a significantly slower rate than those without this combination (Martin et al. 2002a). Although the ligand for KIR3DS1 is not known, this gene shows 97% sequence similarity in the extracellular domain to KIR3DL1, the inhibitory counterpart of KIR3DS1 that binds HLA-B allotypes that have the Bw4 motif (an epitope determined by the sequence at positions 77–83 of the molecule) (Muller et al. 1989). Previous data had suggested the preference of KIR3DL1 for HLA-B Bw4-80I allotypes relative to HLA-B Bw4 allotypes with threonine at this position (Cella et al. 1994; Rojo et al. 1997), a finding that may explain the restriction of resistance to the combination of KIR3DS1 and HLA-B Bw4-80I, specifically. Interestingly, KIR3DS1 in the absence of Bw4-80I showed a significant recessive susceptibility effect on AIDS progression, negating the possibility of an additive protective effect of KIR3DS1 and HLA-B Bw4-80I. This study suggests that KIR3DS1 may be expressed and may bind certain HLA-B Bw4 allotypes in defense against HIV-1, but no functional data to support this contention have been forthcoming. KIR3DS1 in the presence of HLA-B Bw4 allotypes as a whole also showed significant protection in clearance of hepatitis C virus (HCV) infection, an effect that persisted even after multiple variable analysis of another protective *KIR/HLA* compound genotype that was observed in the same study (Khakoo et al. 2004) (see below).

Inhibitory KIR may promote the maintenance and accumulation of memory CD8+ T cells, as suggested by phenotypes observed in KIR2DL3/HLA-Cw3 transgenic mice (Ugolini et al. 2001). These data support the hypothesis that expression of inhibitory KIR (and perhaps other inhibitory NK cell receptors) protects CD8+ T cells from apoptosis in the face of excessive TCR stimulation. A potentially adverse element of inhibitory KIR expression on CD8+ T cells is suggested by the observation that inhibitory KIR expressed by Epstein–Barr virus (EBV)-specific or HIV-specific CD8+ T cells expanded in vitro hinder viral specific cytotoxicity of infected cells (De Maria et al. 1997; De Maria and Moretta 2000; Vely et al. 2001). A similar situation may apply to NK cells; while inhibitory KIR protect from self reactivity, these same molecules could dampen NK response in times of need. In this regard, the entire NK cell population of a child suffering from recurrent infections, particularly CMV, was shown to express KIR2DL1 on a genetic background of two *HLA-C* group 2 alleles, ligands for KIR2DL1 (Gazit et al. 2004). Symptoms observed in this child were virtually identical to those described in other patients who have NK cell deficiency (Biron et al. 1989). This case emphasizes the importance of considering KIR expression levels in disease association studies and understanding the mechanisms regulating KIR expression in general, a topic covered in the chapter by Gumá et al. in this volume.

Inhibition mediated by specific KIR/HLA combinations has also been implicated in the outcome of HCV infection (Khakoo et al. 2004) based on a genetic study of these loci among individuals who either cleared the virus or had persistent infection. The presence of alleles encoding the inhibitory KIR2DL3 and its HLA-C group 1 ligands was shown to associate with HCV clearance, and this effect appeared to be codominant; two complete pairs of *KIR2DL3* and *HLA-C* group 1 (i.e., homozygosity of *KIR2DL3* and *HLA-C* group 1; *KIR2DL3/KIR2DL3:C1/C1*) was strongly associated with viral clearance, whereas one complete pair was relatively neutral, and no complete pairs of *KIR2DL3/C1* associated with viral persistence. The binding affinity of KIR2DL3 for HLA-C group 1 allotypes is measurably lower than that of KIR2DL2 and KIR2DL1 for their cognate ligands (group 1 and group 2 allotypes, respectively) (Winter et al. 1998), resulting in transmission of weaker inhibitory signals to the effector cell. In HCV infection, we proposed that two copies of *KIR2DL3* and *HLA-C* group 1 preclude the stronger inhibitory signals mediated by KIR2DL1 and KIR2DL2, lowering the threshold for effector cell activation through stimulatory receptors (Fig. 4). The protective effect of *KIR2DL3/KIR2DL3:C1/C1* was quite significant among intravenous drug users and needle-stick cases, individuals who would be expected to have received a low-dose viral inoculum. However, this genotype was not significantly protective among patients receiving transfusions, where an expected high-dose inoculum may very well overwhelm any contribution of KIR to the innate immune response. Protection was observed across two ethnic groups, Caucasian and African American nontransfused patients, supporting a direct effect of this compound genotype on HCV clearance rather than simply marking a neighboring disease locus through linkage disequilibrium. This was the first genetic epidemiological study to suggest the importance of inhibitory receptor affinity for cognate ligand in human disease.

Several studies have indicated the importance of NK cells in *Plasmodium falciparum* infection (Theander et al. 1987; Orago and Facer 1991;

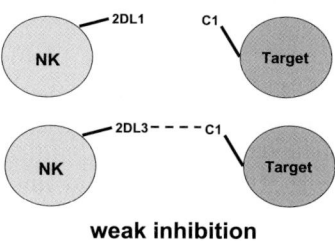
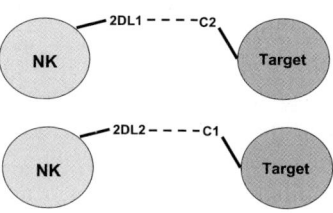

Fig. 4 Model illustrating protective and susceptible genotypes in resolution of HCV infection. In the presence of two copies of *KIR2DL3*, *KIR2DL1* (which is present in virtually all individuals), and *HLA-C* group 1 homozygosity (*upper panel*) there is a weak inhibitory signal relative to the stronger inhibitory signal conferred by the presence of *KIR2DL2*, *KIR2DL1* and *HLA-Cw* group heterozygosity (*lower panel*). The weaker inhibitory signal results in a lower threshold for effector cell activation through stimulatory receptors

Artavanis-Tsakonas and Riley 2002), and a significant association between *KIR* genotype and NK responsiveness to infected red blood cells has been reported(Artavanis-Tsakonas et al. 2003). This study implicated an allele of *KIR3DL2*, *KIR3DL2*002*, in protection against *P. falciparum* because at least one copy of this allele was observed in 5 of 7 high responders compared to 3 of 16 low/nonresponders, representing the first assignment of a specific *KIR* allele association with response to an infected target cell.

4.4
KIR Contribution to Maternal–Fetal Bonding

The most prominent leukocyte in the uterine mucosal lining during pregnancy (the decidua) is a distinct population of NK cells that make close contact with invading fetal extravillous trophoblast (EVT) cells (for reviews of NK cell biology during pregnancy, see Moffett-King 2002; Trundley and Moffett 2004). Entry of fetal EVT into the decidua and walls of the maternal spiral arteries ensures the essential exchange of nutrients and gases between the maternal and fetal circulations. Activation of uterine NK (uNK) cells elicited by interactions between uNK cell receptors and their ligands expressed on the surface of the EVT promotes development of a healthy maternal–fetal interface supportive of fetal growth (Moffett-King 2002). Inadequate blood exchange due to insufficient EVT invasion into the maternal spiral arteries results in poor placental perfusion, a disorder known as preeclampsia, and associates with significant morbidity and mortality in both mother and fetus (Roberts 2003).

EVT express an unusual combination of HLA class I molecules, HLA-G, HLA-E and HLA-C (Hiby et al. 1999; King et al. 2000a,b), and they do not express the polymorphic HLA-A and HLA-B that are found on most other nucleated cells of the body (Goodfellow et al. 1976). Uterine NK cells are distinct from blood-derived NK cells in that a greater proportion of uNK express KIR molecules that bind HLA-C allotypes relative to NK cells circulating in the periphery (Hiby et al. 1997; Verma et al. 1997). Alterations in KIR expression among women with diseases of the reproductive tract, including endometriosis, adenomyosis, and anembryonic pregnancy, have been described (Chao et al. 1999; Wu et al. 2000; Maeda et al. 2002, 2004; Yang et al. 2004), generating further speculation of a potential role for these molecules in disease pathogenesis of the uterus. Understanding the interactions between these receptor-ligand pairs during pregnancy and their role in securing harmonious interactions between the mother and her hemiallogeneic fetus has obvious implications in diagnosis, prevention, and treatment of diseases associated with pregnancy.

Cellular HLA-G expression is almost exclusively limited to EVT in pregnancy (McMaster et al. 1995). HLA-G has been shown to bind soluble KIR2DL4 (Cantoni et al. 1998; Rajagopalan and Long 1999), a receptor displaying properties of both activating and inhibitory receptors, provoking suspicions that this receptor-ligand interaction may confer some protection against maternal NK or T cell-mediated rejection of the fetus. The ubiquitous expression of KIR2DL4 in virtually all NK cells (Rajagopalan and Long 1999) (all other *KIR* genes are expressed in some, but not all, NK clones within a given individual) further suggests that KIR2DL4 may have a unique biological function that is of particular importance relative to other KIR. Nevertheless, a woman has been described who is missing the *KIR2DL4* gene completely and who has had several children (Gomez-Lozano et al. 2003), indicating that the gene is not absolutely essential for normal pregnancy.

Several alleles of *KIR2DL4* have been identified, some of which are characterized by a single nucleotide deletion that results in the elimination of exon 6 during mRNA production (Witt et al. 2000). To test the possibility that risk of developing preeclampsia may in part be a function of *KIR2DL4* variability, 45 women who experienced preeclampsia and 48 normotensive control subjects were subtyped for *KIR2DL4* alleles (Witt et al. 2002). No significant differences in *KIR2DL4* allele frequencies (or *KIR* gene frequencies) were observed. These data do not rule out the possibility of an important role for KIR2DL4 in maintenance of a healthy pregnancy, a function that may be provided by all known *KIR2DL4* alleles.

HLA-C is the only polymorphic class I molecule expressed by EVT, and it is also the only known NK cell receptor ligand on EVT that is recognized differentially by maternal uNK cells, an interaction that depends on the maternal *KIR* and the fetal *HLA-C* genotypes. Combinations of maternal *KIR* and fetal *HLA-C* genotypes are likely to confer a range of uNK cell effects, from relatively strong activation to strong inhibition, just as would be predicted in the periphery mediated by KIR and self MHC class I. The possibility that combinations of maternal KIR and fetal HLA-C ligands may differentially affect risk of preeclampsia was tested in 401 mother-infant pairs, including 200 women with preeclampsia and 201 women with normal pregnancies. The frequency of the *AA* genotype (i.e., those encoding either 0 or 1 expressed activating KIR) was significantly higher among preeclamptic mothers relative to mothers with healthy pregnancies, specifically when the baby carried at least one *HLA-C* group 2 allele (Hiby et al. 2004). This receptor-ligand combination is likely to convey strong inhibitory signals to the uNK cell for two reasons: (a) AA genotypes encode either 0 or 1 activating KIR expressed on the NK cell surface, and (b) the inhibitory KIR2DL1, which is present on all A haplotypes, binds HLA-C group 2 allotypes with very high affinity, sending strong inhibitory signals to the NK cell relative to that observed with KIR2DL3 (also encoded on the A haplotype) and its HLA-C group 1 ligands (Winter et al. 1998; Maenaka et al. 1999; Vales-Gomez et al. 2000; Fan et al. 2001). This situation is reminiscent of the protection conferred by relatively weak inhibitory signals proposed in HCV clearance (Khakoo et al. 2004). Furthermore, the frequency of preeclampsia in mothers with babies who carried at least one *HLA-C* group 2 allele was inversely correlated with the number of distinct activating receptor genes present in the mother's genome. These data cast the role of uNK cells in a new light, one in which stimulation of maternal NK cell activity mediated by appropriate KIR interactions with ligands on the fetal EVT results in proper maturation of the placenta and the healthy coexistence of mother and fetus (Parham 2004).

5
Summary

The *KIR* locus lies at the extreme end of the gene conservation spectrum (the end with least conservation, that is) where genes, especially functionally redundant sets of genes, are allowed to transform at their own free will, relatively speaking. The very fact that they have this privilege suggests that most of the variability observed is not absolutely essential, nor will any new variant have high probability of being outright deadly (though there is a selection bias in this latter measurement); rather the variability represents a means for the innate immune system to remain fluid, delicately contributing to disease outcome as positively as possible. These considerations imply that, for the most part, disease associations with *KIR* variants are expected to be somewhat weak, as is rather common for most variable genes involved in immune responsiveness. Indeed, the strength of the genetic associations described herein for *KIR* and their ligand groups is similar to that previously reported for *HLA* class I alleles and the majority of diseases with which they have been associated, particularly infectious diseases. Given the extent of *KIR* locus variability and the function of their protein products in both innate and acquired immunity, one might reasonably predict that they may influence the outcomes to most multigenic diseases that directly or indirectly involve the immune response. [Although no involvement of *KIR* in terms of presence or absence of several *KIR* genes was observed in celiac disease (Moodie et al. 2002) despite genome-wide linkage studies pointing to 19q13.4 (Zhong et al. 1996), the region in which the *KIR* gene cluster maps. This study did not rule out the possibility of allelic effects of *KIR* loci on disease, a possibility that has not been thoroughly explored for any disease to date.] So, in general, the good news for disease gene hunters is that the *KIR* locus is almost always a strong candidate in the quest for associated genetic variation; the fly in the ointment is the likelihood of small effects conferred by a very complex polymorphic locus, a problem that is only overcome by securing sizeable, clinically well-defined disease cohorts.

Only a handful of diseases have been studied for genetic associations with *KIR* variability to date (summarized in Table 2), impeding our ability to identify common threads of *KIR* involvement across diseases that share some etiological characteristics. Nevertheless, parallels may be emerging, such as the consistent observation of activating *KIR* genotypes with risk of developing autoimmune disease (Yen et al. 2001; van der Slik et al. 2003; Luszczek et al. 2004; Momot et al. 2004; Nelson et al. 2004; Suzuki et al. 2004) and their protection against two infectious diseases (Martin et al. 2002a; Khakoo et al. 2004). Although *KIR2DL3* and *HLA-C* group 1 had the strongest protective effect

Table 2 Summary of KIR/HLA genotype and disease associations

Disease	KIR/HLA ligand association	Effect	Population	Comments	Reference
Autoimmune					
1) Psoriatic Arthritis	KIR2DS1/KIR2DS2; HLA-Cw group homozygosity	Susceptibility	Caucasian: 366 cases; 299 controls	–	Martin et al. 2002b; Nelson et al. 2004
2) Psoriasis	KIR2DS1/HLA-Cw*06	Susceptibility	Polish: 116 cases; 123 controls	Small numbers	Luszczek et al. 2004
	KIR2DS1; KIR2DL5; KIR haplotype B	Susceptibility	Japanese: 96 cases; 50 controls	Small numbers	Suzuki et al. 2004
3) Rheumatoid vasculitis	KIR2DS2/HLA-Cw*03	Susceptibility	Caucasian: 30 cases; 76 controls	Small numbers but corroborated by KIR expression analysis	Yen et al. 2001
4) Scleroderma	KIR2DS2+/KIR2DL2-	Susceptibility	German: 102 cases; 100 controls	Small numbers	Momot et al. 2004
5) IDDM	KIR2DS2/HLA-Cw group 1	Susceptibility	Dutch: 149 cases; 207 controls	–	van der Slik et al. 2003
6) Celiac disease	None	–	UK Caucasian: 101 cases; 133 controls	19q13.4 previously identified as a candidate region	Moodie et al. 2002

Table 2 (continued)

Disease	KIR/HLA ligand association	Effect	Population	Comments	Reference
Infectious					
1) HIV-1	KIR3DS1/HLA-B-Bw480I	Slows progression	Caucasian: $N>1000$	–	Martin et al. 2002a
2) HCV	i) KIR2DL3/HLA-Cw group 1 homozygosity	Resolution of infection	Caucasian and African American: $N = 1023$	KIR3DS1/Bw4 effect was weak	Khakoo et al. 2004
	ii) KIR3DS1/HLA-Bw4	Resolution of infection			
3) P. falciparum	KIR3DL2*002	High response to iRBC	European, Asian, African: $N = 27$	In vitro study. Response of NK cells from normal blood donors to iRBC	Artavanis-Tsakonas et al. 2003
Cancer					
1) Malignant melanoma	KIR2DL2/2DL3; HLA-Cw group 1	Susceptibility	Bulgarian: 50 cases; 54 controls	Small numbers	Naumova et al. 2004
2) Leukemia	i) KIR2DL2	Susceptibility	Belgian: 96 cases; 148 controls	The AB1 and AB9 phenotypes contain all inhibitory KIR genes	Verheyden et al. 2004
	ii) AB1 and AB9 KIR phenotypes				

Table 2 (continued)

Disease	KIR/HLA ligand association	Effect	Population	Comments	Reference
Pregnancy					
Preeclampsia	Mothers with AA KIR genotype; fetus with HLA-Cw group 2	Susceptibility	UK: 200 cases; 201 controls	–	Hiby et al. 2004
	KIR2DL4 polymorphism	None	Australian: 45 cases; 48 controls	Small numbers	Witt et al. 2002

on resolution of HCV, *KIR3DS1/HLA-B Bw4* was also protective against HCV just as *KIR3DS1/HLA-B Bw4-80I* was protective against AIDS progression. These studies pique interest in haplotypes encompassing *KIR3DS1*, because the expression of KIR3DS1 has been questioned, raising the possibility that another *KIR* gene or combination of genes on *KIR3DS1* positive haplotypes may be responsible for the protection observed in these diseases. (This would also have to involve *Bw4* or alleles in LD with *Bw4*, because the *KIR3DS1* protection noted in both HIV and HCV disease was contingent on the presence of *HLA-B Bw4* or a subset of these alleles.) Two genetic epidemiological studies (Hiby et al. 2004; Khakoo et al. 2004) have confirmed the notion that not all inhibitory signals mediated by the various KIR are of equal weight, a property that was recognized through functional studies previously (Winter and Long 1997). Perhaps more intriguing than the similarities in *KIR* associations among this limited sample of diseases are the differences in *KIR/HLA* genetic profiles putatively used to attain one of only two outcomes, activation or inhibition of effector cells, a characteristic that is entirely predictable of a multigenic, functionally closely related, highly polymorphic family of genes.

Acknowledgements This project has been funded in whole or part with Federal funds from the National Cancer Institute, National Institutes of Health, under Contract No. NO1-CO-12400. We would like to thank Dr. Arman Bashirova for helpful comments and assistance with figures and Teresa Covell for properly formatting the manuscript.

References

Allan DS et al. (1999) Tetrameric complexes of human histocompatibility leukocyte antigen (HLA)-G bind to peripheral blood myelomonocytic cells. J Exp Med 189:1149–1156

Artavanis-Tsakonas K et al. (2003) Activation of a subset of human NK cells upon contact with *Plasmodium falciparum*-infected erythrocytes. J Immunol 171:5396–5405

Artavanis-Tsakonas K, Riley EM (2002) Innate immune response to malaria: rapid induction of IFN-γ from human NK cells by live *Plasmodium falciparum*-infected erythrocytes. J Immunol 169:2956–2963

Bagot M et al. (2001) $CD4^+$ cutaneous T-cell lymphoma cells express the p140-killer cell immunoglobulin-like receptor. Blood 97:1388–1391

Bakker AB, Phillips JH, Figdor CG, Lanier LL (1998) Killer cell inhibitory receptors for MHC class I molecules regulate lysis of melanoma cells mediated by NK cells, γδ T cells, and antigen-specific CTL. J Immunol 160:5239–5245

Battistini L et al. (1997) Phenotypic and cytokine analysis of human peripheral blood γδ T cells expressing NK cell receptors. J Immunol 159:3723–3730

Baxter AG, Smyth MJ (2002) The role of NK cells in autoimmune disease. Autoimmunity 35:1–14

Biassoni R et al. (1995) Amino acid substitutions can influence the natural killer (NK)-mediated recognition of HLA-C molecules. Role of serine-77 and lysine-80 in the target cell protection from lysis mediated by "group 2" or "group 1" NK clones. J Exp Med 182:605–609

Biron CA, Byron KS, Sullivan JL (1989) Severe herpesvirus infections in an adolescent without natural killer cells. N Engl J Med 320:1731–1735

Biron CA, Nguyen KB, Pien GC, Cousens LP, Salazar-Mather TP (1999) Natural killer cells in antiviral defense: function and regulation by innate cytokines. Annu Rev Immunol 17:189–220

Brooks AG et al. (1999) Specific recognition of HLA-E, but not classical, HLA class I molecules by soluble CD94/NKG2A and NK cells. J Immunol 162:305–313

Cantoni C et al. (1998) p49, a putative HLA class I-specific inhibitory NK receptor belonging to the immunoglobulin superfamily. Eur J Immunol 28:1980–1990.

Carbone E et al. (1999) Recognition of autologous dendritic cells by human NK cells. Eur J Immunol 29:4022–4029

Carrington M, Cullen M (2004) Justified chauvinism: advances in defining meiotic recombination through sperm typing. Trends Genet 20:196–205

Cella M, Longo A, Ferrara GB, Strominger JL, Colonna M (1994) NK3-specific natural killer cells are selectively inhibited by Bw4-positive HLA alleles with isoleucine 80. J Exp Med 180:1235–1242.

Cerwenka A, Lanier LL (2001) Ligands for natural killer cell receptors: redundancy or specificity. Immunol Rev 181:158–169

Chambers BJ, Salcedo M, Ljunggren HG (1996) Triggering of natural killer cells by the costimulatory molecule CD80 (B7-1). Immunity 5:311–317

Chao KH, Wu MY, Chen CD, Yang JH, Yang YS, Ho HN (1999) The expression of killer cell inhibitory receptors on natural killer cells and activation status of CD4+ and CD8+ T cells in the decidua of normal and abnormal early pregnancies. Hum Immunol 60:791–797

Colonna M et al. (1992) Alloantigen recognition by two human natural killer cell clones is associated with HLA-C or a closely linked gene. Proc Natl Acad Sci USA 89:7983–7985

Cooke GS, Hill AV (2001) Genetics of susceptibility to human infectious disease. Nat Rev Genet 2:967–977

De Maria A et al. (1997) Expression of HLA class I-specific inhibitory natural killer cell receptors in HIV-specific cytolytic T lymphocytes: impairment of specific cytolytic functions. Proc Natl Acad Sci USA 94:10285–10288.

De Maria A, Moretta L (2000) HLA-class I-specific inhibitory receptors in HIV-1 infection. Hum Immunol 61:74–81

Diefenbach A, Raulet DH (2001) Strategies for target cell recognition by natural killer cells. Immunol Rev 181:170–184

Djeu JY, Blanchard DK (1988) Lysis of human monocytes by lymphokine-activated killer cells. Cell Immunol 111:55–65

Dorothee G et al. (2003) Functional and molecular characterization of a KIR3DL2/p140 expressing tumor-specific cytotoxic T lymphocyte clone infiltrating a human lung carcinoma. Oncogene 22:7192–7198

Fan QR, Long EO, Wiley DC (2001) Crystal structure of the human natural killer cell inhibitory receptor KIR2DL1-HLA-Cw4 complex. Nat. Immunol. 2:452–460.

Faure M, Long EO (2002) KIR2DL4 (CD158d), an NK cell-activating receptor with inhibitory potential. J Immunol 168:6208–6214

Ferrini S et al. (1994) T cell clones expressing the natural killer cell-related p58 receptor molecule display heterogeneity in phenotypic properties and p58 function. Eur J Immunol 24:2294–2298

Flodstrom M, Shi FD, Sarvetnick N, Ljunggren HG (2002) The natural killer cell—friend or foe in autoimmune disease? Scand J Immunol 55:432–441

Flores-Villanueva PO et al. (2001) Control of HIV-1 viremia and protection from AIDS are associated with HLA-Bw4 homozygosity. Proc Natl Acad Sci USA 98:5140–5145.

Fujimiya Y et al. (1986) Natural killer-cell immunodeficiency in patients with chronic myelogenous leukemia. I. Analysis of the defect using the monoclonal antibodies HNK-1 (LEU-7) and B73.1. Int J Cancer 37:639–649

Fukushima Y et al. (1998) Increased expression of human histocompatibility leukocyte antigen-G in colorectal cancer cells. Int J Mol Med 2:349–351

Gao X et al. (2001) Effect of a single amino acid change in MHC class I molecules on the rate of progression to AIDS. N Engl J Med 344:1668–1675.

Gardiner CM et al. (2001) Different NK cell surface phenotypes defined by the DX9 antibody are due to KIR3DL1 gene polymorphism. J Immunol 166:2992–3001.

Gati A et al. (2004) Analysis of the natural killer mediated immune response in metastatic renal cell carcinoma patients. Int J Cancer 109:393–401

Gazit R et al. (2004) Expression of KIR2DL1 on the entire NK cell population: a possible novel immunodeficiency syndrome. Blood 103:1965–1966

Geldhof AB, Moser M, De Baetselier P (1998) IL-12-activated NK cells recognize B7 costimulatory molecules on tumor cells and autologous dendritic cells. Adv Exp Med Biol 451:203–210

Gilbertson SM, Shah PD, Rowley DA (1986) NK cells suppress the generation of Lyt-2+ cytolytic T cells by suppressing or eliminating dendritic cells. J Immunol 136:3567–3571

Gladman DD, Rahman P (2001) Psoriatic Arthritis. In: Ruddy S, Harris ED, Sledge CB, Budd RC, Sergent JS (eds) Kelly's Textbook of Rheumatology. W.B. Saunders Co, Philadelphia, pp 1071–1079

Gomez-Lozano N, de Pablo R, Puente S, Vilches C (2003) Recognition of HLA-G by the NK cell receptor KIR2DL4 is not essential for human reproduction. Eur J Immunol 33:639–644

Gomez-Lozano N, Gardiner CM, Parham P, Vilches C (2002) Some human KIR haplotypes contain two KIR2DL5 genes: KIR2DL5A and KIR2DL5B. Immunogenetics 54:314–319.

Goodfellow PN, Barnstable CJ, Bodmer WF, Snary D, Crumpton MJ (1976) Expression of HLA system antigens on placenta. Transplantation 22:595–603

Groh V, Wu J, Yee C, Spies T (2002) Tumour-derived soluble MIC ligands impair expression of NKG2D and T-cell activation. Nature 419:734–738

Guerra N et al. (2000) Killer inhibitory receptor (CD158b) modulates the lytic activity of tumor-specific T lymphocytes infiltrating renal cell carcinomas. Blood 95:2883–2889

Guethlein LA, Flodin LR, Adams EJ, Parham P (2002) NK cell receptors of the orangutan (*Pongo pygmaeus*): a pivotal species for tracking the coevolution of killer cell Ig-like receptors with MHC- C. J Immunol 169:220–229.

Gumperz JE, Litwin V, Phillips JH, Lanier LL, Parham P (1995) The Bw4 public epitope of HLA-B molecules confers reactivity with natural killer cell clones that express NKB1, a putative HLA receptor. J Exp Med 181:1133–1144.

Hansasuta P et al. (2004) Recognition of HLA-A3 and HLA-A11 by KIR3DL2 is peptide-specific. Eur J Immunol 34:1673–1679

Hershberger KL, Shyam R, Miura A, Letvin NL (2001) Diversity of the killer cell Ig-like receptors of rhesus monkeys. J Immunol 166:4380–4390.

Hiby SE, King A, Sharkey A, Loke YW (1999) Molecular studies of trophoblast HLA-G: polymorphism, isoforms, imprinting and expression in preimplantation embryo. Tissue Antigens 53:1–13

Hiby SE, King A, Sharkey AM, Loke YW (1997) Human uterine NK cells have a similar repertoire of killer inhibitory and activatory receptors to those found in blood, as demonstrated by RT-PCR and sequencing. Mol Immunol 34:419–430

Hiby SE et al. (2004) Combinations of maternal KIR and fetal HLA-C genes influence the risk of preeclampsia and reproductive success. J Exp Med 200:957–965

Hoelsbrekken SE et al. (2003) Cutting edge: molecular cloning of a killer cell Ig-like receptor in the mouse and rat. J Immunol 170:2259–2263

Hsu KC, Chida S, Dupont B, Geraghty DE (2002a) The killer cell immunoglobulin-like receptor (KIR) genomic region: gene-order, haplotypes and allelic polymorphism. Immunol Rev 190:40–52

Hsu KC, Liu XR, Selvakumar A, Mickelson E, O'Reilly RJ, Dupont B (2002b) Killer Ig-like receptor haplotype analysis by gene content: evidence for genomic diversity with a minimum of six basic framework haplotypes, each with multiple subsets. J Immunol 169:5118–5129

Kaklamanis L, Hill A (1992) MHC loss in colorectal tumours: evidence for immunoselection? Cancer Surv 13:155–171

Karre K, Ljunggren HG, Piontek G, Kiessling R (1986) Selective rejection of H-2-deficient lymphoma variants suggests alternative immune defence strategy. Nature 319:675–678.

Katz G et al. (2004) MHC class I-independent recognition of NK-activating receptor KIR2DS4. J Immunol 173:1819–1825

Khakoo SI et al. (2000) Rapid evolution of NK cell receptor systems demonstrated by comparison of chimpanzees and humans. Immunity 12:687–698.

Khakoo SI et al. (2004) HLA and NK cell inhibitory receptor genes in resolving hepatitis C virus infection. Science 305:872–874

King A et al. (2000a) HLA-E is expressed on trophoblast and interacts with CD94/NKG2 receptors on decidual NK cells. Eur J Immunol 30:1623–1631

King A et al. (2000b) Surface expression of HLA-C antigen by human extravillous trophoblast. Placenta 21:376–387

Kogure T et al. (2001) Effect of interleukin 2 on killer cell inhibitory receptors in patients with rheumatoid arthritis. Ann Rheum Dis 60:166–169

Lanier LL (1998) NK cell receptors. Annu Rev Immunol 16:359–393

Lanier LL (2001a) Face off—the interplay between activating and inhibitory immune receptors. Curr Opin Immunol 13:326–331

Lanier LL (2001b) On guard—activating NK cell receptors. Nat Immunol 2:23–27
Lefebvre S et al. (2002) Specific activation of the non-classical class I histocompatibility HLA-G antigen and expression of the ILT2 inhibitory receptor in human breast cancer. J Pathol 196:266–274
Ljunggren HG, Karre K (1990) In search of the 'missing self': MHC molecules and NK cell recognition. Immunol Today 11:237–244.
Long EO (1999) Regulation of immune responses through inhibitory receptors. Annu Rev Immunol 17:875–904
Long EO, Rajagopalan S (2000) HLA class I recognition by killer cell Ig-like receptors. Semin Immunol 12:101–108.
Luszczek W et al. (2004) Gene for the activating natural killer cell receptor, KIR2DS1, is associated with susceptibility to psoriasis vulgaris. Hum Immunol 65:758–766
Maeda N et al. (2004) Killer inhibitory receptor CD158a overexpression among natural killer cells in women with endometriosis is undiminished by laparoscopic surgery and gonadotropin releasing hormone agonist treatment. Am J Reprod Immunol 51:364–372
Maeda N, Izumiya C, Yamamoto Y, Oguri H, Kusume T, Fukaya T (2002) Increased killer inhibitory receptor KIR2DL1 expression among natural killer cells in women with pelvic endometriosis. Fertil Steril 77:297–302
Maenaka K et al. (1999) Killer cell immunoglobulin receptors and T cell receptors bind peptide-major histocompatibility complex class I with distinct thermodynamic and kinetic properties. J Biol Chem 274:28329–28334.
Mager DL, McQueen KL, Wee V, Freeman JD (2001) Evolution of natural killer cell receptors: coexistence of functional Ly49 and KIR genes in baboons. Curr Biol 11:626–630.
Mandelboim O et al. (2001) Recognition of haemagglutinins on virus-infected cells by NKp46 activates lysis by human NK cells. Nature 409:1055–1060
Mandelboim O, Wilson SB, Vales-Gomez M, Reyburn HT, Strominger JL (1997) Self and viral peptides can initiate lysis by autologous natural killer cells. Proc Natl Acad Sci USA 94:4604–4609
Martens PB, Goronzy JJ, Schaid D, Weyand CM (1997) Expansion of unusual CD4+ T cells in severe rheumatoid arthritis. Arthritis Rheum 40:1106–1114
Martin MP, Bashirova A, Traherne J, Trowsdale J, Carrington M (2003) Cutting edge: expansion of the KIR locus by unequal crossing over. J Immunol 171:2192–2195
Martin MP et al. (2002a) Epistatic interaction between KIR3DS1 and HLA-B delays the progression to AIDS. Nat Genet 31:429–434
Martin MP et al. (2002b) Cutting edge: susceptibility to psoriatic arthritis: influence of activating killer Ig-like receptor genes in the absence of specific HLA-C alleles. J Immunol 169:2818–2822
Matsui T et al. (2001) Detection of autoantibodies to killer immunoglobulin-like receptors using recombinant fusion proteins for two killer immunoglobulin-like receptors in patients with systemic autoimmune diseases. Arthritis Rheum 44:384–388
Maxwell LD, Wallace A, Middleton D, Curran MD (2002) A common KIR2DS4 deletion variant in the human that predicts a soluble KIR molecule analogous to the KIR1D molecule observed in the rhesus monkey. Tissue Antigens 60:254–258

McMaster MT et al. (1995) Human placental HLA-G expression is restricted to differentiated cytotrophoblasts. J Immunol 154:3771–3778.

McQueen KL, Wilhelm BT, Harden KD, Mager DL (2002) Evolution of NK receptors: a single Ly49 and multiple KIR genes in the cow. Eur J Immunol 32:810–817.

Melioli G et al. (2003) Expansion of natural killer cells in patients with head and neck cancer: detection of "noninhibitory" (activating) killer Ig-like receptors on circulating natural killer cells. Head Neck 25:297–305

Mingari MC et al. (1995) Cytolytic T lymphocytes displaying natural killer (NK)-like activity: expression of NK-related functional receptors for HLA class I molecules (p58 and CD94) and inhibitory effect on the TCR-mediated target cell lysis or lymphokine production. Int Immunol 7:697–703

Moffett-King A (2002) Natural killer cells and pregnancy. Nat Rev Immunol 2:656–663

Momot T et al. (2004) Association of killer cell immunoglobulin-like receptors with scleroderma. Arthritis Rheum 50:1561–1565

Moodie SJ et al. (2002) Analysis of candidate genes on chromosome 19 in coeliac disease: an association study of the KIR and LILR gene clusters. Eur J Immunogenet 29:287–291.

Moretta A et al. (2001) Activating receptors and coreceptors involved in human natural killer cell-mediated cytolysis. Annu Rev Immunol 19:197–223

Moretta A et al. (1995) Existence of both inhibitory (p58) and activatory (p50) receptors for HLA-C molecules in human natural killer cells. J Exp Med 182:875–884.

Moretta L, Bottino C, Pende D, Vitale M, Mingari MC, Moretta A (2004) Different checkpoints in human NK-cell activation. Trends Immunol 25:670–676

Moretta L, Moretta A (2004) Unravelling natural killer cell function: triggering and inhibitory human NK receptors. EMBO J 23:255–259

Muller CA, Engler-Blum G, Gekeler V, Steiert I, Weiss E, Schmidt H (1989) Genetic and serological heterogeneity of the supertypic HLA-B locus specificities Bw4 and Bw6. Immunogenetics 30:200–207

Nakajima H, Tomiyama H, Takiguchi M (1995) Inhibition of γδ T cell recognition by receptors for MHC class I molecules. J Immunol 155:4139–4142

Nakajima T et al. (2003) De novo expression of killer immunoglobulin-like receptors and signaling proteins regulates the cytotoxic function of CD4 T cells in acute coronary syndromes. Circ Res 93:106–113

Namekawa T et al. (2000) Killer cell activating receptors function as costimulatory molecules on CD4+CD28null T cells clonally expanded in rheumatoid arthritis. J Immunol 165:1138–1145

Naumova E, Mihaylova A, Stoitchkov K, Ivanova M, Quin L, Toneva M (2005) Genetic polymorphism of NK receptors and their ligands in melanoma patients: prevalence of inhibitory over activating signals. Cancer Immunol Immunother 54:172–178

Navarro F, Llano M, Bellon T, Colonna M, Geraghty DE, Lopez-Botet M (1999) The ILT2(LIR1) and CD94/NKG2A NK cell receptors respectively recognize HLA-G1 and HLA-E molecules co-expressed on target cells. Eur J Immunol 29:277–283

Nelson GW, Martin MP, Gladman D, Wade J, Trowsdale J, Carrington M (2004) Cutting Edge: heterozygote advantage in autoimmune disease: hierarchy of protection/susceptibility conferred by HLA and killer Ig-like receptor combinations in psoriatic arthritis. J Immunol 173:4273–4276

Norris S et al. (1999) Natural T cells in the human liver: cytotoxic lymphocytes with dual T cell and natural killer cell phenotype and function are phenotypically heterogenous and include Vα24-JαQ and γδ T cell receptor bearing cells. Hum Immunol 60:20–31

Orago AS, Facer CA (1991) Cytotoxicity of human natural killer (NK) cell subsets for *Plasmodium falciparum* erythrocytic schizonts: stimulation by cytokines and inhibition by neomycin. Clin Exp Immunol 86:22–29

Pando MJ, Gardiner CM, Gleimer M, McQueen KL, Parham P (2003) The protein made from a common allele of KIR3DL1 (3DL1*004) is poorly expressed at cell surfaces due to substitution at positions 86 in Ig domain 0 and 182 in Ig domain 1. J Immunol 171:6640–6649

Parham P (2004) NK cells and trophoblasts: partners in pregnancy. J Exp Med 200:951–955

Parolini S et al. (2000) X-linked lymphoproliferative disease. 2B4 molecules displaying inhibitory rather than activating function are responsible for the inability of natural killer cells to kill Epstein-Barr virus-infected cells. J Exp Med 192:337–346

Paul P et al. (1999) Heterogeneity of HLA-G gene transcription and protein expression in malignant melanoma biopsies. Cancer Res 59:1954–1960

Peruzzi M, Parker KC, Long EO, Malnati MS (1996a) Peptide sequence requirements for the recognition of HLA-B*2705 by specific natural killer cells. J Immunol 157:3350–3356

Peruzzi M, Wagtmann N, Long EO (1996b) A p70 killer cell inhibitory receptor specific for several HLA-B allotypes discriminates among peptides bound to HLA-B*2705. J Exp Med 184:1585–1590

Pierson BA, Miller JS (1996) CD56+bright and CD56+dim natural killer cells in patients with chronic myelogenous leukemia progressively decrease in number, respond less to stimuli that recruit clonogenic natural killer cells, and exhibit decreased proliferation on a per cell basis. Blood 88:2279–2287

Poszepczynska-Guigne E et al. (2004) CD158 k/KIR3DL2 is a new phenotypic marker of Sezary cells: relevance for the diagnosis and follow-up of Sezary syndrome. J Invest Dermatol 122:820–823

Rajagopalan S, Long EO (1997) The direct binding of a p58 killer cell inhibitory receptor to human histocompatibility leukocyte antigen (HLA)-Cw4 exhibits peptide selectivity. J Exp Med 185:1523–1528

Rajagopalan S, Long EO (1999) A human histocompatibility leukocyte antigen (HLA)-G-specific receptor expressed on all natural killer cells. J Exp Med 189:1093–1100

Rajalingam R, Parham P, Abi-Rached L (2004) Domain shuffling has been the main mechanism forming new hominoid killer cell Ig-like receptors. J Immunol 172:356–369

Roberts JM (2003) Pre-eclampsia: a two-stage disorder. In: Critchley H, MacLean A, Poston L, Walker J (eds) Pre-eclampsia. RCOG Press, London, UK, pp 66–78

Rojo S, Wagtmann N, Long EO (1997) Binding of a soluble p70 killer cell inhibitory receptor to HLA-B*5101: requirement for all three p70 immunoglobulin domains. Eur J Immunol 27:568–571

Sambrook JG et al. (2005) Single haplotype analysis demonstrates rapid evolution of the killer immunoglobulin-like receptor (KIR) loci in primates. Genome Res 15:25–35

Schottenfeld D, Beebe-Dimmer JL (2005) Advances in cancer epidemiology: understanding causal mechanisms and the evidence for implementing interventions. Annu Rev Public Health 26:37–60

Shah PD, Gilbertson SM, Rowley DA (1985) Dendritic cells that have interacted with antigen are targets for natural killer cells. J Exp Med 162:625–636

Sharma SK, Balamurugan A, Pandey RM, Saha PK, Mehra NK (2003) Human leukocyte antigen-DR alleles influence the clinical course of pulmonary sarcoidosis in Asian Indians. Am J Respir Cell Mol Biol 29:225–231

Shilling HG et al. (2002) Allelic polymorphism synergizes with variable gene content to individualize human KIR genotype. J Immunol 168:2307–2315.

Shilling HG, Lienert-Weidenbach K, Valiante NM, Uhrberg M, Parham P (1998) Evidence for recombination as a mechanism for KIR diversification. Immunogenetics 48:413–416.

Shimizu Y, DeMars R (1989) Demonstration by class I gene transfer that reduced susceptibility of human cells to natural killer cell-mediated lysis is inversely correlated with HLA class I antigen expression. Eur J Immunol 19:447–451.

Sivori S et al. (2000) 2B4 functions as a co-receptor in human NK cell activation. Eur J Immunol 30:787–793

Smith ME, Marsh SG, Bodmer JG, Gelsthorpe K, Bodmer WF (1989) Loss of HLA-A,B,C allele products and lymphocyte function-associated antigen 3 in colorectal neoplasia. Proc Natl Acad Sci USA 86:5557–5561

Spaggiari GM et al. (2002) Soluble HLA class I induces NK cell apoptosis upon the engagement of killer-activating HLA class I receptors through FasL-Fas interaction. Blood 100:4098–4107

Stankiewicz P, Lupski JR (2002) Genome architecture, rearrangements and genomic disorders. Trends Genet 18:74–82

Storkus WJ, Alexander J, Payne JA, Dawson JR, Cresswell P (1989) Reversal of natural killing susceptibility in target cells expressing transfected class I HLA genes. Proc Natl Acad Sci USA 86:2361–2364.

Suzuki Y et al. (2004) Genetic polymorphisms of killer cell immunoglobulin-like receptors are associated with susceptibility to psoriasis vulgaris. J Invest Dermatol 122:1133–1136

Theander TG, Pedersen BK, Bygbjerg IC, Jepsen S, Larsen PB, Kharazmi A (1987) Enhancement of human natural cytotoxicity by *Plasmodium falciparum* antigen activated lymphocytes. Acta Trop 44:415–422

Toneva M et al. (2001) Genomic diversity of natural killer cell receptor genes in three populations. Tissue Antigens 57:358–362.

Tortorella D, Gewurz BE, Furman MH, Schust DJ, Ploegh HL (2000) Viral subversion of the immune system. Annu Rev Immunol 18:861–926

Trowsdale J, Barten R, Haude A, Stewart CA, Beck S, Wilson MJ (2001) The genomic context of natural killer receptor extended gene families. Immunol Rev 181:20–38.

Trundley A, Moffett A (2004) Human uterine leukocytes and pregnancy. Tissue Antigens 63:1–12

Ugolini S et al. (2001) Involvement of inhibitory NKRs in the survival of a subset of memory-phenotype CD8+ T cells. Nat Immunol 2:430–435

Uhrberg M, Parham P, Wernet P (2002) Definition of gene content for nine common group B haplotypes of the Caucasoid population: KIR haplotypes contain between seven and eleven KIR genes. Immunogenetics 54:221–229.

Uhrberg M et al. (1997) Human diversity in killer cell inhibitory receptor genes. Immunity 7:753–763.

Vales-Gomez M, Reyburn H, Strominger J (2000) Molecular analyses of the interactions between human NK receptors and their HLA ligands. Hum Immunol 61:28–38.

Vales-Gomez M, Reyburn HT, Erskine RA, Strominger J (1998) Differential binding to HLA-C of p50-activating and p58-inhibitory natural killer cell receptors. Proc Natl Acad Sci USA 95:14326–14331.

Valiante NM et al. (1997) Functionally and structurally distinct NK cell receptor repertoires in the peripheral blood of two human donors. Immunity 7:739–751.

van der Slik AR, Koeleman BP, Verduijn W, Bruining GJ, Roep BO, Giphart MJ (2003) KIR in type 1 diabetes: disparate distribution of activating and inhibitory natural killer cell receptors in patients versus HLA-matched control subjects. Diabetes 52:2639–2642

Vely F et al. (2001) Regulation of inhibitory and activating killer-cell Ig-like receptor expression occurs in T cells after termination of TCR rearrangements. J Immunol 166:2487–2494

Verheyden S, Bernier M, Demanet C (2004) Identification of natural killer cell receptor phenotypes associated with leukemia. Leukemia 18:2002–2007

Verma S, King A, Loke YW (1997) Expression of killer cell inhibitory receptors on human uterine natural killer cells. Eur J Immunol 27:979–983

Vilches C, Parham P (2002) KIR: diverse, rapidly evolving receptors of innate and adaptive immunity. Annu Rev Immunol 20:217–251

Wechsler J et al. (2003) Killer cell immunoglobulin-like receptor expression delineates in situ Sezary syndrome lymphocytes. J Pathol 199:77–83

Welch AY, Kasahara M, Spain LM (2003) Identification of the mouse killer immunoglobulin-like receptor-like (Kirl) gene family mapping to chromosome X. Immunogenetics 54:782–790

Wilson MJ et al. (2000) Plasticity in the organization and sequences of human KIR/ILT gene families. Proc Natl Acad Sci USA 97:4778–4783.

Winter CC, Gumperz JE, Parham P, Long EO, Wagtmann N (1998) Direct binding and functional transfer of NK cell inhibitory receptors reveal novel patterns of HLA-C allotype recognition. J Immunol 161:571–577.

Winter CC, Long EO (1997) A single amino acid in the p58 killer cell inhibitory receptor controls the ability of natural killer cells to discriminate between the two groups of HLA-C allotypes. J Immunol 158:4026–4028

Witt CS, Dewing C, Sayer DC, Uhrberg M, Parham P, Christiansen FT (1999) Population frequencies and putative haplotypes of the killer cell immunoglobulin-like receptor sequences and evidence for recombination. Transplantation 68:1784–1789.

Witt CS, Martin A, Christiansen FT (2000) Detection of KIR2DL4 alleles by sequencing and SSCP reveals a common allele with a shortened cytoplasmic tail. Tissue Antigens 56:248–257.

Witt CS et al. (2002) Alleles of the KIR2DL4 receptor and their lack of association with pre-eclampsia. Eur J Immunol 32:18–29.

Wu MY, Yang JH, Chao KH, Hwang JL, Yang YS, Ho HN (2000) Increase in the expression of killer cell inhibitory receptors on peritoneal natural killer cells in women with endometriosis. Fertil Steril 74:1187–1191

Yang JH, Chen MJ, Chen HF, Lee TH, Ho HN, Yang YS (2004) Decreased expression of killer cell inhibitory receptors on natural killer cells in eutopic endometrium in women with adenomyosis. Hum Reprod 19:1974–1978

Yawata M et al. (2002) Predominance of group A KIR haplotypes in Japanese associated with diverse NK cell repertoires of KIR expression. Immunogenetics 54:543–550

Yen JH et al. (2001) Major histocompatibility complex class I-recognizing receptors are disease risk genes in rheumatoid arthritis. J Exp Med 193:1159–1167.

Zambello R et al. (2003) Expression and function of KIR and natural cytotoxicity receptors in NK-type lymphoproliferative diseases of granular lymphocytes. Blood 102:1797–1805

Zappacosta F, Borrego F, Brooks AG, Parker KC, Coligan JE (1997) Peptides isolated from HLA-Cw*0304 confer different degrees of protection from natural killer cell-mediated lysis. Proc Natl Acad Sci USA 94:6313–6318

Zhong F et al. (1996) An autosomal screen for genes that predispose to celiac disease in the western counties of Ireland. Nat Genet 14:329–333.

NK Cells in Autoimmune Disease

S. Johansson · H. Hall · L. Berg · P. Höglund (✉)

Microbiology and Tumor Biology Center, Karolinska Institute, Box 280,
17177 Stockholm, Sweden
petter.hoglund@mtc.ki.se

1	Introduction	260
2	NK Cell Biology	261
3	NK Cells in Autoimmune Disease	262
3.1	NK Cells Promoting Disease	263
3.2	NK Cells Protecting from Disease	264
4	Potential Mechanisms Controlling the Function of NK Cells in Autoimmune Conditions	266
4.1	KIR Polymorphisms in Autoimmune Disorders	266
4.2	Tampering with the Activating Pathways	268
5	Concluding Remarks	268
	References	271

Abstract The role of NK cells in autoimmunity has not been extensively studied. Speaking for a disease-promoting role for NK cells in autoimmune diseases are recent results suggesting that IFN-γ production by NK cells may help adaptive immune responses diverge in the direction of a Th1 response. NK cells may also be involved in direct killing of tissue cells, which could lead to acceleration of autoimmunity. However, NK cells have also been shown to protect from some autoimmune diseases. A possible reason for this discrepancy may lie in the capacity of NK cells also to produce Th2 cytokines, which could downregulate the Th1 responses that are common in autoimmune disorders. Thus there is at present no coherent view on the role of NK cells in autoimmunity, and more work is needed to clarify why NK cells in some cases aggravate disease and in some cases protect from disease.

1
Introduction

Autoimmune diseases are controlled by multiple genetic loci and usually modified by a multitude of unknown environmental factors. Insulin-dependent diabetes mellitus (IDDM), also called type 1 diabetes, is one example, others being multiple sclerosis (MS), myasthenia gravis (MG), rheumatoid arthritis (RA), systemic lupus erythematosus (SLE), and Sjögren syndrome (SS). In systemic autoimmunity such as SLE and MG, antibodies normally cause the main damage, with a role for T cells being less clear. In contrast, in organ-specific autoimmune diseases such as IDDM, MS, SS, and RA, organ-infiltrating T cells are believed to be of central importance.

Autoimmunity results from breakdown of immunological tolerance. Both faulty central and peripheral tolerance mechanisms have been implicated, in both cases resulting in escape of autoreactive T cells from normal control. The relative roles of insufficient central versus peripheral tolerance mechanisms in autoimmunity are unclear. Defects in central tolerance, for example, as demonstrated by mutations in the AIRE gene, lead to organ infiltration and functional impairments of organ function (Anderson et al. 2002; Ramsey et al. 2002). Conversely, exaggerated thymic deletion may also result in autoimmunity due to a disrupted balance between thymus-derived regulatory ($CD4^+CD25^+$) and nonregulatory T cells (Hori et al. 2003). Examples of other T cells with regulatory properties are NKT cells (Mars et al. 2004) and $CD8^+CD122^+$ T cells that may also play protective roles in autoimmune conditions (Rifa'i et al. 2004).

Additional players are also important in the induction and subsequent control of immune responses in the periphery. For example, naive T cells must encounter antigen presented as peptides by MHC molecules on specialized antigen-presenting cells (APC) in order to become activated. This occurs in secondary lymphoid organs such as the spleen and lymph nodes. Dendritic cells (DC) are critical players in this game. After activation, both MHC and costimulatory molecules are upregulated on DC and their stimulatory capacity thereby increases. Soluble factors present at the site of T cell activation also dictate the nature of the immune response and determines whether it should be of a Th1 or Th2 type (Dong and Flavell 2001). Many organ-specific autoimmune diseases are dominated by IFN-γ, classifying them as Th1-dominated diseases (Trembleau et al. 1995).

2
NK Cell Biology

NK cells mediate early protection against viruses (Yokoyama et al. 2004). They are also well known for their efficient cytotoxic responses against cancer cells (Smyth et al. 2002) and for their capacity to kill cells coated with antibodies via their expression of the CD16 receptor. However, more focus is currently directed to the immunoregulatory role of NK cells (Raulet 2004). In experimental settings, NK cells are usually derived from human peripheral blood or rodent spleen. In the spleen, they are seen all over the red pulp but rarely in the white pulp (Basse et al. 1992; Rolstad et al. 1986). However, NK cells are also found in other tissues such as lungs (Basse et al. 1992; Stein-Streilein et al. 1983), liver (Basse et al. 1992; Salazar-Mather et al. 1998; Wiltrout et al. 1984), the gastrointestinal tract (Tagliabue et al. 1982) and in the decidua (Moffett et al. 2004). Under inflammatory conditions, NK cells are recruited to sites of inflammation and accumulate at sites of viral replication (Natuk and Welsh 1987) and in growing tumors (Albertsson et al. 2003). Under normal circumstances, rodent NK cells are rare in lymph nodes and resting NK cells recirculate poorly through the lymphatic system (Rolstad et al. 1986). In humans, NK cells appear to be more frequent in peripheral lymphoid tissue (Fehniger et al. 2003; Ferlazzo et al. 2004b).

Human NK cells can be divided into two functionally and phenotypically different subtypes, with $CD56^{dim}$ NK cells making up 90% of blood NK cells. The NK cells found in lymphoid tissue belong to the $CD56^{bright}$ type, which has been described as mainly cytokine producing. Human $CD56^{bright}$ NK cells constitutively express the chemokine receptor CXCR3 that is involved in lymphocyte migration to inflamed lymph nodes as well as to inflamed tissues (Rot and von Andrian 2004). Recent data show that murine NK cells may be recruited from blood into antigen-stimulated lymph nodes in a CXCR3-dependent fashion (Martin-Fontecha et al. 2004). In humans, $CD56^{bright}$ NK cells are found in the T cell region of lymph nodes, where they may interact with DC (Fehniger et al. 2003; Ferlazzo et al. 2004a). Cross talk between purified DC and NK cells is well documented in vitro with purified cells (Ferlazzo et al. 2002, 2004b; Gerosa et al. 2002; Hori et al. 2003), which may result in IFN-γ secretion by NK cells and involve IL-12 and IL-15 (Ferlazzo et al. 2004a). Interestingly, Martín-Fontecha et al. showed that NK cells provide an early source of IFN-γ in the lymph nodes that is necessary for Th1 polarization (Martín-Fontecha et al. 2004). Together, these data propose that NK cells may act as messengers between innate and adaptive immunity in regional lymph nodes.

NK cells can also be recruited across endothelium to nonlymphoid inflamed tissue, where they could participate in inflammatory reactions (Campbell et al. 2001; Fogler et al. 1996). In humans, the minor population of $CD56^{bright}$ NK cells and the major population of $CD56^{dim}$ NK cells express overlapping as well as specific chemokine receptors (Campbell et al. 2001), implying heterogeneity in migratory properties. Whereas only $CD56^{bright}$ NK cells express lymph node-homing receptors, both $CD56^{dim}$ and $CD56^{bright}$ NK cells express chemokine receptors enabling them to migrate into peripheral tissue. Fractalkine, the ligand for CX3CR1, is presented in both membrane-bound and soluble forms (Bazan et al. 1997) and displays adhesive properties, promoting migration and enhancing the cytotoxicity of NK cells (Yoneda et al. 2000). Interestingly, fractalkine is upregulated in both rat and human β cells on IL-1β + IFN-γ treatment (Cardozo et al. 2003), indicating a mechanism for NK cell recruitment into inflamed islets of Langerhans and a possible role in IDDM.

3
NK Cells in Autoimmune Disease

NK cells are not only found at sites of normal immune responses but have also been shown to accumulate in target organs of autoimmunity, for example, in the inflamed joints of RA (Dalbeth and Callan 2002; Tak et al. 1994), in brain lesions of MS (Traugott 1985), in psoriasis lesions (Cameron et al. 2002), and in the inflamed islets of Langerhans in IDDM (Miyazaki et al. 1985; Poirot et al. 2004; and our unpublished data). The presence of NK cells in target organs of autoimmunity, implying a role in disease at this site, is interesting in relation to findings reporting decreased NK cell numbers and impairment of NK cell function in peripheral blood in patients (Cameron et al. 2003; Yabuhara et al. 1996; and reviewed in Baxter and Smyth 2002; Flodström et al. 2002b; Grunebaum et al. 1989). Data from us and others show that rodents with diabetes also have compromised peripheral NK cells (Johansson et al. 2004; Poulton et al. 2001). It is not clear whether the reported alterations in blood NK cells reflect a secondary effect of disease or its treatment or are primary defects involved in the disease pathogenesis. Systemic induction of type 1 IFNs in mice rapidly depletes the spleen from NK cells and induces their migration into the liver (Salazar-Mather et al. 2002 and our observation). One possibility is that inflammatory cues alter the migratory pattern of NK cells and thus redistribute them from the circulation to target organs. This notion would suggest that low NK cell numbers in the blood may still be consistent with a role for NK cells elsewhere in the body.

The availability of mouse models for many human autoimmune diseases would appear to set a stage for analyzing the role for NK cells in these models. However, a general problem with studying NK cell function in vivo is that few markers or genes are expressed solely by NK cells. Many markers overlap with subsets of T cells or NKT cells (Raulet 2004), which makes NK cells difficult to target by knockout technology or by specific antibody depletion. Until now, only a few studies have been done in rodent models of autoimmune diseases in which the authors can confidently state that NK cells are the causative agent of the studied effect. Even so, the studies point toward both protective and disease-promoting effects of NK cells, depending on the disease model.

3.1
NK Cells Promoting Disease

In an experimental model of MG (EAMG), depletion of NK1.1$^+$ cells protected against disease (Shi et al. 2000). Depletion of NK1.1$^+$ cells reduced CD4$^+$ T cell IFN-γ production, whereas the number of CD4$^+$ cells producing TGF-β was increased. Mice depleted of NK1.1$^+$ cells also had reduced levels of pathogenic antibodies against the acetylcholine receptor. By ruling out a role of NK1.1$^+$ CD1-restricted NKT cells with Jα281 or CD1 knockout strains, and by repopulating NK cell-deficient IL-18-knockout mice with NK1.1-expressing cells derived from RAG mice, the authors could demonstrate a central role for NK cells in the pathology of the disease. The effect took place during the priming phase, because depletion of NK cells during later stages of the disease had no effect. To promote disease, NK cells had to produce IFN-γ, as shown by transfer of IFN-γ$^{-/-}$ or control NK cells to NK-deficient mice. Hence, in this study NK cells exacerbated autoimmunity by promoting the development of a Th1 response.

A function of NK cells during later stages of autoimmunity was proposed in a model of virally induced autoimmune diabetes (Flodström et al. 2002a). It was shown that the β cells of the pancreas critically depended on an intact type I interferon response to protect themselves from viral infection. Furthermore, it was proposed that in absence of interferon signaling, β cells became susceptible to NK cell-dependent killing. The study did not address the question of how type I interferons protected from NK cell killing. Speculatively it could be due to upregulation of MHC class I molecules or to upregulation of stress-induced ligands for activating NK cell receptors.

Poirot et al. took a different approach to determine an association between aggressive infiltration in the pancreatic islets and NK cells (Poirot et al. 2004). They compared two mouse strains, BDC2.5/NOD, which develop a mild insulitis but no diabetes, and BDC2.5/B6^{g7}, which rapidly develop both an aggressive form of insulitis and diabetes (Gonzalez et al. 1997). Using a microarray analysis, Poirot et al. found a correlation between expression of NK genes in the infiltrating cells and aggressive insulitis. In addition, a higher frequency of NK cells was demonstrated in aggressive infiltrates compared to mild infiltrates. When NK cells were depleted in two induced models of diabetes, diabetes incidence was decreased, suggesting a role for NK cells in the effector phase also in these models of diabetes. However, both antibodies used to deplete NK cells also recognize other immune cells, which must be taken into consideration when interpreting the data.

3.2
NK Cells Protecting from Disease

The regulatory role for NK cells in immune activation can be achieved either by skewing the immune response toward a Th1 or a Th2 response or by direct inhibition of the immune response. NK cells are capable of producing IL-10 along with IFN-γ, and also immunoregulatory cytokines such as TGF-β, although these properties of NK cells are much less well studied than the prototypic role of NK cells as IFN-γ producers (Gray et al. 1994; Peritt et al. 1998). Furthermore, it has been suggested that NK cells can regulate B cell antibody production via induction of regulatory T cells in a TGF-β-dependent manner (Gray et al. 1994; Horwitz et al. 1999). NK cells can also regulate T cell responses by acting on DC, either by inducing their maturation or by killing them (Ferlazzo et al. 2002, 2004b; Gerosa et al. 2002; Hayakawa et al. 2004; Hori et al. 2003; Piccioli et al. 2002).

MS has been shown to be associated with low NK cell activity (Erkeller-Yusel et al. 1993; Loza et al. 2002; Yabuhara et al. 1996). In a recent paper, Takahashi et al. suggest a protective role for NK cells in humans with MS (Takahashi et al. 2004). NK cells from patients in disease remission expressed high levels of CD95 and were proposed to be NK2 cells, distinguished by secretion of Th2 cytokines such as IL-5 and IL-13 (Takahashi et al. 2001, 2004). Takahashi et al. suggest that those NK cells may control IFN-γ secretion in memory T cells, because depletion of NK cells in ex vivo PBMC increased IFN-γ responses in T cells after stimulation with myelin basic protein (Takahashi et al. 2004). Before disease relapse, NK cells lost their CD95 expression and NK2 phenotype, and thus presumably their regulatory role.

Experimental autoimmune encephalomyelitis (EAE) is a murine model of MS that can be induced in susceptible strains of rats and mice. Matsumoto et al. showed that NK cells were present in the central nervous system of rats at the early stages of EAE. When NK cells were depleted, the disease was aggravated (Matsumoto et al. 1998). Zhang et al. found a similar protective role of NK cells in EAE in mice (Zhang et al. 1997). The regulatory role was independent of CD8$^+$ T cells and NKT cells because the aggravating effect of depleting NK cells was present also in β_2m-deficient mice. Interestingly, NK depletion led to an in vivo increase in production of Th1 cytokines by CD4 T cells and an increased T cell proliferation in vitro when NK-depleted spleen cells were used as antigen-presenting cells. The regulatory role of NK cells in rodent models of EAE is further strengthened by a study of Smeltz et al. showing that NK cells inhibit proliferation of autoreactive T cells from DA rats in vitro (Smeltz et al. 1999).

In SLE, which is another relapsing-remitting disease, low NK cell numbers in the blood are associated with relapses, whereas the NK cell number is restored during remission. However, a low NK activity on a per cell basis is sustained throughout the disease cycle in these patients (Erkeller-Yusel et al. 1993; Yabuhara et al. 1996). Two different mechanistic abnormalities have been associated with the low NK cell activity in SLE patients. The first is a higher frequency of a genetic polymorphism in the FcγIIIR (CD16), resulting in a low-avidity binding of IgG antibodies (Wu et al. 1997). The other mechanistic abnormality affects the expression of the signaling adapter molecule DAP12 (Toyabe et al. 2004). DAP12 is an adapter protein used by several activating NK receptors (but not by CD16) and also by activating receptors on myeloid cells including DC (Colonna 2003; Djeu et al. 2002). Low DAP12 activity was associated with a dysfunctional posttranscriptional editing of mRNA rather than a mutation in the DAP12 gene.

Lpr mice, harboring a mutation affecting Fas expression, display an SLE-like phenotype (Watanabe-Fukunaga et al. 1992). Similar to SLE patients, *lpr* mice have low NK activity, especially in aging mice (Scribner and Steinberg 1988), and Takeda et al. showed an association in time between disease development and cessation of NK activity (Takeda and Dennert 1993). In this model, the disease process could also be accelerated or decelerated by depleting or transferring NK1.1$^+$ cells, respectively. A regulatory role of NK1.1$^+$ cells was seen in vitro, and NK cells from nude mice were also efficient in this respect, making an effect of contaminating NKT cells less likely.

A protective role of NK cells in murine diabetes was recently reported by Lee et al. (Lee et al. 2004). Diabetes in NOD mice can be prevented by administration of complete Freund's adjuvant (CFA). In parallel, CFA induced NK cell trafficking to the blood and spleen, induced IFN-γ production by NK cells, and decreased activation of β cell-specific T cells. Depletion of NK cells abrogated the protective effect of CFA, and addition of sorted NK cells to the depleted mice restored the protective effect. It is somewhat surprising that an increased IFN-γ response in NK cells would be associated with decreased T cell activation, arguing against the T cell-enhancing role of NK cells suggested previously. CFA might induce a unique regulatory cytokine profile in NK cells that are capable, despite the IFN-γ secretion, of downregulating T cell responses.

Todd et al. showed a decrease in intraepithelial NK cell numbers in the gut preceding diabetes onset in the BB rat. These cells normally produce both IFN-γ and IL-4, and the production of these cytokines in the intraepithelial lymphocyte compartment was consequentially reduced (Todd et al. 2004). Intraepithelial NK cells might therefore confer regulatory functions in this model.

4
Potential Mechanisms Controlling the Function of NK Cells in Autoimmune Conditions

4.1
KIR Polymorphisms in Autoimmune Disorders

A potent mechanism to secure NK cell tolerance is their expression of MHC class I-specific inhibitory receptors. On ligation of these receptors, NK functions are downregulated. Consequently, when MHC class I molecules are lost, target cells are killed. This recognition strategy has been termed "missing self" because the lack of the body's self markers leads to NK cell susceptibility (Bix et al. 1991; Hoglund et al. 1988; Karre et al. 1986; Moretta et al. 2002). In humans, inhibitory signals in response to MHC class I encounter are delivered primarily by killer immunoglobulin like (KIR) receptors on NK cells. Given that NK cells can lose tolerance against self cells in case of low MHC class I expression, it has been postulated that genetic polymorphisms in the KIR haplotypes could contribute to risk for autoimmunity.

Humans contain several genes encoding activating and inhibitory forms of KIR. Activating KIRs that contain two extracellular immunoglobulin domains and a short cytoplasmatic tail are designated KIR2DS. The corresponding inhibitory KIRs are called KIR2DL. Ligands for inhibitory KIR2DL receptors are HLA-C molecules that fall into two functional groups: KIR2DL1 binds to HLA-C with a Lys^{80} residue (HLA-Cw4 group), whereas KIR2DL2 and KIR2DL3 recognize HLA-C with an Asn^{80} residue (HLA-Cw3 and related alleles). Inhibitory KIRs can also contain three extracellular domains and are then called KIR3DL. The relative activity of activating and inhibitory KIRs on each NK cell is one parameter, albeit not the only one, that controls the activation of human NK cells (Moretta et al. 2002).

KIR genes are very polymorphic and are also clonally expressed in a stochastic manner on human NK cells. Furthermore, although there are at least 14 described KIR genes, not all genes are present in all individuals. It is thus likely that different NK cells, in the same individual or between individuals, are differentially capable of forming inhibitory KIR-HLA interactions, which may lead to differences in the amount of activating signal needed to trigger effector functions, for example, in autoimmunity. Consistent with this view, Martin et al. showed that the risk for developing psoriatic arthritis was highest among subjects that carried activating KIRs and at the same time lacked HLA-Cw ligands for some of their inhibitory KIRs (Martin et al. 2002; Nelson et al. 2004). Similarly, KIR2DS2 in absence of KIR2DL2 was more common in patients with scleroderma compared to healthy controls (Momot et al. 2004). KIR2DS2 has also been shown to associate with vasculitis in patients with RA (Yen et al. 2001) and with susceptibility to psoriasis vulgaris (Suzuki et al. 2004). In addition, psoriasis vulgaris was found to be associated with KIR2DS1 (Luszczek et al. 2004). These studies point toward activating KIRs conferring a more activated phenotype of immune responses, presumably by decreasing the activation threshold for KIR-expressing lymphocytes. These activating haplotypes thus confer an increased risk of developing autoimmunity. Also in IDDM, increased numbers of activating KIR genes compared to healthy controls have been demonstrated and the association with disease was clearest when combined with presence of HLA-C ligand and in DQ2 and/or DQ8 individuals (van der Slik et al. 2003).

Genetic associations between alleles of NK receptors and risk of developing autoimmune diseases bear a scientific weight, but the functional consequence of these associations is not easily studied. One drawback is that genetic studies do not take into account which cells potentially express the receptors under study. In the case of KIR receptors, they are expressed both by NK and T cells. It is also unknown at which level the KIR/MHC matching may operate. One possibility is in the target organ. Target cells could potentially downmodulate MHC class I molecules because of viral targeting, which could break NK cell tolerance in some NK cells and trigger NK cell-mediated target cell destruction. Alternatively, MHC class I downregulation on other cells in the body could trigger a helper function of NK cells, as has been described in cancer models (Kelly et al. 2002). Future studies will have to be set up to study this question specifically.

4.2
Tampering with the Activating Pathways

NK cell activity is not only regulated by activating signals delivered to KIR receptors but also by target cell expression of ligands for other activating receptors. Tolerance can be broken in cases of induction of those ligands. For example, the NKG2D receptor has several ligands that may be upregulated after cellular stress (Snyder et al. 2004). One such ligand is MIC, alleles of which have been associated with psoriasis vulgaris (Romphruk et al. 2004). In addition, MIC-A and MIC-B alleles have been associated with autoimmune Addison disease (Gambelunghe et al. 1999). It is interesting that HLA and MIC-A polymorphisms may together make up additive risk factors, such as certain HLA-DRB1 and MIC-A haplotypes in Basque families with celiac disease (Bilbao et al. 2002) and DR3-DQ2, MICA5, and MICA5.1 in SLE (Gambelunghe et al. 2004). However, independent associations are also reported, such as that of MIC-A5, DR3-DQ2, or DR4-DQ8 with IDDM where the MIC-A5 association was clearest in patients with young disease onset. No linkage disequilibrium was seen between MIC and class II alleles, that is, a distinct genetic background characterizes the more acute form of early-onset type 1 diabetes (Gambelunghe et al. 2000).

There are also several recent nongenetic studies that support a role for the NKG2D receptor in autoimmunity that could potentially link NK cells to disease pathogenesis. Thus blocking the activating NKG2D receptor in NOD mice prevents disease development, presumably by blocking NK cell or T cell activation induced by the NKG2D ligand RAE-1 expressed by β cells of the pancreas (Ogasawara et al. 2004). In celiac disease, where T cell responses against tissue transglutaminase are effective in the pathogenesis (Dieterich et al. 1997), a role for immune activation through NKG2D has been suggested (Hue et al. 2004; Meresse et al. 2004). Here, as well as in RA (Groh et al. 2003), T cells expressing NKG2D, rather than NK cells, seem to be of primary importance, although the studies have not ruled out a role also for NK cells activated by ligands for NKG2D induced by stress at sites of inflammation.

5
Concluding Remarks

Although adaptive arms of immunity are well-known culprits in autoimmunity, there is likely a similarly important role for innate cells, including NK cells, in those responses (Fig. 1). As far as NK cells are concerned, the current picture shows evidence for both disease-promoting and disease-preventing roles. A closer, comparative dissection of diseases models in which NK cells

a Immunoregulation by NK cells

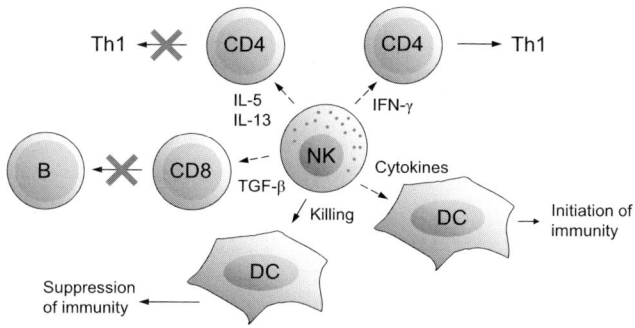

b Target destruction by NK cells

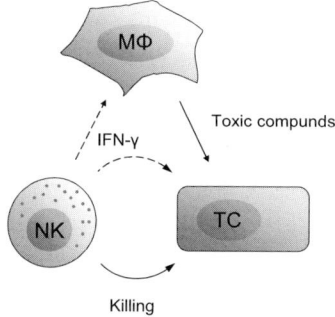

Fig. 1 a Some proposed roles of NK cells as modulators of adaptive immune responses. Immunoregulation such as this could occur anywhere in the body, e.g., blood, secondary lymphoid organs, and target tissues. Key to this complex pattern may be the regulation of cytokine responses in NK cells. The *right* part of the picture reflects disease-promoting roles. For example, IFN-γ may directly stimulate Th1 development in T cells (*upper right*) and this cytokine may also prime DC to become better stimulators (*lower right*). DC may also be killed by NK cells (*lower left*), which would downregulate T cell responses. TGF-β secreted by NK cells has been reported to downregulate Ab production via $CD8^+$ T cells (*middle left*), and NK cells showing a Th2-like cytokine pattern may counteract IFN-γ and downregulate Th1 responses (*upper left*). b In tissues, NK cells could potentially contribute to tissue destruction by direct cytotoxicity, perhaps triggered via activating KIR or by NKG2D. In addition, IFN-γ production by NK cells can activate macrophages to produce toxic compounds, for example, NO and free radicals, and is also by itself, especially in conjunction with monokines such as IL-1 and TNF-α, directly toxic for certain cells, such as the β cells of the pancreas

perform different functions will be important to identify potential differences in NK cell biology that may be responsible for these opposing roles. In humans, low NK cell numbers in the blood are frequently observed, but this is also difficult to interpret because many autoimmune diseases are associated with systemic inflammation that may deplete or affect NK cells. As more and more genetic markers for NK cells become available, genetic studies may be important to study this question further. Prospective studies of NK cell markers, for example, in patients at risk of developing autoimmunity, may be informative. Difficulties in understanding discrepancies in the role of NK cells in autoimmunity may lie in our incomplete understanding of the in vivo biology of NK cells as well as the role of different functional subsets.

To dissect the role of NK cells in autoimmune diseases, we believe that the following aspects of NK cell biology must be studied in greater detail:

1. *The function of NK cells in tissues.* A role for NK cells in tissues and target organs during different phases of autoimmune diseases must be undertaken. In the target organ, NK cells may change their behavior compared to when in the blood. The balance between NK cell functions at different anatomic sites may thus be different in different autoimmune conditions and may explain why NK cells play different roles depending on which disease is studied. This problem includes the question of how NK cells circulate and whether organ-residing NK cells and NK cells in the circulation are the same cell type or distinct subsets.

2. *Intensify the search for functional NK cell subsets.* Just as for T cells, there certainly exists a multitude of NK cell subsets that mediate different effector functions depending on how, where, and when they may be stimulated. Just as for Th1 and Th2 T cells, such subset compositions are likely to be partly genetically determined but may also be a consequence of the local microenvironment to which they home and become activated. An important question will be how functionally distinct NK cell subsets overlap with subsets distinguished by their expression of activating and inhibitory MHC class I-specific receptors, the balance of which is important in autoimmunity.

3. *Explore the genetic paths further.* The emerging genetic analyses of KIR polymorphisms, in particular in relation to polymorphisms of ligands for activating NK cell receptors, should give novel insights into a possible role for a balance between activating and inhibitory signals in autoimmunity. When genetic profiles for different functional subsets are generated, new markers suitable for genetic mapping of NK cells could potentially be developed.

4. *Explore the "NK kinetics" of different diseases.* It is becoming increasingly clear that cells and molecules of the immune system may play different and sometime opposing roles at different ages and different stages of disease. For example, several cytokines have been shown to play completely opposite roles at early and late stages of autoimmunity. Thus differences in time kinetics of critical NK-related events in induction, progression, and final stages of different autoimmune diseases may also hold clues as to why NK cells could play different roles in different diseases.

References

Albertsson PA, Basse PH, Hokland M, Goldfarb RH, Nagelkerke JF, Nannmark U, Kuppen PJ. (2003) NK cells and the tumour microenvironment: implications for NK-cell function and anti-tumour activity. Trends Immunol 24:603–609

Anderson MS, Venanzi ES, Klein L, Chen Z, Berzins SP, Turley SJ, von Boehmer H, Bronson R, Dierich A, Benoist C, Mathis D. (2002) Projection of an immunological self shadow within the thymus by the aire protein. Science 298:1395–1401

Basse PH, Hokland P, Gundersen HJ, Hokland M. (1992) Enumeration of organ-associated natural killer cells in mice: application of a new stereological method. Apmis 100:202–208

Baxter AG, Smyth MJ. (2002) The role of NK cells in autoimmune disease. Autoimmunity 35:1–14

Bazan JF, Bacon KB, Hardiman G, Wang W, Soo K, Rossi D, Greaves DR, Zlotnik A, Schall TJ. (1997) A new class of membrane-bound chemokine with a CX3C motif. Nature 385:640–644

Bilbao JR, Martin-Pagola A, Vitoria JC, Zubillaga P, Ortiz L, Castano L. (2002) HLA-DRB1 and MHC class 1 chain-related A haplotypes in Basque families with celiac disease. Tissue Antigens 60:71–76

Bix M, Liao NS, Zijlstra M, Loring J, Jaenisch R, Raulet D. (1991) Rejection of class I MHC-deficient haemopoietic cells by irradiated MHC-matched mice. Nature 349:329–331

Cameron AL, Kirby B, Fei W, Griffiths CE. (2002) Natural killer and natural killer-T cells in psoriasis. Arch Dermatol Res 294:363–369

Cameron AL, Kirby B, Griffiths CE. (2003) Circulating natural killer cells in psoriasis. Br J Dermatol 149:160–164

Campbell JJ, Qin S, Unutmaz D, Soler D, Murphy KE, Hodge MR, Wu L, Butcher EC. (2001) Unique subpopulations of CD56+ NK and NK-T peripheral blood lymphocytes identified by chemokine receptor expression repertoire. J Immunol 166:6477–6482

Cardozo AK, Proost P, Gysemans C, Chen MC, Mathieu C, Eizirik DL. (2003) IL-1β and IFN-γ induce the expression of diverse chemokines and IL-15 in human and rat pancreatic islet cells, and in islets from pre-diabetic NOD mice. Diabetologia 46:255–266

Colonna M. (2003) TREMs in the immune system and beyond. Nat Rev Immunol 3:445-453
Dalbeth N, Callan MF. (2002) A subset of natural killer cells is greatly expanded within inflamed joints. Arthritis Rheum 46:1763-1772
Dieterich W, Ehnis T, Bauer M, Donner P, Volta U, Riecken EO, Schuppan D. (1997) Identification of tissue transglutaminase as the autoantigen of celiac disease. Nat Med 3:797-801
Djeu JY, Jiang K, Wei S. (2002) A view to a kill: signals triggering cytotoxicity. Clin Cancer Res 8:636-640
Dong C, Flavell RA. (2001) Th1 and Th2 cells. Curr Opin Hematol 8:47-51
Erkeller-Yusel F, Hulstaart F, Hannet I, Isenberg D, Lydyard P. (1993) Lymphocyte subsets in a large cohort of patients with systemic lupus erythematosus. Lupus 2:227-231
Fehniger TA, Cooper MA, Nuovo GJ, Cella M, Facchetti F, Colonna M, Caligiuri MA. (2003) CD56bright natural killer cells are present in human lymph nodes and are activated by T cell-derived IL-2: a potential new link between adaptive and innate immunity. Blood 101:3052-3057
Ferlazzo G, Pack M, Thomas D, Paludan C, Schmid D, Strowig T, Bougras G, Muller WA, Moretta L, Munz C. (2004a) Distinct roles of IL-12 and IL-15 in human natural killer cell activation by dendritic cells from secondary lymphoid organs. Proc Natl Acad Sci USA 101:16606-16611
Ferlazzo G, Thomas D, Lin SL, Goodman K, Morandi B, Muller WA, Moretta A, Munz C. (2004b) The abundant NK cells in human secondary lymphoid tissues require activation to express killer cell Ig-like receptors and become cytolytic. J Immunol 172:1455-1462
Ferlazzo G, Tsang ML, Moretta L, Melioli G, Steinman RM, Munz C. (2002) Human dendritic cells activate resting natural killer (NK) cells and are recognized via the NKp30 receptor by activated NK cells. J Exp Med 195:343-351
Flodström M, Maday A, Balakrishna D, Cleary MM, Yoshimura A, Sarvetnick N. (2002a) Target cell defense prevents the development of diabetes after viral infection. Nat Immunol 3:373-382
Flodström M, Shi FD, Sarvetnick N, Ljunggren HG. (2002b) The natural killer cell— friend or foe in autoimmune disease? Scand J Immunol 55:432-441
Fogler WE, Volker K, McCormick KL, Watanabe M, Ortaldo JR, Wiltrout RH. (1996) NK cell infiltration into lung, liver, and subcutaneous B16 melanoma is mediated by VCAM-1/VLA-4 interaction. J Immunol 156:4707-4714
Gambelunghe G, Falorni A, Ghaderi M, Laureti S, Tortoioli C, Santeusanio F, Brunetti P, Sanjeevi CB. (1999) Microsatellite polymorphism of the MHC class I chain-related (MIC-A and MIC-B) genes marks the risk for autoimmune Addison's disease. J Clin Endocrinol Metab 84:3701-3707
Gambelunghe G, Gerli R, Bocci EB, Del Sindaco P, Ghaderi M, Sanjeevi CB, Bistoni O, Bini V, Falorni A. (2005) Contribution of MHC class I chain-related A (MICA) gene polymorphism to genetic susceptibility for systemic lupus erythematosus. Rheumatology (Oxford) 44:287-292
Gambelunghe G, Ghaderi M, Cosentino A, Falorni A, Brunetti P, Sanjeevi CB. (2000) Association of MHC Class I chain-related A (MIC-A) gene polymorphism with Type I diabetes. Diabetologia 43:507-514

Gerosa F, Baldani-Guerra B, Nisii C, Marchesini V, Carra G, Trinchieri G. (2002) Reciprocal activating interaction between natural killer cells and dendritic cells. J Exp Med 195:327–333

Gonzalez A, Katz JD, Mattei MG, Kikutani H, Benoist C, Mathis D. (1997) Genetic control of diabetes progression. Immunity 7:873–883

Gray JD, Hirokawa M, Horwitz DA. (1994) The role of transforming growth factor β in the generation of suppression: an interaction between CD8+ T and NK cells. J Exp Med 180:1937–1942

Groh V, Bruhl A, El-Gabalawy H, Nelson JL, Spies T. (2003) Stimulation of T cell autoreactivity by anomalous expression of NKG2D and its MIC ligands in rheumatoid arthritis. Proc Natl Acad Sci USA 100:9452–9457

Grunebaum E, Malatzky-Goshen E, Shoenfeld Y. (1989) Natural killer cells and autoimmunity. Immunol Res 8:292–304

Hayakawa Y, Screpanti V, Yagita H, Grandien A, Ljunggren HG, Smyth MJ, Chambers BJ. (2004) NK cell TRAIL eliminates immature dendritic cells in vivo and limits dendritic cell vaccination efficacy. J Immunol 172:123–129

Hoglund P, Ljunggren HG, Ohlen C, Ahrlund-Richter L, Scangos G, Bieberich C, Jay G, Klein G, Karre K. (1988) Natural resistance against lymphoma grafts conveyed by H-2Dd transgene to C57BL mice. J Exp Med 168:1469–1474

Hori S, Takahashi T, Sakaguchi S. (2003) Control of autoimmunity by naturally arising regulatory CD4+ T cells. Adv Immunol 81:331–371

Horwitz DA, Gray JD, Ohtsuka K. (1999) Role of NK cells and TGF-β in the regulation of T-cell-dependent antibody production in health and autoimmune disease. Microbes Infect 1:1305–1311

Hue S, Mention JJ, Monteiro RC, Zhang S, Cellier C, Schmitz J, Verkarre V, Fodil N, Bahram S, Cerf-Bensussan N, Caillat-Zucman S. (2004) A direct role for NKG2D/MICA interaction in villous atrophy during celiac disease. Immunity 21:367–377

Johansson SE, Hall H, Bjorklund J, Hoglund P. (2004) Broadly impaired NK cell function in non-obese diabetic mice is partially restored by NK cell activation in vivo and by IL-12/IL-18 in vitro. Int Immunol 16:1–11

Karre K, Ljunggren HG, Piontek G, Kiessling R. (1986) Selective rejection of H-2-deficient lymphoma variants suggests alternative immune defence strategy. Nature 319:675–678

Kelly JM, Takeda K, Darcy PK, Yagita H, Smyth MJ. (2002) A role for IFN-gamma in primary and secondary immunity generated by NK cell-sensitive tumor-expressing CD80 in vivo. J Immunol 168:4472–4479

Lee IF, Qin H, Trudeau J, Dutz J, Tan R. (2004) Regulation of autoimmune diabetes by complete Freund's adjuvant is mediated by NK cells. J Immunol 172:937–942

Loza MJ, Zamai L, Azzoni L, Rosati E, Perussia B. (2002) Expression of type 1 (interferon γ) and type 2 (interleukin-13, interleukin-5) cytokines at distinct stages of natural killer cell differentiation from progenitor cells. Blood 99:1273–1281

Luszczek W, Manczak M, Cislo M, Nockowski P, Wisniewski A, Jasek M, Kusnierczyk P. (2004) Gene for the activating natural killer cell receptor, KIR2DS1, is associated with susceptibility to psoriasis vulgaris. Hum Immunol 65:758–766

Mars LT, Novak J, Liblau RS, Lehuen A. (2004) Therapeutic manipulation of iNKT cells in autoimmunity: modes of action and potential risks. Trends Immunol 25:471–476

Martin MP, Nelson G, Lee JH, Pellett F, Gao X, Wade J, Wilson MJ, Trowsdale J, Gladman D, Carrington M. (2002) Cutting edge: susceptibility to psoriatic arthritis: influence of activating killer Ig-like receptor genes in the absence of specific HLA-C alleles. J Immunol 169:2818–2822

Martin-Fontecha A, Thomsen LL, Brett S, Gerard C, Lipp M, Lanzavecchia A, Sallusto F. (2004) Induced recruitment of NK cells to lymph nodes provides IFN-γgamma for T_H1 priming. Nat Immunol 5:1260–1265

Matsumoto Y, Kohyama K, Aikawa Y, Shin T, Kawazoe Y, Suzuki Y, Tanuma N. (1998) Role of natural killer cells and TCR γδ T cells in acute autoimmune encephalomyelitis. Eur J Immunol 28:1681–1688

Meresse B, Chen Z, Ciszewski C, Tretiakova M, Bhagat G, Krausz TN, Raulet DH, Lanier LL, Groh V, Spies T, Ebert EC, Green PH, Jabri B. (2004) Coordinated induction by IL15 of a TCR-independent NKG2D signaling pathway converts CTL into lymphokine-activated killer cells in celiac disease. Immunity 21:357–366

Miyazaki A, Hanafusa T, Yamada K, Miyagawa J, Fujino-Kurihara H, Nakajima H, Nonaka K, Tarui S. (1985) Predominance of T lymphocytes in pancreatic islets and spleen of pre-diabetic non-obese diabetic (NOD) mice: a longitudinal study. Clin Exp Immunol 60:622–630

Moffett A, Regan L, Braude P. (2004) Natural killer cells, miscarriage, and infertility. BMJ 329:1283–1285

Momot T, Koch S, Hunzelmann N, Krieg T, Ulbricht K, Schmidt RE, Witte T. (2004) Association of killer cell immunoglobulin-like receptors with scleroderma. Arthritis Rheum 50:1561–1565

Moretta L, Bottino C, Pende D, Mingari MC, Biassoni R, Moretta A. (2002) Human natural killer cells: their origin, receptors and function. Eur J Immunol 32:1205–1211

Natuk RJ, Welsh RM. (1987) Accumulation and chemotaxis of natural killer/large granular lymphocytes at sites of virus replication. J Immunol 138:877–883

Nelson GW, Martin MP, Gladman D, Wade J, Trowsdale J, Carrington M. (2004) Cutting edge: heterozygote advantage in autoimmune disease: hierarchy of protection/susceptibility conferred by HLA and killer Ig-like receptor combinations in psoriatic arthritis. J Immunol 173:4273–4276

Ogasawara K, Hamerman JA, Ehrlich LR, Bour-Jordan H, Santamaria P, Bluestone JA, Lanier LL. (2004) NKG2D blockade prevents autoimmune diabetes in NOD mice. Immunity 20:757–767

Peritt D, Robertson S, Gri G, Showe L, Aste-Amezaga M, Trinchieri G. (1998) Differentiation of human NK cells into NK1 and NK2 subsets. J Immunol 161:5821–5824

Piccioli D, Sbrana S, Melandri E, Valiante NM. (2002) Contact-dependent stimulation and inhibition of dendritic cells by natural killer cells. J Exp Med 195:335–341

Poirot L, Benoist C, Mathis D. (2004) Natural killer cells distinguish innocuous and destructive forms of pancreatic islet autoimmunity. Proc Natl Acad Sci USA 101:8102–8107

Poulton LD, Smyth MJ, Hawke CG, Silveira P, Shepherd D, Naidenko OV, Godfrey DI, Baxter AG. (2001) Cytometric and functional analyses of NK and NKT cell deficiencies in NOD mice. Int Immunol 13:887–896

Ramsey C, Winqvist O, Puhakka L, Halonen M, Moro A, Kampe O, Eskelin P, Pelto-Huikko M, Peltonen L. (2002) Aire deficient mice develop multiple features of APECED phenotype and show altered immune response. Hum Mol Genet 11:397–409

Raulet DH. (2004) Interplay of natural killer cells and their receptors with the adaptive immune response. Nat Immunol 5:996–1002

Rifa'i M, Kawamoto Y, Nakashima I, Suzuki H. (2004) Essential roles of CD8+CD122+ regulatory T cells in the maintenance of T cell homeostasis. J Exp Med 200:1123–1134

Rolstad B, Herberman RB, Reynolds CW. (1986) Natural killer cell activity in the rat. V. The circulation patterns and tissue localization of peripheral blood large granular lymphocytes (LGL). J Immunol 136:2800–2808

Romphruk AV, Romphruk A, Choonhakarn C, Puapairoj C, Inoko H, Leelayuwat C. (2004) Major histocompatibility complex class I chain-related gene A in Thai psoriasis patients: MICA association as a part of human leukocyte antigen-B-Cw haplotypes. Tissue Antigens 63:547–554

Rot A, von Andrian UH. (2004) Chemokines in innate and adaptive host defense: basic chemokinese grammar for immune cells. Annu Rev Immunol 22:891–928

Salazar-Mather TP, Lewis CA, Biron CA. (2002) Type I interferons regulate inflammatory cell trafficking and macrophage inflammatory protein 1α delivery to the liver. J Clin Invest 110:321–330

Salazar-Mather TP, Orange JS, Biron CA. (1998) Early murine cytomegalovirus (MCMV) infection induces liver natural killer (NK) cell inflammation and protection through macrophage inflammatory protein 1α (MIP-1α)-dependent pathways. J Exp Med 187:1–14

Scribner CL, Steinberg AD. (1988) The role of splenic colony-forming units in autoimmune disease. Clin Immunol Immunopathol 49:133–142

Shi FD, Wang HB, Li H, Hong S, Taniguchi M, Link H, Van Kaer L, Ljunggren HG. (2000) Natural killer cells determine the outcome of B cell-mediated autoimmunity. Nat Immunol 1:245–251

Smeltz RB, Wolf NA, Swanborg RH. (1999) Inhibition of autoimmune T cell responses in the DA rat by bone marrow-derived NK cells in vitro: implications for autoimmunity. J Immunol 163:1390–1397

Smyth MJ, Hayakawa Y, Takeda K, Yagita H. (2002) New aspects of natural-killer-cell surveillance and therapy of cancer. Nat Rev Cancer 2:850–861

Snyder MR, Weyand CM, Goronzy JJ. (2004) The double life of NK receptors: stimulation or co-stimulation? Trends Immunol 25:25–32

Stein-Streilein J, Bennett M, Mann D, Kumar V. (1983) Natural killer cells in mouse lung: surface phenotype, target preference, and response to local influenza virus infection. J Immunol 131:2699–2704

Suzuki Y, Hamamoto Y, Ogasawara Y, Ishikawa K, Yoshikawa Y, Sasazuki T, Muto M. (2004) Genetic polymorphisms of killer cell immunoglobulin-like receptors are associated with susceptibility to psoriasis vulgaris. J Invest Dermatol 122:1133–1136

Tagliabue A, Befus AD, Clark DA, Bienenstock J. (1982) Characteristics of natural killer cells in the murine intestinal epithelium and lamina propria. J Exp Med 155:1785–1796

Tak PP, Kummer JA, Hack CE, Daha MR, Smeets TJ, Erkelens GW, Meinders AE, Kluin PM, Breedveld FC. (1994) Granzyme-positive cytotoxic cells are specifically increased in early rheumatoid synovial tissue. Arthritis Rheum 37:1735–1743

Takahashi K, Aranami T, Endoh M, Miyake S, Yamamura T. (2004) The regulatory role of natural killer cells in multiple sclerosis. Brain 127:1917–1927

Takahashi K, Miyake S, Kondo T, Terao K, Hatakenaka M, Hashimoto S, Yamamura T. (2001) Natural killer type 2 bias in remission of multiple sclerosis. J Clin Invest 107:R23–R29

Takeda K, Dennert G. (1993) The development of autoimmunity in C57BL/6 lpr mice correlates with the disappearance of natural killer type 1-positive cells: evidence for their suppressive action on bone marrow stem cell proliferation, B cell immunoglobulin secretion, and autoimmune symptoms. J Exp Med 177:155–164

Todd DJ, Forsberg EM, Greiner DL, Mordes JP, Rossini AA, Bortell R. (2004) Deficiencies in gut NK cell number and function precede diabetes onset in BB rats. J Immunol 172:5356–5362

Toyabe SI, Kaneko U, Uchiyama M. (2004) Decreased DAP12 expression in natural killer lymphocytes from patients with systemic lupus erythematosus is associated with increased transcript mutations. J Autoimmun 23:371–378

Traugott U. (1985) Characterization and distribution of lymphocyte subpopulations in multiple sclerosis plaques versus autoimmune demyelinating lesions. Springer Semin Immunopathol 8:71–95

Trembleau S, Germann T, Gately MK, Adorini L. (1995) The role of IL-12 in the induction of organ-specific autoimmune diseases. Immunol Today 16:383–386

van der Slik AR, Koeleman BP, Verduijn W, Bruining GJ, Roep BO, Giphart MJ. (2003) KIR in type 1 diabetes: disparate distribution of activating and inhibitory natural killer cell receptors in patients versus HLA-matched control subjects. Diabetes 52:2639–2642

Watanabe-Fukunaga R, Brannan CI, Copeland NG, Jenkins NA, Nagata S. (1992) Lymphoproliferation disorder in mice explained by defects in Fas antigen that mediates apoptosis. Nature 356:314–317

Wiltrout RH, Mathieson BJ, Talmadge JE, Reynolds CW, Zhang SR, Herberman RB, Ortaldo JR. (1984) Augmentation of organ-associated natural killer activity by biological response modifiers. Isolation and characterization of large granular lymphocytes from the liver. J Exp Med 160:1431–1449

Wu J, Edberg JC, Redecha PB, Bansal V, Guyre PM, Coleman K, Salmon JE, Kimberly RP. (1997) A novel polymorphism of FcγRIIIa (CD16) alters receptor function and predisposes to autoimmune disease. J Clin Invest 100:1059–1070

Yabuhara A, Yang FC, Nakazawa T, Iwasaki Y, Mori T, Koike K, Kawai H, Komiyama A. (1996) A killing defect of natural killer cells as an underlying immunologic abnormality in childhood systemic lupus erythematosus. J Rheumatol 23:171–177

Yen JH, Moore BE, Nakajima T, Scholl D, Schaid DJ, Weyand CM, Goronzy JJ. (2001) Major histocompatibility complex class I-recognizing receptors are disease risk genes in rheumatoid arthritis. J Exp Med 193:1159–1167

Yokoyama WM, Kim S, French AR. (2004) The dynamic life of natural killer cells. Annu Rev Immunol 22:405–429

Yoneda O, Imai T, Goda S, Inoue H, Yamauchi A, Okazaki T, Imai H, Yoshie O, Bloom ET, Domae N, Umehara H. (2000) Fractalkine-mediated endothelial cell injury by NK cells. J Immunol 164:4055–4062

Zhang B, Yamamura T, Kondo T, Fujiwara M, Tabira T. (1997) Regulation of experimental autoimmune encephalomyelitis by natural killer (NK) cells. J Exp Med 186:1677–1687

Subject Index

2B4 10, 11, 29, 39, 40, 92–95, 97–103, 106, 107, 109, 110, 178

activating and inhibitory receptor 229
activating KIR 227
acute coronary syndromes (ACS) 234
AIDS 239
antibody dependent cellular cytotoxicity (ADCC), FcγRIIIA 6
autoimmunity
– KIR genes in 266
– NK cell prevention 264
– NK cell promotion of 263
– NK cells in 259–271
– NK cells in target organs of 262, 270
– Th1 and Th2 responses in 260

B lymphocyte activator macrophage expressed (BLAME) 92–94, 96, 97, 108
BCR/ABL protooncogene 159, 168

c-kit 167
c-SMAC 25–28, 41
c-SMIC 36
Ca^{2+} mobilization 9, 12
CCR5 163
CD112 179
CD144 178
CD150 91–98, 106–109
CD155 179

CD2 91–94, 97, 99, 102–104, 107–109
CD2 subset 1 (CS1) 92, 93, 96–98, 104, 105, 110
CD2-like receptor activating cytotoxic cells (CRACC) *see* CS1
CD226 179
CD229 92, 93, 96, 97, 104
CD244 *see* 2B4
CD314 179
CD3ζ 6, 27, 28, 38, 39, 42, 177
CD48 92–95, 97, 99–103, 106, 107, 109, 110, 178
CD58 92–94, 97, 102, 105, 108, 109
CD59 178
CD84 92, 93, 95, 97, 98, 108
CD84-homologue 1 (CG84-H1) 92, 94, 97, 107
CD94 35, 191
CD94/NKG2 receptors 3
Cdc42 27, 32–35
central supramolecular activation cluster (c-SMAC) 25
chronic myelogenous leukemia 237
cNKIS 25–27, 36, 38, 41
component WASP 27
CRACC *see* CS1
CRTAM 12
CX3CR1 163
cytomegalovirus
– m04 186
– m06 186
– m144 187, 188
– m145 186, 188, 193
– m152 186, 188, 192, 193
– m155 186, 188, 192, 193

- m157   195, 196
- UL16   187, 192
- UL18   187, 188
- UL40   191
- US11   186
- US2   186
- US3   186
- US6   186

DAP10 (KAP10)   7, 27–29, 31, 33, 34, 179, 190, 192
DAP12 (KARAP)   6, 27, 28, 31, 33, 34, 42, 177, 190–192, 196
dendritic cells   260, 261
- NK cell interaction with   261
DNA methylation   70
DNAM-1   12, 179, 180

EAT-2   *see* Ewings sarcoma activated transcript-2
EAT-2 (EWS-activated transcript 2)   11
Epstein-Barr virus (EBV)   98, 101, 106, 109
ERK   29, 30, 32, 35, 42
evolution of the KIR locus   231
Ewings sarcoma activated transcript-2 (EAT-2)   94–96, 98, 99, 101, 104–106, 108
EWS-activated transcript 2 (EAT-2)   11
exist   27
extravillous trophoblast (EVT)   242

FcεRIγ   27
Fcγ   177
FcγRIIIA   6
FcRγ   6
Flt3-L   160
Fyn   26, 28, 40, 41

γ   27, 28, 42
GTPases   29, 31–34

H60   192
HCV infection   240

hepatitis C virus (HCV) infection   239
HIV-1   239
HLA-B allotypes   230
HLA-C allotypes   230

ICAM-1   13
IFNγ
- NK cell production of   259, 261, 263, 266
ILT2   35, 36
immune synapse (IS)   9, 13
immunoreceptor tyrosine-based motifs
- ITAM – immunoreceptor tyrosine-based activation motifs   6, 8–10
- ITIM – immunoreceptor tyrosine-based inhibitory motifs   2–6
- ITSM – immunoreceptor tyrosine-based switch motifs   11
immunoreceptor tyrosine-based switch motif (ITSM)   95–99, 104, 105, 110
inhibitory KIR   227
iNKIS   25, 36–39
integrin β2, LFA-1   11–13
integrins   11
interferon gamma   160
interleukin 12   160
ITAM   27, 29–34
- containing   28
ITAMS   38
ITIM   36, 37, 39, 42
ITSM   39
- sequences   40

JNK   32

killer cell immunoglobulin-like receptor (KIR)   226
kinases   8
KIR   31, 35–39, 42
- diversity   232
- expression   233
- gene profiles   226

- genes 226
- genotype 226
- haplotypes 226, 227
KIR – killer immunoglobin.like receptors 3–5, 7, 8
KIR2DL4 28, 42

LAT 26, 38, 40, 41, 179
Lck 26, 28, 36
leukemia 238
leukocyte receptor complex (LRC) 226
LFA-1 13
ligands for activating NK molecules
- CD48 178
- MICA, MICB 179
- NCR-ligands (NCR-L) 177
- Nectin-2 (CD112) 179
- PVR (CD155) 179, 180
- ULBPs 179
linkage disequilibrium (LD) 231
lipid rafts 26, 28, 35, 39–41
LIR-1 188
LIR1 35, 36
Ly108 see NK-T-B-antigen
Ly49 3–5, 7, 8, 35, 36, 39
Ly49D 28
Ly49H 194, 196
LY49I 194
Ly49I 196
Ly49P 194, 197
lymph nodes
- NK cells recruitment to 261
lymphoproliferative disease of granular lymphocytes 238

malignant melanoma 237
MAPKs 32
MEF$^{-/-}$ mice 71
melanoma cell lines 237
MHC (major histocompatibility complex) class I 2–5, 7, 8
MHC class I (MHC I)-specific receptors 175
MHC class I receptors 60, 61
MICA 179, 192
MICB 179, 192

microtubule organizing center (MTOC) 9
missing self 24
missing-self 2, 6
mitogen-activated protein kinase (MAPK) 29
MULT1 192, 193

Natural cytotoxicity receptors (NCR) 177
NCR 178
NCR (natural cytotoxicity receptors) 3, 6
NCR-L 177
Nectin-2 179
Nectins, nectin-like molecules (Necl) 12
- receptors – DNAM-1, Tactile, CRTAM 12
NF-κB 33, 34
NF-AT 33
NK activating molecules
- 2B4 (CD144) 178
- CD59 178
- DNAM-1 (CD226) 179, 180
- natural cytotoxicity receptors (NCR) 177, 178
- NKG2D (CD314) 179
- NKp80 178
- NTB-A 178
NK cell activation 233
NK cell control of viral infections 238
NK cells
- activating receptors 268
- adoptive transfer of 263, 265
- and Th1 cytokines 259, 261, 263, 264, 266, 270
- and Th2 cytokines 259, 264, 270
- depletion of 263, 265
- in autoimmunity 259–271
- in lymph nodes 261
- inhibition my MHC class I 266
NK immune synapse (NKIS) 25
NK MHC I-specific receptors 175
NK-LDGL 30

NK-T-B-antigen   92, 93, 95, 96, 105–107, 109, 110
NKG2A   35, 36, 190, 191
NKG2D   7, 28, 31–33, 179, 190–192
NKG2C   190–192
NKIS   36
NKp30   165
NKp80   178
nonallelic homologous recombination (NAHR)   226
NTB-A   178

p-SMAC   25, 41
p38   32, 35, 42
peripheral tissue
- NK cell migration to   262, 270
- NK cells in   262, 270
    CD56 expression on   262
phosphatase   2, 10, 11, 39
- SHIP-1   11
- SHP-1   10, 13
- SHP-2   10, 11
phosphatidylinositol   9
- P13K – phosphatidylinositol 3-kinase   9, 10
phosphoITIM   38
phospholipase C (PLCγ1, PLCγ2)   9
phospholipases   9
PI3K   31, 32, 38–40
Plasmodium falciparum infection   240
preeclampsia   243
pregnancy   241
proportional   35
psoriasis vulgaris (PV)   235
psoriatic arthritis (PsA)   234
PTK   24, 26, 28, 29, 38, 40, 41
PTP   24, 26, 35, 37, 38
PVR   179, 180

RA vasculitis   233
Rac   32–34
RAE-1   192, 193
Ras   30, 32, 42
- family   29
receptors, the previously mentioned YINM motif on DAP10 becomes phosphorylated on ligation of NKG2D [10], thereby establishing a membrane-proximal binding   31
rheumatoid arthritis (RA)   233
Rho family   29, 31–34

SAP   40, 41
- also known as SH2D1A   40
SAP   *see* SH2D1A, *see* signaling lymphocyte activation associated molecule
SAP (also termed SH2D1A)   178
scleroderma   234
SH2 domain-containing inositol 5   39
SH2D1A   *see* signaling lymphocyte activation molecule associated molecule
SH2D1A (SAP)   11
SHIP   39–41
SHIP-null mice   63
SHP   26, 27, 35, 36
SHP-1   38, 41
SHP-2   35–37, 41, 42
signaling adaptor proteins   6, 7
signaling lymphocyte activation molecule (SLAM)   *see* CD150
signaling lymphocyte activation molecule associated molecule (SAP)   94–102, 104–106, 108–110
signaling polypeptides
- CD3zeta (e.g. CD3ζ)   177
- DAP10   179
- DAP12   177
- Fcgamma (e.g. Fcγ)   177
- LAT   179
- SAP (also termed SH2D1A)   178
SLAM   *see* CD150
SLP-76   26, 31, 36, 38, 41
SMIC   36
soluble HLA class I   237
Src   38, 40
- family   26
- kinases   31
stochastic   59, 67

Syk 26, 28, 29, 31, 38
synapse 162

Tactile 12
TCF-1-null mice 62
Toll-like receptors (TLR) 13
triggering receptor expressed on myeloid cells-2 (TREM2) 160
type 1 diabetes 234
type 1 interferon 158
tyrosine kinase 8–13
tyrosine phosphorylation 8–13

ULBP 179, 192
uterine NK (uNK) cells 242

variegated expression 61, 64, 65, 67–70, 72
variegated gene expression 59
Vav 29, 31–34, 38

WASP 26, 35

X-linked lymphoproliferative disease (XLP) 91, 98–100, 105, 106, 110, 178
X-linked lymphoproliferative disorder (XLP) 11
X-linked proliferative disease (XLP) 41

ZAP-70 26, 28, 29, 31, 36, 38

Current Topics in Microbiology and Immunology

Volumes published since 1989 (and still available)

Vol. 253: **Gosztonyi, Georg (Ed.):** The Mechanisms of Neuronal Damage in Virus Infections of the Nervous System. 2001. approx. XVI, 270 pp. ISBN 3-540-67617-1

Vol. 254: **Privalsky, Martin L. (Ed.):** Transcriptional Corepressors. 2001. 25 figs. XIV, 190 pp. ISBN 3-540-67569-8

Vol. 255: **Hirai, Kanji (Ed.):** Marek's Disease. 2001. 22 figs. XII, 294 pp. ISBN 3-540-67798-4

Vol. 256: **Schmaljohn, Connie S.; Nichol, Stuart T. (Eds.):** Hantaviruses. 2001. 24 figs. XI, 196 pp. ISBN 3-540-41045-7

Vol. 257: **van der Goot, Gisou (Ed.):** PoreForming Toxins, 2001. 19 figs. IX, 166 pp. ISBN 3-540-41386-3

Vol. 258: **Takada, Kenzo (Ed.):** Epstein-Barr Virus and Human Cancer. 2001. 38 figs. IX, 233 pp. ISBN 3-540-41506-8

Vol. 259: **Hauber, Joachim, Vogt, Peter K. (Eds.):** Nuclear Export of Viral RNAs. 2001. 19 figs. IX, 131 pp. ISBN 3-540-41278-6

Vol. 260: **Burton, Didier R. (Ed.):** Antibodies in Viral Infection. 2001. 51 figs. IX, 309 pp. ISBN 3-540-41611-0

Vol. 261: **Trono, Didier (Ed.):** Lentiviral Vectors. 2002. 32 figs. X, 258 pp. ISBN 3-540-42190-4

Vol. 262: **Oldstone, Michael B.A. (Ed.):** Arenaviruses I. 2002. 30 figs. XVIII, 197 pp. ISBN 3-540-42244-7

Vol. 263: **Oldstone, Michael B. A. (Ed.):** Arenaviruses II. 2002. 49 figs. XVIII, 268 pp. ISBN 3-540-42705-8

Vol. 264/I: **Hacker, Jörg; Kaper, James B. (Eds.):** Pathogenicity Islands and the Evolution of Microbes. 2002. 34 figs. XVIII, 232 pp. ISBN 3-540-42681-7

Vol. 264/II: **Hacker, Jörg; Kaper, James B. (Eds.):** Pathogenicity Islands and the Evolution of Microbes. 2002. 24 figs. XVIII, 228 pp. ISBN 3-540-42682-5

Vol. 265: **Dietzschold, Bernhard; Richt, Jürgen A. (Eds.):** Protective and Pathological Immune Responses in the CNS. 2002. 21 figs. X, 278 pp. ISBN 3-540-42668X

Vol. 266: **Cooper, Koproski (Eds.):** The Interface Between Innate and Acquired Immunity, 2002. 15 figs. XIV, 116 pp. ISBN 3-540-42894-X

Vol. 267: **Mackenzie, John S.; Barrett, Alan D. T.; Deubel, Vincent (Eds.):** Japanese Encephalitis and West Nile Viruses. 2002. 66 figs. X, 418 pp. ISBN 3-540-42783X

Vol. 268: **Zwickl, Peter; Baumeister, Wolfgang (Eds.):** The Proteasome-Ubiquitin Protein Degradation Pathway. 2002. 17 figs. X, 213 pp. ISBN 3-540-43096-2

Vol. 269: **Koszinowski, Ulrich H.; Hengel, Hartmut (Eds.):** Viral Proteins Counteracting Host Defenses. 2002. 47 figs. XII, 325 pp. ISBN 3-540-43261-2

Vol. 270: **Beutler, Bruce; Wagner, Hermann (Eds.):** Toll-Like Receptor Family Members and Their Ligands. 2002. 31 figs. X, 192 pp. ISBN 3-540-43560-3

Vol. 271: **Koehler, Theresa M. (Ed.):** Anthrax. 2002. 14 figs. X, 169 pp. ISBN 3-540-43497-6

Vol. 272: **Doerfler, Walter; Böhm, Petra (Eds.):** Adenoviruses: Model and Vectors in Virus-Host Interactions. Virion and Structure, Viral Replication, Host Cell Interactions. 2003. 63 figs., approx. 280 pp. ISBN 3-540-00154-9

Vol. 273: **Doerfler, Walter; Böhm, Petra (Eds.):** Adenoviruses: Model and Vectors in VirusHost Interactions. Immune System, Oncogenesis, Gene

Therapy. 2004. 35 figs., approx. 280 pp. ISBN 3-540-06851-1

Vol. 274: **Workman, Jerry L. (Ed.):** Protein Complexes that Modify Chromatin. 2003. 38 figs., XII, 296 pp. ISBN 3-540-44208-1

Vol. 275: **Fan, Hung (Ed.):** Jaagsiekte Sheep Retrovirus and Lung Cancer. 2003. 63 figs., XII, 252 pp. ISBN 3-540-44096-3

Vol. 276: **Steinkasserer, Alexander (Ed.):** Dendritic Cells and Virus Infection. 2003. 24 figs., X, 296 pp. ISBN 3-540-44290-1

Vol. 277: **Rethwilm, Axel (Ed.):** Foamy Viruses. 2003. 40 figs., X, 214 pp. ISBN 3-540-44388-6

Vol. 278: **Salomon, Daniel R.; Wilson, Carolyn (Eds.):** Xenotransplantation. 2003. 22 figs., IX, 254 pp. ISBN 3-540-00210-3

Vol. 279: **Thomas, George; Sabatini, David; Hall, Michael N. (Eds.):** TOR. 2004. 49 figs., X, 364 pp. ISBN 3-540-00534X

Vol. 280: **Heber-Katz, Ellen (Ed.):** Regeneration: Stem Cells and Beyond. 2004. 42 figs., XII, 194 pp. ISBN 3-540-02238-4

Vol. 281: **Young, John A. T. (Ed.):** Cellular Factors Involved in Early Steps of Retroviral Replication. 2003. 21 figs., IX, 240 pp. ISBN 3-540-00844-6

Vol. 282: **Stenmark, Harald (Ed.):** Phosphoinositides in Subcellular Targeting and Enzyme Activation. 2003. 20 figs., X, 210 pp. ISBN 3-540-00950-7

Vol. 283: **Kawaoka, Yoshihiro (Ed.):** Biology of Negative Strand RNA Viruses: The Power of Reverse Genetics. 2004. 24 figs., IX, 350 pp. ISBN 3-540-40661-1

Vol. 284: **Harris, David (Ed.):** Mad Cow Disease and Related Spongiform Encephalopathies. 2004. 34 figs., IX, 219 pp. ISBN 3-540-20107-6

Vol. 285: **Marsh, Mark (Ed.):** Membrane Trafficking in Viral Replication. 2004. 19 figs., IX, 259 pp. ISBN 3-540-21430-5

Vol. 286: **Madshus, Inger H. (Ed.):** Signalling from Internalized Growth Factor Receptors. 2004. 19 figs., IX, 187 pp. ISBN 3-540-21038-5

Vol. 287: **Enjuanes, Luis (Ed.):** Coronavirus Replication and Reverse Genetics. 2005. 49 figs., XI, 257 pp. ISBN 3-540-21494-1

Vol. 288: **Mahy, Brain W. J. (Ed.):** Foot-and-Mouth-Disease Virus. 2005. 16 figs., IX, 178 pp. ISBN 3-540-22419X

Vol. 289: **Griffin, Diane E. (Ed.):** Role of Apoptosis in Infection. 2005. 40 figs., IX, 294 pp. ISBN 3-540-23006-8

Vol. 290: **Singh, Harinder; Grosschedl, Rudolf (Eds.):** Molecular Analysis of B Lymphocyte Development and Activation. 2005. 28 figs., XI, 255 pp. ISBN 3-540-23090-4

Vol. 291: **Boquet, Patrice; Lemichez Emmanuel (Eds.)** Bacterial Virulence Factors and Rho GTPases. 2005. 28 figs., IX, 196 pp. ISBN 3-540-23865-4

Vol. 292: **Fu, Zhen F (Ed.):** The World of Rhabdoviruses. 2005. 27 figs., X, 210 pp. ISBN 3-540-24011-X

Vol. 293: **Kyewski, Bruno; Suri-Payer, Elisabeth (Eds.):** CD4+CD25+ Regulatory T Cells: Origin, Function and Therapeutic Potential. 2005. 22 figs., XII, 332 pp. ISBN 3-540-24444-1

Vol. 294: **Caligaris-Cappio, Federico, Dalla Favera, Ricardo (Eds.):** Chronic Lymphocytic Leukemia. 2005. 25 figs., VIII, 187 pp. ISBN 3-540-25279-7

Vol. 295: **Sullivan, David J.; Krishna Sanjeew (Eds.):** Malaria: Drugs, Disease and Post-genomic Biology. 2005. 40 figs., XI, 446 pp. ISBN 3-540-25363-7

Vol. 296: **Oldstone, Michael B. A. (Ed.):** Molecular Mimicry: Infection Induced Autoimmune Disease. 2005. 28 figs., VIII, 167 pp. ISBN 3-540-25597-4

Vol. 297: **Langhorne, Jean (Ed.):** Immunology and Immunopathogenesis of Malaria. 2005. 8 figs., XII, 236pp. ISBN 3-540-25718-7

Printing: Krips bv, Meppel
Binding: Stürtz, Würzburg